The Profession of Ophthalmology

Practice Management, Ethics, and Advocacy

Executive Editor

David W. Parke II, MD

Section Editors

David A. Durfee, MD (practice management)
Charles M. Zacks, MD (ethics)
Paul N. Orloff, MD (advocacy)

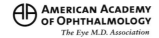

**AMERICAN ACADEMY
OF OPHTHALMOLOGY**
The Eye M.D. Association

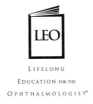

LEO

LIFELONG
EDUCATION FOR THE
OPHTHALMOLOGIST®

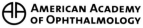
**AMERICAN ACADEMY
OF OPHTHALMOLOGY**
The Eye M.D. Association

655 Beach Street
Box 7424
San Francisco, CA 94120-7424

Portions of this work are derived from *Starting a Medical Practice*, second edition, ©2003
American Medical Association, with permission granted by the American Medical As-
sociation. All editorial decisions regarding inclusion of portions of *Starting a Medical
Practice* are solely those of the American Academy of Ophthalmology.

The authors state the following financial relationships:
David W. Parke II, MD: affiliated with Alcon, Medem, Novartis, OMIC, and Zeiss
Michael J. Parshall: affiliated with Health Care Group
Derek Preece: affiliated with BSM Consulting Group

The other authors state that they have no significant financial interest or other relationship
with the manufacturer of any commercial product mentioned in the text that they contributed
to this publication or with the manufacturer of any competing commercial product.

Library of Congress Cataloging-in-Publication Data

The profession of ophthalmology : practice management, ethics, and advocacy / executive
editor,
David W. Parke II.
      p. ; cm.
   Includes index.
   ISBN 1-56055-494-0 (softcover)
   1. Ophthalmology—Practice. 2. Ophthalmology—Vocational guidance. 3. Ophthalmol-
ogy—Moral
and ethical aspects. 4. Patient advocacy.
   [DNLM: 1. Ophthalmology—organization & administration. 2. Practice Management,
Medical. 3.
Ophthalmology—ethics. 4. Vocational Guidance. WW 21 P964 2005] I. Parke, David W. II.
American Academy of Ophthalmology.

   RE72.P76 2005
   617.7'0068—dc22
                        2005005204

Academy Staff

Advocacy/Governmental Affairs
> Catherine G. Cohen, *Vice-President*
> DeChane Dorsey, *Health Policy*
> Bob Palmer, *State Governmental Affairs*
> Michael Levitt, *Manager, State Governmental Affairs*

Clinical Education
> Richard A. Zorab, *Vice-President*
> Hal Straus, *Director of Publications*
> Kim Torgerson, *Publications Editor*
> Ruth Modric, *Production Manager*

Office of the Executive Vice-President
> Gail Schmidt, *Director, Ophthalmic Society Relations*

Ophthalmic Practice and Services
> Jane Aguirre, *Vice-President*
> Robert Stein, *Executive Director, American Academy of Ophthalmic Executives*
> Mara Pearse Burke, *Ethics Program Manager*

Preface

A professional position is distinguished from a nonprofessional one in large measure by the concept of "professionalism" and professional obligations. This concept extends far beyond the unique set of knowledge and skills that defines the operational scope of the profession and includes ideas about the application of the profession and the interaction of the profession with society. The application of complex professional knowledge and skills while maintaining an ethos of professionalism has become particularly challenging in today's social and economic climate. However, as the medical ethicist Pellegrino noted in an editorial to the *Journal of the American Medical Association*, " . . . any ethic changeable by fortuitous social, economic, political or legal fiat ultimately ceases to be a viable ethic." (Pellegrino, ED. Ethics. *JAMA*. 1996;275:1807–1809).

For decades, graduate medical education in ophthalmology and continuing postgraduate education in ophthalmology have been focused largely on the scientific aspects of the profession—on the body of ophthalmologic knowledge and skills and their application in the physician–patient interaction. Over the past quarter century, while ophthalmology residency training has remained generally a 36-month process, the science and skills of ophthalmology have exploded in complexity. Molecular genetics, phacoemulsification, immunomodulation, pars plana vitrectomy—all have emerged largely in the last quarter century.

The environment of medical practice has likewise undergone a revolution. Viewed retrospectively, the physician–patient relationship in the past was delightfully simple. Health care was an individual matter and a straightforward transaction. The individual patient chose to come to a physician; the physician provided care to the patient; a bill was rendered to and paid by the patient (or by an insurance company at billed charges or at a nominal discount from the charges). Relations between practicing physicians and corporations were minimal. Relations between physicians and pharmaceutical and equipment corporations occurred locally through "detailers" or "representatives" or on the floor of the American Academy of Ophthalmology's Annual Meeting. Surgery was performed at nonprofit institutions. Interaction with the government concerning professional matters engaged a relatively small fraction of our profession.

Graduate medical education in ophthalmology thus did not concern itself greatly with the business of medical practice or with nonscientific questions about the physician's role beyond caring for patients—that is, with the physician's role in society and the larger considerations of professionalism and biomedical ethics.

Our training programs, our profession, and our patients can no longer afford that luxury. Regardless of whether an ophthalmologist starts a solo practice, joins colleagues in a small group, or joins an academic faculty, he or she must understand the different payor mechanisms, personnel management issues, compliance obligations of a myriad of federal regulations, and ethical and legal questions surrounding professional marketing. Corporate relationships engender many perceived and real issues of conflict of interest. State and federal policy, legislation, and regulations affect every physician in every aspect of professional life.

In fact, the Accreditation Council for Graduate Medical Education (ACGME) in its General Competencies has included subjects pertaining to the environment of care and the "nonscientific" process of care, subjects that must be addressed by all residency programs. According to the ACGME, all residents are required to demonstrate the competencies based on appropriate educational experiences incorporating specific knowledge, skills, and attitudes.

Specifically, the general competencies under patient care include:

- Communication skills as they reflect basic principles of medical ethics
  - ➤ Communicate effectively and demonstrate caring and respectful behaviors when interacting with patients and their families.
  - ➤ Counsel and educate patients and their families.
- An obligation to employ effective interpersonal skills and a commitment to lifelong learning and application of information technology:
  - ➤ Work with health care professionals, including those from other disciplines, to provide patient-focused care.
  - ➤ Use information technology to support patient care decisions and patient education.

The general competencies under professionalism state that residents must demonstrate a commitment to carrying out professional responsibilities, adherence to ethical principles, and sensitivity to a diverse patient population. Residents are expected to:

- Demonstrate respect, compassion, and integrity; a responsiveness to the needs of patients and society that supersedes self-interest; accountability to patients, society, and the profession; and a commitment to excellence and ongoing professional development.
- Demonstrate a commitment to ethical principles pertaining to provision or withholding of clinical care, confidentiality of patient information, informed consent, and business practices.
- Demonstrate sensitivity and responsiveness to patients' culture, age, gender, and disabilities.

The general competencies for systems-based practice state that residents must demonstrate an awareness of and responsiveness to the larger context and system of health care and the ability to effectively call on system resources to provide care that is of optimal value. Residents are expected to:

- Understand how their patient care and other professional practices affect other health care professionals, the health care organization, and the larger society and how these elements of the system affect their own practice.
- Know how types of medical practice and delivery systems differ from one another, including methods of controlling health care costs and allocating resources.

- Practice cost-effective health care and resource allocation that does not compromise quality of care.
- Advocate for quality patient care and assist patients in dealing with system complexities.
- Know how to partner with health care managers and health care providers to assess, coordinate, and improve health care and know how these activities can affect system performance.

Historically, the American Academy of Ophthalmology's *Basic and Clinical Science Course* (BCSC) has been used by most ophthalmology residency training programs as an important part of the didactic curriculum. The many volumes in this series do a superb job of organizing and presenting the science of ophthalmology. The series does not (nor was it ever intended to) deliver a curriculum on the application of that knowledge in the practice environment in the profession of ophthalmology. Yet that is now what the ACGME requires.

Pragmatically, this implies that the ophthalmologist residency graduate is not only expected to be clinically competent in the correct application of clinical knowledge and skills in solving the patient's medical problem; the graduate is also expected to apply that ability in a way that is cost-effective, efficient, ethical, and sensitive to the patient and to societal and professional imperatives. The material in this volume is not designed simply to respond to ACGME requirements, but also to empower the ophthalmologist through the development of the profession and professionalism, and to address the socioeconomic challenges presented by the practice of ophthalmology.

Accordingly, this volume is divided into three parts:

- *Practice management.* The business of managing and leading a medical practice goes well beyond the boundaries of this part. This part will, however, provide an ophthalmologist beginning practice with a blueprint for practice organization and business operations. The information may also be of value to many more experienced practitioners seeking to measure their practice against current recommendations and guidelines. It presents the art and the method of the structured application (or business) of the science of medicine. The most capable ophthalmologist will fail patients if he or she does not possess the business skills to develop a sustainable business model from which to apply his or her medical training.
- *Ethics.* The American Academy of Ophthalmology and the profession of ophthalmology has been well served by a robust Code of Ethics—the only medical code of ethics to be formally approved by the Federal Trade Commission. The Academy's Ethics Committee has developed this part to deal not only with abstract principles of ethics but also with real-life ethics questions.
- *Advocacy.* Advocacy on behalf of patients' best health care interests may take two forms: (1) direct patient advocacy, and (2) professional advocacy when the interests of the profession and its practitioners and the interests of the patient are congruent. Physicians and organized advocacy are not a natural mix. Physicians choose to practice medicine in general to advance science and to have an effect on the lives of individual patients. Our profession is data driven, and many physicians assume

that policy will follow data. Some dismiss advocacy as a "dirty" subjugation of clear data and obvious fact by influence—and not worth their time or resources. This part attempts to demonstrate that advocacy is not only critical for physicians and their practices but it is a set of knowledge and skills that can, if applied effectively, have a profound influence on the practice of medicine.

You may ask, "What are practice management, ethics, and advocacy doing in the same volume?" The answer is that they are all integral aspects of the profession of ophthalmology and of the practical real-world application of ophthalmologic clinical knowledge and skills. Correctly applied, all enhance the value of the ophthalmologist to his or her patients and community. The American Academy of Ophthalmology is organized into three Senior Secretariats—for Education, Advocacy, and Ophthalmic Practice. Ophthalmic Practice includes both the Ethics Committee and the Practice Management Secretariat. Quite obviously, the Academy believes not only in the importance of each area represented in this volume but also in their relationship to clinical education. Through these committees and secretariats, the Academy serves as a resource to all ophthalmologists as we advance our profession—to better serve our patients.

This volume is dedicated to our trainees and graduates, with the hope that it will help them deliver care more efficiently, ethically, and effectively. Our profession's promise and our communities' future depend on all ophthalmologists' active advocacy on behalf of patients everywhere.

David W. Parke II, MD
Executive Editor
Oklahoma City, Oklahoma

Acknowledgments

Many individuals helped create this volume. Project leaders David W. Parke II, MD, and Jane Aguirre in particular would like to acknowledge the following contributing authors. Practice management: David A. Durfee, MD (section lead); Michael J. Parshall; and Derek A. Preece. Ethics: Charles M. Zacks, MD (section lead); Christie L. Morse, MD; and Samuel Packer, MD. Advocacy: Paul N. Orloff, MD (section lead); Cynthia A. Bradford, MD; Stephen A. Kamenetzky, MD; Mark C. Maria, MD; Robin M. Pellegrino; William R. Penland, MD; William L. Rich, MD; Kenneth D. Tuck, MD; and Ruth D. Williams, MD.

The following physicians reviewed portions of the content: Randolph Johnston, MD; Thomas J. Liesegang, MD; and Harry A. Zink, MD.

This book benefited immensely from a broad review of a variety of groups. We appreciate the review and the residency-training expertise of the following individuals: Louis Cantor, MD; Anthony Arnold, MD; Bartley Mondino, MD; and Andrew Lee, MD. We appreciate the review and practice management expertise of the American Academy of Ophthalmic Executives (AAOE) Board of Directors: Gaye Baker; Ricky Bass, MBA, MHA; Ann Hulett, COE, CMPE; John Segal, MBA; Walter Underwood, MBA; and Ann Warn, MD, MBA. This book also benefited from the review of the members of the Young Ophthalmologists Committee: Gail Schwartz, MD; Ravi Goel, MD; Richard Grostern, MD; Jennifer Smith, MD; Stephen Whiteside, MD; Charissa Wong, MD; and Dianna M. Seldomridge, MD.

Many thanks to the American Medical Association for permission to derive portions of this work from *Starting a Medical Practice*, second edition.

Finally, we wish to acknowledge two independent contractors: developmental editor Margaret Petela, without whose talents and hard work this book would never have been published in a timely fashion, and Jeff Van Bueren, who did his usual excellent copyediting job.

PART I

The Business of Ophthalmology Practice

Ophthalmology practice in today's world is challenging, exciting, difficult at times, and complex. Yet, unlike the science of ophthalmology, the business of ophthalmology receives relatively little attention during formal ophthalmologic training. Put another way, an ophthalmologist completing residency or fellowship training may be extraordinarily well prepared to care for individual patients, but may fail to master the business of delivering that care and ultimately not serve his or her career or patients as well as possible. While these issues are paramount for the ophthalmologist beginning practice, every ophthalmologist is impacted by issues of professional management. This volume should benefit all ophthalmologists regardless of the stage of their careers.

The early stages of your ophthalmology career involve important decisions that will affect the entire course of your career. The chapters in Part I of this book give you an overview of some of the main issues you will encounter as you embark on your career as an ophthalmologist. You will also get practical guidance about the options you have in starting out and managing your practice. If you are considering the recruitment of a young ophthalmologist, this will provide you with an overview of the transaction from that person's perspective.

Chapters 1–3 present processes and resources for getting a job or establishing your medical practice. By strategically mapping out an action plan and timeline, you will be able to approach your decision making systematically, in accordance with your goals and desired results. These chapters will help you in evaluating practice opportunities, managing the interview process, and negotiating your contract.

Once you have signed the contract or decided to set up your own practice, you will want to be aware of the business issues involved. Although you may have a knowledgeable administrator to help you in this area, ultimate responsibility for professional success is yours. Chapters 4–11 explore topics not often taught in medical school: financial management, regulations and licensing, risk management, insurance, personnel, marketing, and information technology. Individually and collectively, all of these subjects must be carefully considered and the knowledge well applied in order to run your practice efficiently and effectively.

Chapter 12 examines how to foster your ongoing professional development and how to assess the progress of your practice.

CHAPTER 1

Evaluating Practice Opportunities

As you contemplate your first ophthalmology practice, the questions that must be asked and answered seem overwhelming. What kind of practice would best suit you? How much can you expect to be paid? Where do you want to practice? How many patients are available, and what are their eye care needs? How do you find out about open positions, and how do you know whether the practice is a sound and stable one?

In addition to these purely professional and business-oriented questions, you need to consider what might be most *personally* satisfying to you. What situation will meet not only your own needs but also those of your family? Decisions made now will affect you professionally and personally for years to come, and they cannot be taken lightly. This chapter offers tips and tools to help you determine the answers to these complex questions and considerations so that you can make the most informed choices from the outset.

Preparations During Residency

Your preparations to enter into practice begin during residency and gain momentum during your final residency year. The timeline in Table 1-1 can help you plan the sequence of events leading to your first position in ophthalmology. It is important that you prepare well ahead of time because the processing of your practice documents (particularly medical license application and professional liability insurance) may take several months, and most hospitals and insurers require that you have that license before you apply for privileges and panel membership.

Types of Practices

Perhaps the most important initial question to answer is, "What type of practice setting will you find most personally compatible and satisfying?" Is it an academic/university setting or a private practice? Should you join a group? If you think you would be comfortable in a group practice, what appeals to you—a single-specialty ophthalmology group, a multispecialty ophthalmology group, or a diversified multispecialty group? Will you practice comprehensive ophthalmology, or will you concentrate on your subspecialty?

Practice settings differ in important ways. For the advantages and disadvantages of five types of practice settings, see Table 1-2.

Every practice, regardless of its size, is a complicated, service-oriented business. A single-specialty or multispecialty ophthalmology group practice may be a million-

Table 1-1 Timeline for Starting to Practice

During residency	Review your strengths, weaknesses, and desires to determine the type of practice best for you. Decide whether or not to pursue additional subspecialty training.
By 12 months before end of training	Decide on specific practice type to pursue, such as solo private practice, group practice, or academic environment. Research and decide on acceptable geographic locations. Contact offices fitting your practice type and geographic goals to ascertain their needs and interest. Send cover letter and curriculum vitae to interested offices.
By 6 months before end of training	Interview with practices. Review the offers received. Request a written contract from your top one or two practices. Have an attorney review the formal employment contracts. Sign an employment agreement with your choice of practice. Apply for your state medical license. Apply for your state drug registration. Apply for your DEA license.
By 4 months before end of training	Apply for hospital privileges. Apply for Medicare and Medicaid numbers. Apply for acceptance on insurer panels. Apply for professional liability insurance.
By 2 months before end of training	Arrange for housing at new location. Arrange for moving your household goods. Make other personal arrangements involving family.
By 1 month before end of training	Complete new employee forms. Complete health insurance forms.
After commencement of new employment	Meet all practice staff members. Meet hospital and surgery center staff members. Meet referring doctors. Participate in talks, screenings and other public events to become known in the community. Participate in hospital meetings and committees. Build relationships with patients. Show interest in and participate in practice meetings. Through your positive actions, build your reputation as a caring and competent ophthalmologist.

dollar—or multimillion dollar—business with many expenses. Most physicians, however, are more skilled in the clinical aspects of their practices than they are in the business aspects. Although this is changing, this lack of focused business acumen may be reflected in the way the practice recruits you and how it manages itself. To help you in considering the group practice option, refer to the "Group Practice Questionnaire" in Appendix I.

Many facets of medical practice management are changing as physicians recognize the need to function as business people to survive the increased competition and reduced reimbursements. It is becoming more common to see higher-level administrators in ophthalmology practices hired to handle the myriad of day-to-day complexities of managing the business aspects of practice, from personnel management to risk-bearing managed care contracting. As ophthalmology and mixed-practice medicine groups are growing, this trend is likely to continue. In today's dynamic health care environment, medical

Table 1-2 Types of Practice Settings

Practice Type	Characteristics	Considerations
Institutional practice	HMO/employment Hospital/employment Academic/faculty practice	In this setting you are trading the potential risk/value of equity for the risk/value of an employment contract and no commitment of capital. You also trade administrative control for more distributed leadership and management.
Group practice—single or multisubspecialty	Full-spectrum "eye care" Vision care, optical, and dispensing Comprehensive ophthalmology Anterior segment/refractive/cataract Retina and vitreous Cornea/external disease Glaucoma Oculoplastics Neuro-ophthalmology Pediatrics	This practice model may position itself as the "total eye care" provider or the single subspecialty practice with (by virtue of size) market clout. Like the institutional and multispeciality practice models, it requires some loss of individual management control.
Private practice—comprehensive ophthalmology	Most common type of practice Includes starting your own practice or joining an existing solo practice	These practices usually offer most ophthalmology services that the physicians feel comfortable providing and refer subspecialty care to other doctors.
Solo subspecialty practice	Any subspecialty large enough to support a practice, probably a referral practice	Establishment of a new, solo subspecialty referral practice depends on a careful assessment of referral catchment area demand for service.
Multispecialty group practice	Combines primary care physicians with specialists to offer all or most of the health care services needed by patients	These groups tend to be much larger than typical ophthalmology groups and generally nonproceduralists with all the attendant benefits and (particularly compensation) complexities.

practices (particularly ophthalmology practices) must adapt to accommodate a variety of market forces. As a result, many ophthalmology practices are becoming larger and more "full service."

Of course, larger organizations also tend to be more complicated and expensive to operate and manage. A university faculty practice group, for instance, is generally a large group with a complex mission involving non–revenue-generating components such as teaching and research. Those mission components may or may not be completely supported by the parent institution through an overhead charge called the *Dean's Tax,* which is applied to the group's clinical revenues. The staff-model health maintenance organization (HMO) group is, paradoxically, in both the health insurance and health care provider roles, and has to balance the care with the costs of care in order to remain solvent. These staff model groups also tend to have shareholders as owners and professional managers. Generally both of these factors lead to there being less control by any one physician.

Smaller organizations, while able to be more responsive, tend to be more at risk when reimbursements change, and they may not be able to afford new technology or services due to their smaller scale of practice.

Compensation

Many ophthalmologists seeking their first position focus inordinately on the issue of personal compensation. Certainly compensation is a critical issue. Ask yourself, however, "Would I turn away from my basic ethical principles for an additional $50,000 a year?" or "Would I choose to work for someone I do not like and do not trust for an additional $50,000 a year?" Hopefully, the answer to these questions is "no." The implication is that cultural or nonfinancial issues have to be satisfied as well as do the financial ones. In fact, some professional management consultants believe these considerations must be satisfied before any discussion of compensation takes place.

Compensation varies with each practice model. Most notably, academic opportunities may offer a more moderate monetary compensation package, but they are perceived as prestigious and may offer a rewarding opportunity to pursue scientific or research interests and to participate in the training of physicians. However, with time, compensation in the academic environment has become increasingly governed by clinical incentives, effectively narrowing the gap with private practice.

In comparison, a private practice may offer you a substantially higher compensation package, but work and productivity expectations are usually also significantly higher.

A large group, regardless of the practice setting, usually has a defined pay range, particularly for new associates. Since it is always adding or replacing physicians, it has to stay within the limits of compensation that it has paid to newly hired associates, a concept called *internal equity*. If compensation is an important factor for you, your goal during the interview process is to influence where you fall in that range, although the group's internal equities may leave you with little negotiating room. More and more large groups are recognizing that there is little purpose in disadvantaging the high revenue generator by putting a ceiling on clinical earnings.

Because a larger organization tends to have greater financial resources and more predictable revenues, it is more capable of paying a higher base salary. At the same time, it may be less willing to share profits with you through bonuses or other compensation arrangements because of higher overhead or the need to adequately compensate less-significant revenue generators (whose services are valued by the greater physician group). On the other hand, some large groups may have a very adequate reward structure in place through either direct or deferred compensation. The smaller the practice setting, the greater the likelihood the employer will pay a smaller base with a generous incentive-compensation. Thus, the employee shares some of the financial risk associated with the smaller employer, but he or she is also positioned to enjoy the upside rewards.

Compensation is *always* a two-way street. The amount and the manner in which you are initially paid depends on how well you promote yourself to your potential employer and how well the potential employer promotes itself to available candidates, in addition to other factors such as the reason the practice is recruiting at the time you are interviewing. This is simple economics, based on the law of supply and demand. Young ophthalmologists looking for positions are the supply; the employers are the demand. Both parties are usually trying to "sell" something to the other. If the demand outstrips the supply, compensation tends to rise; if there is excess supply, compensation tends to be moderated.

Your long-term compensation depends on your ability to produce what is most important to your practice. In private practice, that usually means how well you produce income. In academic settings, that can mean obtaining research contracts.

When evaluating practice opportunities it is critical to take the long-term view. It makes little economic sense to focus on the initial 1- or 2-year guarantee and to ignore the longer-term earnings potential. The box "Factors to Consider in Evaluating a Practice Opportunity" lists a few additional considerations to help you put the economic opportunity presented into perspective.

Factors that are key to the group's ability to compensate a new associate are often driven by the reasons for recruiting as well as by the practice's location. These are important factors in the supply-and-demand equation. If the group is recruiting to replace

---

✓ KEY POINT

Compensation is ultimately determined based on your initial ability to "sell yourself" and your negotiation process, including the trade-offs you are willing to make.

Factors to Consider in Evaluating a Practice Opportunity

- Geographic location, both regional and local
- Office building location, style, layout
- Available technology and practice amenities
- Lifestyle demands (eg, work hours and productivity expectations)
- Market share, competitive position, and reputation in its service area
- Referral patterns of the practice and caseload type and mix
- Effectiveness executing its business plan
- Building style, amenities, equipment, and so forth
- Co-ownership and employment terms offered
- Governance structure
- Need for physicians and reasons for the need (eg, workload, practice expansion, physician departure or death)
- Ability to fit in professionally and personally with existing practice physicians
- Quality of existing practice physicians

a very busy departing physician, it has an acute need to replace that doctor. The group presumably has both the economic ability to compensate a new doctor without risk to the partners' income and the willingness to share the patient workload with the new associate. Therefore, that group might be able to offer an above-market package to the new associate who is immediately available. If the group is adding a new doctor because of practice growth, there is a greater risk to the partners' income if the new associate is, in the partners' view, overcompensated, or they may still be unsure whether patient workload will justify another full-time doctor.

The laws of supply and demand apply to both the employer and employee when finding and securing a position in a practice. Therefore, both candidate and employer are affected by the number of ophthalmology residents and fellows seeking practice opportunities each year, and by the overall economic conditions within the profession (reimbursement trends, practice consolidations, and new technological innovations), much of which is beyond the control of either the candidate or the employer.

If a high guaranteed salary level is important to you, then you may have to be flexible about location, bonus potential, or other benefits. Alternatively, you might be offered a great compensation package to join the practice, only to discover that your annual salary increases will be small or nonexistent, or that the buy-in terms are either oppressive or not offered at all. (Co-ownership is not always a part of the agreement and it is usually not automatic.) Therefore, you will want your contract to define the options, timing, and costs associated with a possible future equity transfer.

Table 1-3 shows nationwide average starting salary ranges as of 2004. These salary ranges do not reflect other elements of compensation, such as bonuses, insurance, paid expenses, personal leave time, and the like. Other important issues, such as the overall desirability of the practice or the situation itself, are not considered.

Geographic and Demographic Influences

Expect starting salaries in highly desirable metropolitan areas to be at the low end of the scale, and starting salaries in rural or more difficult hiring areas to be generally higher. Also, be very careful about comparing your offer to offers your colleagues receive. The

Table 1-3 Nationwide Average Starting Salary Ranges

Subspecialty	Starting Salary Range*
Comprehensive ophthalmology	$95,000–$140,000
Anterior segment (fellowship trained)	$100,000–$150,000
Glaucoma	$110,000–$180,000
Cornea/refractive	$120,000–$220,000
Retina and vitreous	$150,000–$240,000
Pediatrics	$100,000–$180,000
Oculoplastics	$110,000–$140,000

* Starting salaries vary broadly by region and according to local demographics. Salaries are slightly higher for Board-certified candidates. Most private practice ophthalmology associates also have bonus potential.
  Source: The Healthcare Group, 2004.

facts of the actual practice situations will dictate the financial offer and contract terms, and few situations are really comparable.

In addition, consider taking the long-term view of any offer you receive. While a particular opportunity may not represent the highest offer you might receive, your research will reveal that with some opportunities—in the long run—you may be better off starting with a lower salary in exchange for other opportunities in the future. Be sure these other options are addressed in the agreement.

There is no single source of information on what population base is needed to support an ophthalmology practice on average. Clearly, an ophthalmology practice is very dependent on the age of the patients and on the age of the population within a reasonable distance of the practice. It is also dependent in part on the number of optometrists in the region and on their referral pattern for ophthalmologic care. Nonetheless, as a very rough estimate of the need for your talents in an area, you might consider that, generally, an average comprehensive ophthalmology practice probably needs a universe of about 20,000 people. This is influenced greatly however, by both the age of the population and the managed care environment (high HMO penetration).

Demographic issues are very important to ophthalmologists' success. With increasing age comes the onset of cataracts, macular degeneration, diabetes, and other eye problems. Consider that the ratio of ophthalmologists required for a "Medicare population" is generally four to six times that of a "commercial population." The census bureau counts the Medicare population and computes the percentage that population represents in a given geographic area. Nationally, the Medicare population is 12.8% of the total population. Any market that has a higher percentage is "better" for ophthalmologists. Any market with over 20% Medicare population is excellent.

Another good demographic indicator to consider is how well similarly situated "parallel" practices look. For example, cardiology, urology, and orthopedic practices generally rely on an older population for patients. How many of these parallel practitioners are in the area? How does the number of physicians in those parallel practices compare to the ophthalmologists in the area?

There are dozens of questions you might ask yourself about these topics before you can construct even an initial "A list" of location choices. The suggestions in the box "Questions to Ask Yourself About Geography, Demographics, and Opportunities" can help get you started on this process.

Personal Preferences and Needs

Along with the other considerations discussed, your personal preferences and needs will help determine which practice opportunity is likely to suit you. Some relevant issues to consider are listed in the box "Questions to Ask Yourself About Your Personal Preferences."

It is imperative to realize that economics is only one (and frequently not the major) factor in choosing a practice setting. No matter how good the economics are, if you are not personally and professionally satisfied, the match is not a good one. Factors such as the community, the interpersonal relationships and collegiality, the professionalism and

Questions to Ask Yourself About Geography, Demographics, and Opportunities

- How many other ophthalmologists are practicing in the same area?
- Is the area overserved? Underserved?
- To what extent have managed care plans penetrated the area and how has that penetration altered the area patient demographics and/or referral patterns?
- Is the population growing, and are there favorable demographics for your subspecialty?
- How do you differentiate your practice?
- What about the practice competitors? How busy are they? How do they compare to your potential employer? How do they differentiate or market themselves?
- Can you successfully compete with a rival practice? How?
- Will you be able to be credentialed with the local payors?
- What are the sources of referrals in the practice?
- How do you know there is a shortage in your practice area?
- Is there a reason for the undersupply of physicians?
- How will those factors affect your practice if you locate there? Can you live with this situation?

Questions to Ask Yourself About Your Personal Preferences

- In what kind of environment will your "ideal" practice be found?
- How hard do you want to work? At what pace?
- How much control do you want to have over practice decisions?
- How many other physicians do you want to work with in the practice?
- Do you prefer a large office staff, including allied health personnel, or do you prefer to do most things yourself?
- What feels to be the most natural fit for you?
- Do you want to be involved with teaching or research?

quality of the practice, and the opportunity to have governance input may ultimately be more important. If the culture does not fit you, the money may be irrelevant.

Consider both your priorities and the trade-offs you are realistically willing to make, and be clear about your economic, geographic, practice setting, and other preferences, and their relative importance to you. Completing the questionnaire in Table 1-4 can help you assess the kind of practice that is compatible with some of your personal characteristics.

Involving Your Family and Other Advisors

In making your decisions, be sure to involve your spouse or partner, family members, and others close to you whom your decision will strongly affect, as well as trusted advisors and friends. Ask these others for their take on your personal preferences for your work

> **✓ KEY POINT**
>
> **Each practice option has trade-offs. The goal is to find a practice situation that is best suited to you and satisfies most of your personal and professional needs.**

Table 1-4 Job-Seeker's Self-Assessment Tool

Circle the answer to each question that most closely represents your characteristics and then total the circled responses for each column. The column with the most responses circled represents the practice setting that may be most compatible with your working style. Recognize that this is an oversimplification and that there are numerous permutations of every major practice type.

Question	Sole Proprietor	Partnership or Group Practice— Co-Ownership	Employment— No Ownership
Do you want *complete* control over your business environment and do you feel comfortable with all business decisions such as hiring and firing, and buying equipment?	Yes	Somewhat	No
Are you comfortable making difficult business decisions?	Yes	Somewhat	No
Are you organized and detail oriented with regard to business issues?	Yes	Somewhat	No
Are you comfortable taking financial risk?	Yes	Somewhat	No
Do you perform well having your clinical utilization monitored?	No	Somewhat	Yes
Do you enjoy marketing and networking?	Yes	Somewhat	No
Are you willing to compromise on difficult issues?	No	Somewhat	Yes
Do you enjoy managing and leadership?	Yes	Somewhat	No
Are you good at containing expenses?	Yes	Somewhat	No
Is getting the maximum possible compensation important to you?	Yes	Somewhat	No
Can you focus on business issues and profits in addition to patient care?	Yes	Somewhat	No
Totals:			

environment, and how it might affect both you and them. This will help ensure that everyone whose input is important is considered and will reduce the chances of creating a situation in which someone is unhappy later.

The Search for Practice Opportunities

Unless you are a real risk-taker, you will probably not start out by establishing a new practice in a highly competitive city. When they are starting out, most residents join or purchase an established practice. Since most practices are really no better at finding candidates than candidates are at finding available positions, you will need to conduct the broadest possible search to find the largest variety of alternatives from which to choose. The box "Sources for Finding Opportunities" lists some of these options, and describes ways in which they might help you. You will most likely find a practice that is a good match if you:

- Know what you are looking for
- Start your search early
- Keep an open mind
- Talk to as many people as possible
- Search as broadly as possible
- Separate your needs from your wants

Do this within your expressed criteria and priorities. Remember, you cannot make a good choice if you fail to look at all of your options.

Using Recruiters

Some recruiters will say that they will "represent" you and handle your practice search. If you are approached this way, ask the recruiter how much you have to pay for this service. If you do not have to pay the recruiter, will he or she actually be working for you? Remember that recruiters refer you only to practices that have agreed to pay their fee. That represents a relatively small number of the available opportunities.

Sources for Finding Opportunities

American Academy of Ophthalmology	The Academy's Annual Meeting features the Professional Choices Job Fair designed to bring practices with open positions together in the same setting with physicians seeking employment. The Professional Choices online job board is maintained throughout the year. Visit www.aao.org/professionalchoices. This site is also a good resource to learn about practices for sale.
Attending physicians, professors, and advisors	Ask them about their own and their friends' practices, and about former residents and fellows now in practice who might be looking for associates.
Medical school	Some schools maintain active lists of practice opportunities (to join or purchase practices that have become available).
Print or online advertisements	Opportunities are listed in such publications as *Ophthalmology*, *EyeNet*, and other ophthalmic magazines and trade journals (including Professional Choices online).
Hospital administrators and surgery center operators	Often hospital and surgery center administrators are aware of practices that are recruiting additional doctors; if location is critical, administrators in your preferred location can help you develop a "most likely" list of target practices.
Office staff	Technicians, photographers, and other office staff you work with may have maintained contact with past co-workers in other practices. Ask them if they will have their colleagues advise them if they know of practice opportunities for physicians where they work.
Recruiters	Recruiters can be a good source of free information about who is looking, where they are looking, and what levels of salary they are paying.
Pharmaceutical and equipment representatives	These representatives have contact with many practices and may have knowledge of opportunities in their market area.
Colleagues and friends	You and your colleagues will likely interview with some practices that are not really a good match for you, but that might be right for someone else. Pass these opportunities on to others, and invite colleagues to do the same.
Contacts for employment in an academic setting	Your department Chair or fellowship director will have knowledge of open positions. The newsletter of the Association of University Professors of Ophthalmology (AUPO), available from your Chair, also lists some open positions. If you have a specific geographic or department interest, it helps to specifically query your Chair or contact that department directly. While they may not have posted an open position, the availability of an interested candidate may spur recruitment. Academic positions also can be found on the Academy web site (www.aao.org) in the Professional Choices area described above. These positions are listed in all major ophthalmic journals, and they are also available through the AUPO.

CHAPTER 2

The Interview Process

The interviews you will experience in seeking your first practice opportunity are far different from any you have had before. The practice is seeking a close match with its culture, and an offer will be based as much on subjective as on objective factors. This chapter will help you present yourself as a desirable candidate and get the position that is the most suitable match for success.

The Established Practice

Most new physicians join established practices. Being sure you join the one that is right for you depends first on whether you recognize the right practice opportunity when you encounter it, and second on how well you "connect" with the practice and stimulate their interest in you. To achieve the first goal, start by using Table 2-1 to winnow the less stable practices from your list of possibilities. The next section, "Presenting Yourself Effectively," helps you achieve the second goal.

Presenting Yourself Effectively

As described above, you need to evaluate various characteristics of the practice you are considering joining. To present yourself effectively, you also need to know what employers are seeking. The list below presents just a few major characteristics that favorably impress potential employers:

- Excellent training record
- Experience
- Ability and willingness to respond effectively to practice demands
- Ability and willingness to promote the practice (for example, by means of specialized or new skills, or by reputation brought to the employer)
- Personality and ability to "fit in" with other members of the practice
- Ability and willingness to relate to patients and to build a patient following
- Board certification and/or fellowship status

Making Contact with a Prospective Employer

To pursue an opportunity with an existing practice, start by sending a cover letter and a copy of your curriculum vitae (CV) to the practice. Do this either as your initial contact with the practice or as a follow-up step after you have met someone who might be interested in employing you.

Table 2-1 Characteristics of a Well-Run Practice

To help you assess each of the practices you are considering joining, rate each from 1 to 5 for each characteristic in this table, then total the responses. Practices with scores less than 30 may need significant restructuring to be viable in the future, so keep that in mind if you decide to accept a position there.

KEY:

1 = Poor or nonexistent   2 = Fair   3 = Average   4 = Above average   5 = Excellent

Characteristic	Score (1–5)
Office location: easy to find, ease of access, central to population, etc.	_____
Office facility: attractiveness of building exterior and interior, clear signs, etc.	_____
Office organization: clear roles for staff, written job descriptions, policies and procedures, clear supervision structure, etc.	_____
Staff longevity: have any employees been with the practice a number of years, or is there constant turnover?	_____
Staff morale: do the employees seem to enjoy working there?	_____
Physician morale: what is the attitude of the owner(s) and other physicians toward the practice? Do the physicians enjoy working together?	_____
Insurance situation: are the doctors in the practice on the key insurance panels? Will you be able to get on those panels?	_____
Billing situation: how many days outstanding are in the accounts receivable?	_____
Competitive situation: how is the practice competing with other practices in the market?	_____
Demand for your services: how far into the future are the practice's current doctors booked? Less than a week indicates minimal excess demand and a longer time building your practice. More than a month means the practice is losing patients who could help build your practice.	_____
Total:	_____

Cover Letter

Send your cover letter and CV directly to the practice administrator or the managing physician responsible for the search. Call the practice if you have any doubt at all about the person's correct name, how to spell it, or his or her title or position in the practice.

Your cover letter should contain at least the following information:

- Your full name, address, and home phone number
- How you learned the practice is looking for an ophthalmologist with your subspecialty
- Why you are interested in the position (from the area, looking for a position in a similarly situated practice, etc)
- Your professional and personal objectives
- Your medical-training status, when you will be finished (or when you finished), and a description of your training experience (number of cases performed, prominent teachers, technology/procedures skills)

✓ **KEY POINT**

First impressions last. Ensure that your cover letter and CV have no typographic errors or misspelled names and are presented in a clean, easy-to-read format. Be certain you have included all of the information discussed in the "Cover Letter" section. A compelling cover letter without your phone number will not produce the result you desire.

- A request for a telephone interview to learn more about the practice and its physicians
- Your Board status
- How, when, and at what phone number you can be reached

Figure 2-1 shows a sample cover letter.

Curriculum Vitae

Your CV is a recitation of how you have spent the last 10 or more years of your life. It must be neat, accurate, and complete. It must answer the "who, why, when, where, and how" of your past medical training and work experience. Truly, your CV is *sales* literature that describes you and what you offer. Figure 2-2 presents a sample CV.

Your CV should include the following elements:

- Your full name, address, home and work phone numbers, e-mail address, and pager number
- All of your medical training, including where you trained, when you trained, and with whom you trained (particularly if notable) since college
- All the honors you ever earned, even if not medically related
- Any research or articles that you have published, worked on, or collaborated on, even if not medically related
- Any special personal or professional interests that you have or wish to pursue
- A list of the states in which you are currently licensed to practice

Also consider having more than one CV for the different audiences you may approach. For example, while a five-page CV reciting all of your research and written projects is ideal for an academic-based practice, it may not be the image you wish to present if you are considering a private practice at a community hospital, because it may send a different message about your professional interests and goals.

Have your CV professionally prepared and check it very carefully for typographic errors. Print it on good-quality, traditionally colored (white or beige) stationery. Alternatively, it is appropriate to send your CV to the prospective employer by e-mail. If you fax your CV, make sure it is printed on white paper so that it looks as good as possible when printed on the receiver's fax machine.

The Telephone Interview

Suppose that you have sent out your letters and CVs and someone interested in speaking to you has just paged you or left you a message. Call back quickly, even if all you do is

---

Rhonda M. Smith, MD
4270 Ridge Lane
Philadelphia, PA 04040

August 14, 2005

Michael J. Foreman, MD
Ophthalmology Associates, PA
20 Twenty-First Street
Philadelphia, PA 04040

Dear Dr. Foreman:

William Edelman, MD, suggested I contact you to see if you are looking for an associate this year. Dr. Edelman spoke highly of your practice and its aggressive approach to providing a full range of eye care services. I am currently board eligible in ophthalmology and am completing a one-year glaucoma fellowship with Dr. Preser at Wills Eye Medical Center. I will complete my fellowship in July of this academic year, and I am looking for a full-time position thereafter.

I am very interested in joining a progressive ophthalmology practice where I may offer subspecialist services. Such a practice would enable me to take advantage of my professional interest in the treatment and management of the glaucoma patient.

I was raised in the Philadelphia suburb of Bryn Mawr, and I am actively pursuing opportunities in the Philadelphia area. My family still resides in Philadelphia, and I am very familiar with the city.

I am interested in speaking with you about your practice and any possible job availability, either with you or another practice that you may know is looking for an associate. I have enclosed my Curriculum Vitae for your consideration.

Please feel free to contact me at (123) 456-7890 or at my home in the evening, (123) 202-2020, to discuss your practice and my qualifications. I look forward to speaking with you.

Sincerely,

Rhonda M. Smith

Rhonda M. Smith, MD

Figure 2-1 Sample cover letter.

say that it is inconvenient to speak at that exact moment. Ask to schedule a telephone interview at a more relaxed but specific time for both of you.

Schedule the call for a block of time during which you have a period of uninterrupted time to talk. Do not try to do other things at the same time; you will sound distracted, and you will not likely make the best impression.

Preparing for and Conducting the Interview

Prior to the conversation, compile a list of questions you wish to have answered. Research the community and refresh yourself on the facts so you can show that you have "done your homework." Plan to discuss the following areas.

CURRICULUM VITAE

Rhonda M. Smith, MD
4270 Ridge Lane
Philadelphia, PA 04040
(123) 202-2020 (H)
(123) 456-1234 (F)
rsmith@abc.com

EDUCATION

Doctor of Medicine
University of Pennsylvania School of Medicine, Philadelphia,   1997–2001
Pennsylvania
Bachelor of Science in Biology
University of Maryland, College Park, Maryland   1993–1997

RESIDENCY

General Ophthalmology
State University Of New York At Buffalo, Buffalo, New York   2001–2003

FELLOWSHIP

Glaucoma Fellowship
George Preser, MD, Wills Eye Hospital   2003–2004

HONORS
- Administrative Chief Resident   2003–2004
- Ellen T. Ross Teaching Resident of the Year   2002–2003
- Amy S. Noble Award for Outstanding Medical Student   2001
- Alpha Omega Alpha   2001
- William D. Smith Aware for Distinction in Biology   1997
- Phi Beta Kappa   1993–1997

CERTIFICATIONS
- National Boards Part 3   2003
- Board Eligible - General Surgery   June 2004
- Advanced Trauma Life Support Instruction   2003–Present
- Advanced Cardiac Life Support   2003

PROFESSIONAL AFFILIATIONS
- American College of Surgeons (Candidate Group)
- American Medical Association (Residents Forum)
- New York State Medical Society
- Pennsylvania Medical Society

LICENSURE
- New York
- Pennsylvania
- DEA

PUBLICATIONS

Guarino J, Marone L, Moenning S, et al. Ultrasound evaluation of blunt abdominal trauma. Annuals of Ophthalmology. 2001;75:234–238.

Corcoran J, Sweeney D, Decker P, et al. The influence of retinal translocation. New England Journal of Medicine. 2002;82:89–95.

PERSONAL INTERESTS
- Snow skiing, tennis, jogging, aerobics, gourmet cooking

REFERENCES
- Available upon request

Figure 2-2 Sample curriculum vitae.

- The type and size of the practice (eg, number of offices, doctors, and specialties, or presence of ambulatory surgery centers)
- Why the practice is recruiting (eg, turnover, growth, disability, or new service)
- What clinical, business, and interpersonal skills are being sought
- What long-term plans the practice has

Take lots of notes. This will help you to keep the facts straight, especially if you plan to speak with the usual number of prospective employers (most candidates consider only three to at most eight practices). You will then be able to compare practices in a meaningful way, based on commonly solicited information.

Right from the start, do your best to impress the interviewing person or group. You may not get another chance. The group is no different than you in that it will only consider a handful of candidates at any given time. Express your enthusiasm for the opportunity, and reiterate your strongest "selling points," your training, and how well you match the group's hiring criteria. Of course, be cordial, tactful, and communicative, and thank each interviewer for his or her time.

Ask for the names of former associates of the practice and why they left. You should ask if there are former associates you can speak with about the practice's culture and operations. You should also be prepared to identify former associates by asking staff in other practices. You will want to know if, and why, a number of associates may have passed through a particular practice. You may want to ask if the practice has ever had lawsuits involving former associates, and what issues led to any legal actions. There may be valuable lessons in this line of inquiry, but keep in mind most practices would be reluctant to share this information. You may get a better result by asking staff in other practices in the same town.

Following Up

Immediately after the telephone interview, send a note, even if you are *not* planning to pursue an interview. Neatly handwritten notes are better than typewritten notes (or e-mail), assuming your handwriting is legible. Your goal is to leave a good impression and to either terminate or continue this process with this group.

If you are interested in moving forward in the interview process, then remind the person you spoke with about the high points of your conversation, including when you talked and what your special talents are. Describe your interest in the practice opportunity. This is a good time to request an in-person interview to meet the physician(s) and to see the practice. Again, remind the contact person how to reach you (phone and pager numbers and/or e-mail address), ideal times to call, and provide other helpful information. Be sure to clarify who is expected to take the next step, and when. Always end by thanking your contact for his or her time and interest.

✓ KEY POINT

Always follow up every telephone interview with a note. You may be surprised how such a simple acknowledgment may make you stand out from your peers, and keeps the process moving.

✓ KEY POINT

You had a successful initial telephone interview with a practice representative, and you have been invited for an in-person interview, or extended phone interview with other practice members. Be aware that sometimes the prospective employer pays the reasonable costs associated with interviewing, but not always; find out in advance.

Even if you are not interested in pursuing further discussions with the prospective employer, you should still send a follow-up note showing your appreciation for the interest shown in you, and letting the practice know your thoughts on the opportunity.

The In-Person Interview

Your in-person interview is your most important opportunity to assess a practice. It is one of the few times that you will be face to face with your potential associates and colleagues. You will have the opportunity to ask important questions, observe the practice in operation, and see how people in the practice interact among themselves and with patients. This is the time to gather the information you need to make an informed decision about joining the practice and to influence the offer (Figure 2-3).

Your in-person interview is an ideal opportunity for you to display your medical knowledge and skills, as well as your opinions and your views of patient care. But, most important, both you and the practice members should consider how you would fit into the practice in terms of personality, philosophy of medicine, and your personal, medical, and professional style. You should assess the practice members in those terms, because they will assess you in those same terms.

In a good interview, both sides are open, honest, and fair in the way they present themselves. Ideally, you are a candidate of interest to the practice, and the practice is an interesting opportunity for you. Both sides, though, are usually also on their "best behavior," so being thorough in asking questions enables you to collect all the information you need to make the right decision.

Understanding the Interview Process

Practices approach the interviewing process in many different ways, depending upon their location, the number of attractive candidates they have to interview, and their reasons for recruiting and their experience with the recruitment process.

In urban areas, where medical schools and teaching programs are common, there is often an overabundance of new candidates and experienced physicians looking for a change. A practice may have a series of interviews with various types of candidates. The process may start with a brief meeting and then proceed to more in-depth meetings during the second (and possibly third) interviews. In more remote areas, where travel to the practice is more costly in terms of both time and money, a practice may complete the entire interview process with you in one in-depth meeting. Recognizing which type of situation you are facing will help you to plan and organize your time.

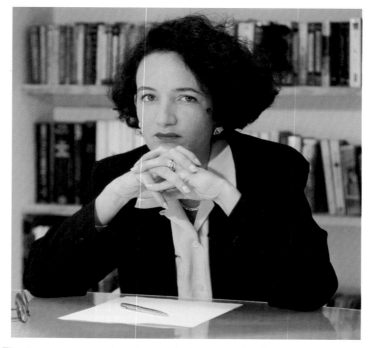

Figure 2-3 The in-person interview is an ideal opportunity for you to display your medical knowledge and skills. Be mindful that both sides want the interview to be successful; the practice is eager to conclude its search for a new associate, and you are likely eager to find a good opportunity so you can return to concentrating on your program and skills.

While there are no hard and fast rules to which your interview must conform, any good interview will include at least the following elements:

- Meetings with all the practice physicians relevant to the position, including the senior and associate physicians
- Meetings with key administrative and support personnel of the practice
- Introductions to a number of practice staff
- An opportunity to see the physician(s) interacting with patients, in both the office and the facilities in which they operate
- A complete tour of the main practice office(s) where you will be practicing
- A community tour, which may be accompanied by a Realtor, so you have an opportunity to investigate housing options and learn about the social and financial climate of the community, the school systems, and other important community features
- A social meeting, such as a relaxed dinner with the physicians, at which you will have an opportunity to talk more candidly with the doctor(s) and with their spouse(s), and they with you
- A tour of the hospital or ambulatory surgery facilities

Know the agenda for your interview; as necessary, ask for that agenda to be modified so that you have time to conduct a thorough search for information about the practice, its physician(s), its environment, and any other important factors.

Ask if the practice is planning to pay all or part of your expenses. If the practice is financing these costs, find out if the practice will pay your expenses directly or if you are expected to submit receipts after the meeting.

Depending upon the practice location, you may want to have your spouse or partner accompany you on at least one of these visits, as his or her input will no doubt affect your final practice selection. However, do not presume to bring anyone to any tour or interview who has not been invited, especially if the practice is paying the costs of your visit. Always find out, in advance, whenever possible and appropriate, whether your spouse, partner, or fiancée is invited to attend the interview; if so, ask whether his or her agenda will differ from yours. Unless you are planning a single, extended, practice interview, the best time for your spouse to accompany you would be on a second interview, when an employer begins to talk seriously about hiring you. Again, be sure to clarify that this is appropriate beforehand.

Preparation

No matter how many times you have been through the process, an interview is a stressful situation. However, proper preparation will improve your performance during an interview. After the interview has been scheduled and before it takes place, attend to the following activities:

1. Prepare a list of questions that relate to the factors that are important to you or that address matters you may wish to have clarified, based on your discussions with other practices.
2. Confirm the date and time of your meetings and all of your travel arrangements, allowing enough time in the event of delayed planes, missed connections, or just getting lost.
3. If traveling to another city, confirm your hotel arrangements before you leave, and make sure you have accurate directions to both your hotel and to the practice.
4. Review your notes from your telephone conversation with the practice in order to reacquaint yourself with the particulars of the practice.
5. With these details out of the way, focus on making important preparations for the interview; think about what you are going to say, how you will present your points, and most importantly, what you bring to this practice opportunity.

The box "Commonly Asked Interview Questions" lists some that you are likely to hear at the interview; be sure to give some thought before the interview to how you will answer them. Although the nuances of the questions you are asked may differ, in some form or manner, from those that you anticipate, typically the same kinds of information are being sought. Remember that the questions you need to answer may be asked either directly or indirectly. Carefully consider your responses in advance. Include substantive evidence to support any contentions (eg, give an example of how you took a leadership role in a project, or how you dealt with a conflict).

Commonly Asked Interview Questions

These questions are all designed to encourage you to talk about yourself and to reveal "what makes you tick." The practice will want to know what prejudices and expectations you already have about your professional career and, if you can express it, why you feel that way.

- How or why did you choose to pursue medicine as a career? Why ophthalmology?
- Why did you choose your subspecialty area of practice (if any)?
- What do you like or dislike most about ophthalmology?
- What are your long-term practice and personal goals?
- Why do you think you would like to be in this type of practice setting?
- How do you think you can contribute to the practice?
- What is your general philosophy of practice?
- Why should we consider you for this opportunity?
- What do you think your references will say about you?
- Where do you want to be in 5 years?
- How do you plan to grow your practice?

Professional and Personal Responses

A common request is "Tell me about yourself." This comment is so broad that it needs to be broken down into its two basic components: the professional and the personal responses.

Address the professional component rather simply with why you chose a career in medicine, what attracted you to this specialty, what your basic training interests are, and what practice goals you have.

On the personal side, your answers should include where you grew up, your family background, your outside interests and hobbies, and your personal goals.

Be sure that you volunteer information about yourself. Beyond your being a good clinician, your prospective employer wants to know that you will be able to get along in the practice personally and professionally, that you are trustworthy, and that you are easy to work with. Can you handle the pace? Do you have the skills and capacity to do the difficult cases? Be prepared to qualify your experience (eg, "I performed 75 cataract extractions last year.").

Questions to Ask Practice Representatives

Your questions to the physicians in the practice—just as their questions addressed to you—should be open-ended and require thorough, well-reasoned responses. Be tactful in what you ask, and how you phrase each question. Do not be too aggressive; your goal is to be perceived as collegial, not adversarial.

Divide your questions into two basic areas: clinical and business. Ask the clinical questions first, before any business issues are discussed. You need to find out if your approach to patient care is the same as the group's approach. A good starting question is "Tell me about your patients." This will lead to a discussion of the types of pathology that present to the practice and what treatment guidelines and protocols are used. Practices vary widely, and some physicians are more aggressive than others about embracing new technology and medicines. You should know how your approach to patient care compares to the group's approach. Once you have learned about the clinical issues, then you can go on to the business questions. Good questions you might ask are in the box "Questions for the Practice." The responses to these questions should generate a comprehensive discussion. Your purpose is to see whether the overall opinions and views of the senior doctors are similar to your views, and whether there is a basic philosophical agreement (or disagreement) between you and the prospective employer.

Interview Tips for Success

In the interview, allow the practice representative to lead. If the interviewer starts by asking you what you want to know, you might ask the interviewer to describe the practice's patients. In other words, focus first on the clinical issues and then move to business issues. The most obvious thing you have in common with the interviewer is the clinical issue, and it is a good way to "break the ice" and promote a good discussion.

After the initial information has been gathered, the discussion should move on to more specific areas, including proposed salary, benefits, call schedule, and terms for co-ownership, if any.

Remember, in an interview, your goal is to develop your assessment of the available opportunity. This cannot be accomplished unless an offer is made to you. It would be very unusual to receive an offer after the first interview. If you wish to pursue this practice,

---

Questions for the Practice

- Why are you looking for a new associate?
- How long have you been recruiting?
- How do you intend to help your new associate become busy? Productive? How will you measure performance?
- Tell me about the practice's primary competition? How is this practice similar to or different from its competitors?
- Of the previous associates who were successful in the practice, what characteristics and skills contributed to their success?
- What are the long-term plans for the practice? How often are these plans reviewed? How has the practice started to move toward these goals?
- What is a typical day/week in the practice like for the physicians?
- Does the practice use outside advisors? How?
- How are practice decisions made?
- How often do the owners meet?
- What is the competitive environment like?
- I offer the following skills to you (*outline them*). How will my skills add value to this practice?
- What do you expect from me to grow my practice, and what can I expect from you to support this goal?

make that wish known. You will be able to acquire additional information in subsequent contact with the practice. Only then will you have all the information you need to make your decision.

Equally important to the substance of the interview are the style and tone that both sides project during this stage of the process. Remember that the physician(s) and administrator(s) interviewing you are your potential colleagues, not your adversaries. At the same time, however, these people are not your close friends, so avoid being overly familiar. Overall, be polite, friendly, and open—not guarded—in your presentation.

At some point later in the interview, you might offer a few suggestions of what you are able to do for, or contribute to, the practice. Examples include making presentations to physicians, schools and retirement communities; developing new markets; obtaining clinical trials; expanding subspecialty practice; and describing other positive steps you are willing to take to contribute to the success of the practice.

After the initial interview you may wish to present to the practice a video or DVD of selected surgical procedures you have performed. This will demonstrate your abilities to the practice.

Salary is only one element of the broader financial package picture; other significant elements include the length of guaranteed employment, benefits offered, terms of co-ownership, and overall potential income as a partner. The answers to these questions are more completely and appropriately communicated at the time an offer is made. For more information on co-ownership, see "Buying Into the Practice (Co-Ownership)" in Chapter 3.

Finally, take a look at suggestions and caveats in the box "How to Shine at an Interview." By being prepared for this event—one of the most important in your career—you can be assured of appearing comfortable and confident when it matters most.

Interviewing for an Academic Position

Much of the information in the preceding sections is as relevant to the interview process for an academic position as it is for private practice. There are some important distinctions, however. First, the department Chair will want you to articulate your career objectives. How do you view your role not only in patient care but also in teaching (at all levels), research (clinical and/or bench research), and administration/professional organization leadership? Second, the Chair will need to understand what resources you require such as laboratory space, research technicians, access to a biostatistician, and computer resources. Third, the Chair will ask you how you intend to integrate your clinical skills into the department. To what degree will you limit the scope of your practice? How will you interface with other department clinicians?

At the interview, try to understand at least the broad brushstrokes of department finance. Is it fiscally sound? What are the major revenue sources? To what extent does the department control its billing and collection processes or are they centralized at the medical school/practice plan level? How is research funded? What is the process for negotiation of compensation? How does the Chair see the department evolving? What role does he or she see you playing?

How to Shine at an Interview

- Be yourself—show the practice what you are like so it can determine whether or not you will fit with their corporate and clinical culture.
- Present yourself well by wearing professional attire, using a nice smile, making eye contact, and using a firm handshake.
- If the practice opportunity, community, and personal chemistry between you and the interviewers seem to interest you, let them know, and tell them what you think about this opportunity.
- Express any areas of concern. This is a good opportunity to demonstrate that you have carefully reviewed the opportunity and you have identified some areas of concern; however, be careful not to appear overly negative in this inquiry process.
- Promote yourself.
- Once you have learned what the practice is looking for, and if you have the required characteristics, demonstrate to the decision makers that you possess the skills, training, and personality traits they need.
- Reinforce your statements with specifics, such as case counts, videos or DVDs of selected surgical cases, events, letters of references, awards, and honors.
- Do not *initiate* salary or financial discussions.
- One of the surest ways to make the wrong impression is to bring up the question of salary or the financial picture of the practice prematurely.
- Wait for the practice to initiate the discussion regarding the financial particulars, to guard against appearing too aggressive.

The interview process itself is also somewhat different from the private practice model. Typically, the process begins during the summer or early fall of your final year of fellowship and concludes by late February. Many Chairs conduct preliminary interviews at the Annual Meeting of the American Academy of Ophthalmology. Prospective candidates will be brought in at the department's expense for a day or two of interviews that will include meetings with many of the faculty. Typically a second visit will also include your spouse and will be more in depth—including compensation discussions.

The Second and Subsequent Interviews

The interview process that progresses to a job offer always includes more than one interview. While the first interview allows the practice representatives and the candidate to learn about each others' goals and expectations, it would be during the subsequent interview(s) where salary discussions would likely be more appropriate. You can leave the wrong impression if you initiate salary discussions too soon in the process. Ideally, wait for the practice representative(s) to initiate the salary discussions.

Also, during the subsequent interviews you may wish to ask the following more probing questions:

- Have any physicians (associates or partners) ever left the practice? Why? Has a physician's departure ever led to litigation or violation of restrictive covenants?
- May I see the practice's income statements and balance sheets for the last 2 years?
- What does your accounts receivable ledger look like? What about the accounts receivable aging report? How many days in receivables do you have?
- Have there been ophthalmologists in this practice who have expected an equity position and then not been offered that opportunity?

Next Steps

In time, all of the dedicated thought and work you have put into finding and participating in interviews will lead to a good match. The next chapter helps you navigate what looks like the promise of a successful marriage: an offer to join the practice.

CHAPTER 3

Your Initial Contract

Imagine this positive scenario: You are presented with an offer to join a practice, and you are accepting the offer. You and the physicians in the group have reached a verbal agreement on the basic terms. You have sent the practice a letter confirming your understanding of the offer and the exact relationship you will have with the practice as an employee, potential co-owner, partner, or otherwise.

This chapter describes the importance of a written agreement and what it should cover. The written agreement (employment contract) spells out your responsibilities, compensation, vacation, fringe benefits, disability, business expenses, and the like. The details to be addressed range from basics such as contract length, compensation scale, and bonuses, to ways in which you will be remunerated when you leave the practice. By clarifying everyone's expectations when you join a practice, you will prevent the frustration that often results later if (or when) the circumstances change.

What an Agreement Contains

Three phases of the employment relationship are often defined in the agreement. The first phase may define your employment as "at-will" initially, meaning the practice may terminate you at any time. The second phase would be more or less the second to the fifth year, spelling out the process for working toward partner status. The third phase would define the terms of a possible or eventual partner contract.

As an agreement is drafted, be sure to have your own attorney review it and guide you in finalizing it (see Figure 3-1 as well as "A Second Opinion" at the end of this chapter). The practice will likely involve its lawyer in the early stages of its recruitment process, to draft the terms of the proposed employment relationship. While this pre-planning is good, be sure that all of the terms you feel are important are addressed to your satisfaction before you sign a contract.

> ✓ **KEY POINT**
>
> **In spite of changes to the business of health care, some practices still do business on a handshake. While that trust is admirable, it is not advisable. Many people forget the exact terms to which they agreed and time often distorts one's perception of what happened.**

> **✓ KEY POINT**
>
> **Your written agreement with the practice should be in plain, easy-to-understand language, and free of ambiguity. In any event, have your own attorney review the agreement before you sign it.**

Be wary when anyone tells you "Do not worry about what the contract says, that's not the way we do it." A contract is a legally binding recitation of the mutual intent and understanding of the parties. While it is true that you may never really look at it again, its real purpose is to be certain that each party performs by the agreed rules when certain events occur. It can be your best protection, or your worst nightmare, when things go wrong. Therefore, review it carefully, and be certain your rights are protected.

Fortunately, a practice usually sends you its offer of terms (contract) in writing soon after a successful interview. Recognize that different types of practices will have different contractual requirements. For example, an academic practice might include in its contract teaching and research expectations, and the like.

Getting the Details Spelled Out

The Term of Employment

Your agreement (or employment contract) should clearly specify the starting date for your employment with the practice. This is especially important if your contract contains a buy-in (co-ownership) provision, because your starting date is usually used as a measuring date thereafter. For more information on co-ownership, see "Buying Into the

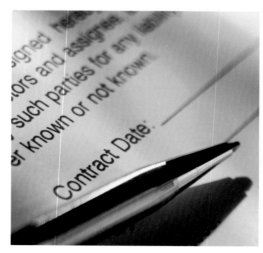

Figure 3-1 Get your offer in writing, and be sure to have an attorney review it and guide you. Be certain your rights are protected.

Practice" later in this chapter. Term is also important as a measuring point for salary and benefits increases.

Be sure you know what happens at the end of the contract term. Do you have to renegotiate a new contract? Is the term guaranteed? Does the contract automatically renew, or must you enter into a new one?

Be wary of 1-year term agreements. You will be in a much weaker negotiating position once you have started to work for the practice. Try to have a 2- to 4-year contract, with annual increases in salary, bonuses, benefits, and other perquisites agreed on.

Termination

Believe it or not, not all contracts provide for termination by the employee prior to the end of the term. While no one can make you work, an employer may be able to sue you for damages if you leave early.

Your agreement should have some statement about how your employment can be terminated by *either* party. Therefore, if you decide that you do not want to continue working for the employer, the question is not *may* you leave early, but *how* you go about doing it.

Termination points should include the following:

- How much notice do you have to give to the practice?
- Can you terminate your employment for any reason, or only if the employer breaches the agreement first?
- If the practice wants to discontinue your employment, how much notice does it have to give you?
- Can the employer terminate your employment without cause?
- Will you be expected to work after you have been given notice? If so, will you be paid during that time?
- Is your employment "at will," meaning that either you or the practice can terminate it at any time or for any reason? Or, is termination only for cause?

"For cause" employment termination is often immediately upon some egregious action, such as committing a felony, becoming uninsurable at standard rates, breaching a material (important) part of the contract, or committing any action of similar severity. Be leery of "for cause" language in your contract that includes "acts harmful to the employer or actions determined in the sole discretion of the employer." These loose provisions essentially reduce the employment to an "at will" arrangement. Your goal, of course, is to have your contract state that the employer may only terminate your employment immediately "for cause" or on 90 days written notice, but you can quit for any reason on 90 days notice and you are paid in the interim if you work. Recognize, however, that more and more contracts contain a "termination without cause" provision.

What other factors apply to employment termination? For example, if your contract contains a bonus provision, will you still be paid that bonus if you are not employed through, or at the end of, the contract term?

Be sure your contract addresses the following issues:

- If my employment terminates, is the bonus I am due prorated? If yes, is it prorated through the date of notice or the date of effective termination?
- When will that bonus be paid? What verification will I be given of the amount ultimately due?

This notice provision can be a particularly important question if you (and your family) are relocating to a new area of the country or if your contract has a restrictive covenant (covenants are covered later in this chapter). If your employment is terminated, how long would it realistically take for you to find a new position, particularly if you must move again and relocate your family?

Compensation Scale

It is typical to go through an employment period of 2–3 years before being offered a co-ownership interest (co-ownership is covered later in this chapter). It is therefore important that you have the salary (compensation) terms spelled out clearly for *each* year in which you will be an employee of the practice. Annual increases in (base) salary must be spelled out in the contract in specific terms.

Incentives and Bonuses

Some practices after the first year may transition the new associate to fully incentivized compensation based on productivity (the so-called "eat what you kill" model). However, typically, incentives and bonuses are paid in *addition* to base (fixed) salary. These incentives are generally offered to induce young ophthalmologists to attract patients to the practice, to work hard for the practice (and therefore also for yourself), and to reward you for your financial contribution and work effort on behalf of the practice. Bonuses are of three different types: gross production, net income, and fully discretionary.

Gross Production Some practices pay bonuses based on a percentage of the income you generate (measured in either charges or collections with collections being preferred) for the practice in excess of a predetermined amount (known as *required revenues*). In some subspecialty areas, particularly refractive surgery and retina, it is common to see higher required revenues than for other subspecialty areas, as the reimbursement per work unit for those subspecialties is higher.

Most threshold bonus amounts are about 2.5–4 times your base pay each year and are a function of the practice's overhead. This bonus method is best for you if your income is predictable (eg, you are being hired to replace a physician who is leaving). But this approach may work against you if it promotes competition among the practice physicians for patients. In the latter case, because you likely cannot control patient assignment, this bonus method may not be right for you.

Know the practice's payor methods (discounted fee, cash, capitation fee [or *set fee*], and so on). Know how (or if) the practice will be able to credit your collection efforts if it receives capitated payments.

The important issues about this bonus type that you should address in the contract include the following:

- Will I start to receive my bonus monthly, quarterly, or annually once I achieve the required revenues?
- What production data will I have access to? How often?
- How will patients be assigned?
- How will my productivity be measured for patients of managed care plans or those who do not pay a fee for each unit of work?

While the timing of bonus payments should be spelled out in the bonus calculation section of the contract, issues related to how "production" is actually measured or how patient assignments are made may not be spelled out. In any event, you must feel comfortable that this bonus allocation will work for you.

Net Income Approach This bonus approach comes in many forms. The most typical states that, to the extent the "net income" in the practice exceeds, for instance, 100% of the previous year's net income, then you are entitled to some portion of that excess. This is a relatively common threshold, but one that obviously cannot be calculated until the end of the year, when all of the income and expenses are known.

Notice that this bonus method does not create competition among physicians by tying an associate's bonus to his or her individual production. It stresses "group" success. However, any extraordinary expenses of the group (even if not directly related to your employment), may reduce your entitlement to a bonus. For example, if the group opens a new office, those new expenses may lower everyone's available net income, therefore reducing your bonus potential.

If you are offered an incentive bonus based on a net income calculation, know how the terms are defined and understand the expectations and assumptions underlying the practice physicians' belief that the net income goal is achievable. After all, an incentive bonus that cannot be achieved is no incentive at all.

Your contract should also meet the following criteria:

- Clarify all terms related to how net income is defined.
- Indicate when your bonus will be paid.
- Assure that expenses for extraordinary items (eg, opening new offices, retiring senior physicians) will not be considered deductions to net income.

Of course, this bonus method works best when your services are really needed and they expand the range of services of the group. They do not work well when you are being hired so senior physicians can work less.

Fully Discretionary Bonus While a fully discretionary bonus is not as common as the other bonus approaches, some practices do still retain the right to determine, based upon the individual merit of each situation, whether or not a physician will earn a bonus. Therefore, these practices will offer a competitive base salary with no stated incentive. The contract will instead stipulate that, to the extent that the Board of Directors of the corporation (or the partners in the partnership) determine, you may be paid a bonus.

Ophthalmology, like other fields, is rapidly changing and subject to large variations in income and expense depending on a variety of market factors. Refractive surgery fees range from $300–$2000 per eye in many areas. The associated technology, marketing, and operational costs vary only slightly. Thus, the difference between the fees is the surgeon's income. Photodynamic therapy for macular degeneration has a completely different revenue/expense ratio than other retina services. Many practices are creating hybrid compensation models that combine work effort and profitability measures for the services the doctors perform as the basis for compensation.

In the bonus methods discussed so far, some issues must still be addressed. These include:

- How will I track how I am doing compared to my bonus targets? Will I be given monthly updates on my performance, productivity, or profitability?
- How will collections be allocated if we deal with managed care plans or have capitated contracts?
- How will patients be assigned to me? Do I have any control over these assignments?
- What other factors will be considered in determining my "contribution" to the practice?
- How is other compensation treated, such as fees related to medical or legal deposition compensation, and speaker honorariums?

If you are expected to generate a defined level of income, ask the practice what assumptions it makes about the following areas:

- Arriving at that threshold figure
- How realistic it is believed to be
- How the practice plans to market your services to help increase your workload
- Why the practice feels it needs an associate
- Whether the (productivity) incentive will create any competition among the practice's physicians

Business Expenses

Typically, a practice pays at least some portion of the general business expenses that you can expect to incur, including:

- Professional liability insurance
- Professional society dues (sometimes only up to a predetermined limit)
- Professional journals and books (sometimes only up to a predetermined limit)
- Hospital staff fees
- Professional travel and education (CME) and at least some costs related to your successfully attaining your basic and/or specialty board certification, if you do not already have it (sometimes only up to a predetermined limit)
- Cellular phones, pagers, personal digital assistants, and other electronic devices (if used)
- All items necessary for you to practice (staff, equipment, and an office)

Be sure your contract clarifies the answers to these questions:

- Are there any limits on the amounts related to these expenses?
- If so, are they determined annually?
- What if you exceed these limits?
- Does the practice pay the expense, or do you pay it personally and then seek reimbursement?
- How do you seek reimbursement?
- What happens if you leave the employment relationship earlier than the contract specifies? Will you have to refund any of these costs?

Malpractice Insurance

There are two basic forms of malpractice insurance: *occurrence* and *claims made.* An occurrence policy is a form of insurance that provides coverage for all claims arising from medical incidents that occur while the policy is in force, regardless of when the claim is ultimately reported. A claims-made policy is a form of insurance that provides coverage to an insured only if the policy is in force both on the date the incident causing the claim occurs and on the date the claim is first reported to the carrier. For additional information, see "Professional Liability Insurance (Malpractice Insurance)" in Chapter 8.

If you already have claims-made malpractice coverage that you will cancel when you join the group, you will need to purchase malpractice insurance that covers you in the event of future claims on past acts, known as *tail coverage,* to cover any potential litigation stemming from actions prior to the new group coverage taking effect.

While your practice may pay the costs of the premiums for your malpractice insurance policy, you must resolve in your employment contract which party is responsible for payment of the tail coverage if the practice will purchase claims-made coverage for you. Always attempt to have the employer pay the tail coverage. After all, your employer is the one who received the advantage from the lower cost. Also, on employment termination, most employers keep your accounts receivable so they have a source of income to fund this payment.

In some cases, the premium for a tail is not charged. Often, in cases of death or disability, a tail is provided free of charge. Also, when a physician retires the premium may be waived if he or she has been insured for a certain number of years and meets any other requirements of the carrier. Make sure to ask the carrier for details of what circumstances will qualify you for a free tail policy.

✓ KEY POINT

According to recent studies, the typical ophthalmologist can expect to be sued at least once during a career. Therefore making the best current and long-term coverage decisions about malpractice coverage is imperative in order to protect the practice you will spend your career building.

Remember, your malpractice insurance is personal to you. It makes no difference that the practice happens to pay the premiums; under most state laws, the policy is treated as yours. Therefore, your failure to pay the tail may lead to uncovered claims, difficulty in obtaining future insurance coverage, or even loss of your license to practice medicine in that state. If you lose your license in one state, you may also lose it elsewhere.

As you can see, malpractice insurance is critically important to protecting your financial resources. You can find additional information in *Protecting Your Practice: What You Need to Know About Insurance,* a guide published by the American Academy of Ophthalmic Executives (see Appendix I).

Employee Fringe Benefits

The practice that you are joining may offer fringe benefits to its physician-employees. Typically, some combination (or all) of the following benefits are offered:

- Payment of basic health and major medical insurance for you (and usually also for your family)
- Group term life insurance
- Payment or reimbursement for your disability insurance premiums
- Coverage under the retirement plans of the practice, after some waiting period (usually not more than 24 months)
- Moving and relocation expenses (generally capped, if paid at all)

The law for fringe benefits changes from time to time, so know what benefits are offered when you join a practice, particularly since these benefits may constitute salary trade-offs. Also note the tax treatment of these benefits. Life insurance, where the practice pays the premiums but the beneficiary is your spouse or your estate, will be taxable when your beneficiary receives it. If you buy this policy personally, then your spouse or estate will receive the policy amount tax-free.

Disability insurance is treated similarly. If the practice pays the premiums, then you are considered to have received the policy amounts in lieu of wages, and therefore in a taxable manner. Conversely, if you pay the policy personally, then you will receive the benefit amounts tax-free if you become disabled. Given your tax-bracket, both policies have significant tax implications, and, in any event, you should probably purchase your own policies, even if the practice provides the insurance for you.

Note that retirement plan deductions are tax-deferred. This means that you contribute income before payment of tax. When you receive those funds, the income will be taxed at the ordinary income rates in effect at that time for your income tax bracket. Most retirement plans also have penalties for early withdrawal of funds.

If the practice has a retirement plan, find out what happens when you are eligible to participate in the plan. Will the contribution made on your behalf be *in addition* to your compensation or *in lieu of* a portion of what you receive?

While many of these benefits are negotiable, you must still understand what is being offered and the tax implication involved, so you may realistically compare contract offers.

Vacation and Leave of Absence

Typically, as a new physician, you will be offered 3–4 weeks of paid vacation during the first 12 months of employment, plus another week of absence to take continuing medical education courses, to attend professional society meetings, or to take your boards. If you have completed a fellowship and had 4 weeks of paid leave, then expect 4 weeks as leave during your initial year. This period of absence may be expressed in terms of a total amount of time off or it may be more precisely allocated between "vacation" and "professional absence."

Whatever amount of paid time off you have in your first year of employment, that amount usually phases up, over the length of time you spend with the practice, to something less than a full partner share while you are still an employee.

If you know that you will be taking an extended leave for additional training, promised family commitment, maternity or paternity leave or otherwise, have that leave of absence addressed in the contract. Then it clearly will be paid leave, and your benefits will continue during your absence.

Your offer should address the following:

- Will unused absence be compensated if not taken?
- Can unused leave be accrued from year to year?
- How much time may be taken consecutively?

Sick Pay

Sick pay is really a misnomer. Usually, the concern is not that you may be sick, but instead that you may be disabled or seriously hurt. Know what time and compensation you will receive if you are absent for a particularly long period of time. Most typically, at least 15–30 annual days of sick pay is offered. Absence in excess of what is allowed is usually without pay, although your benefits will likely continue, as you are still an employee of the practice.

Due to an extended illness or injury, you would become eligible for state disability insurance coverage and/or private disability insurance. You need to understand whether the practice will offer you only long-term disability (often with a waiting period of 60 days or more) or will offer a short-term disability policy (usually with a waiting period of 7–30 days). If the practice does not offer a short-term disability policy, you should investigate obtaining such a policy for yourself.

Generally count on pregnancy-related leave to be treated as sick leave, unless your contract states otherwise or the practice has a separate maternity leave policy. Thus, while federal laws may permit more (uncompensated) leave than the practice, you may find that a significant portion of a prolonged leave will be uncompensated.

Also know that federal laws, such as the Americans with Disabilities Act and the Family Medical Leave Act, may apply to male and female physicians if you or any immediate family member is seriously sick or disabled.

Increasingly, practices are combining vacation and sick leave into one category called paid time off (PTO), which makes time available for any personal need for time off.

Your contract should also be clear on these issues:

- What are the terms of the family leave policy (pay, amount, length of compensated leave, notice)? What happens when you return to work? Is your bonus prorated for your period of absence?
- How is maternity leave handled? What about paternity leave?
- Can the practice terminate your employment if you are sick for an extended period of time?

Covenants

Most employment contracts will have one or more obligations imposed (covenants). These are formal, enforceable agreements between the two parties. Pay strict attention to any covenants. Generally covenants are of two types: *restrictive* and *nonsolicitation*.

Restrictive Covenant A restrictive or "noncompete" covenant is a *promise* that you will limit your actions in some way as to not affect your employer's practice after you leave. Therefore, "competition" must be defined in the contract.

Restrictive covenants are becoming more prevalent as the competition for patients and payor contracts increases, and practices take greater risk in recruiting associates who might leave and take with them many practice referral sources, patients, payor contracts, and business contracts.

The general law regarding restrictive covenants is that they must be reasonable in *time* (ie, the duration of the restriction), *scope* (ie, exactly what you are prohibited from doing), and *place* (ie, the geographic area in which the restriction applies), and they may not violate the public interest.

If the contract you are offered has a restrictive covenant, try to have that restriction either eliminated or reduced. If you cannot negotiate this point, try to negotiate a fee to "buy out" of the covenant, often referred to as *liquidated damages*.

A common restrictive covenant might state: "You shall not, for a period of two (2) years after your employment with the practice ends, render any competitive services at any office, hospital or other facility within a five (5) mile radius of any office maintained by the employer on the date your employment terminates." Often, covenant language has been extended to include mandatory resignation of the associate's facility privileges as well. This may require you to seek another hospital affiliation, and not all hospital staffs are open. Further, such a covenant forces you to replace your physician referral base.

As many practices consider the covenant to be critical to your employment, you may be faced with the difficult decision of agreeing to the covenant or forgetting the whole contract. Consider whether (based on what you know about the practice) this restriction is reasonable. In making this determination, review these factors:

- What are the state laws on restrictive covenants?
- How many physicians are practicing your same specialty or subspecialty within a reasonable traveling distance? Within the restricted area? Note that the fewer competitors for this practice, the more difficult this covenant may be for the practice to enforce, for public interest reasons.

- For how long would you be restricted from practicing in this area? A year or two may be acceptable, but more than 5 years is probably not.
- How is "competitive practice" defined? Could you remain on your local hospital staff? Could you continue to admit patients to hospitals within the restricted area? What about emergency care?
- Does the practice have similar restrictions on its other physicians?
- Does the restriction amount to an unfair burden upon you?
- Can you remain a participating or on-panel physician with any payors you joined while with the practice? Can you continue as a subcontractor for any arrangements entered into by your employer?

Have a lawyer who is familiar with medical practice contracting review your agreement and guide you.

Do not sign an agreement relying on the possibility that the covenant may, at a later date, be unenforceable. That may not be true. These covenants are extremely expensive to litigate (often costing more than $50,000), so consider carefully what to do, and seek good legal advice.

The general rule is that liquidated damages may not amount to a penalty. This has often been interpreted to mean that such damages may not exceed twice your most recent year's compensation (salary and bonus).

Nonsolicitation Covenant It is common for the practice to state that its patient lists are proprietary information. Therefore, if you depart from the practice for any reason (even if you are fired), you may not solicit from the practice any patient or any member of any patient's household, any referral source, or any employee. Usually, you are also prohibited from soliciting any patient contract or any practice business relationship (such as an HMO or a joint-venture arrangement) for some period of time (usually 1–2 years) after the termination of your employment.

When you see these clauses, know that they are usually enforceable, even in states where the restrictive covenant itself may not be enforceable. Recognize, however, that these solicitation covenants may not interfere with your doctor-patient relationship, if you leave the practice and the patient requests to have his or her chart transferred. The purpose of these clauses is to prohibit you from taking a patient list and soliciting everyone on the list to come to your new practice.

Be sure that your contract resolves these issues:

- Can you tell patients you are in the course of treating that your employment is being terminated?
- What and how can you tell patients you formerly treated?
- What will patients and/or referral sources be told about why you left the practice? Do you have input into any letters that will be sent notifying others of your departure from the practice?
- Can you remain on panel with any managed care payors you joined while an employee? What can you tell managed care organizations about your employment termination?

- What are the practice's remedies if you breach one of these provisions? Does the remedy depend on which provision you breach? How does it differ?
- If the practice *may* seek an injunction, must it? Who pays if the practice prevails?

The Ethics Committee of the American Academy of Ophthalmology has guidelines regarding the relocation of a physician. (See Part II for more information about ethics in ophthalmology.) The guidelines include, but are not limited to, a large print sign at the reception desk stating the practice change, a general mailing to all patients mentioning the change, and so on. The reception staff should be made aware of the change so that they can inform patients who call regarding the specifics of the change. There should be no time designation as to current or past patients. Patients calling to make an appointment with the departing ophthalmologist must be notified of the change. Patients who make the decision to move to another practice should, following receipt of an appropriately signed record release form, have their records copied, and ready for pickup or delivery to the alternate practice as expeditiously as possible to assure continuity of care.

To circumvent these measures limits a patient's autonomy in making informed decisions about his or her medical eye care. If a patient is unable to locate a departing ophthalmologist because of a communication failure with the original practice, the patient can claim abandonment by both the practice and the departing ophthalmologist. Ultimately, it is imperative to keep patients informed and to keep their best interests foremost.

Senior Doctor's Untimely Death or Disability

If you are joining a physician in a solo practice, you should be interested in knowing what will happen to the practice if the senior physician dies or becomes permanently disabled before you become a co-owner. This issue is not always spelled out for you, but it should be.

You clearly do not want the physician's estate to sell the practice to someone else while you are an employee. However, you do not want to be forced to buy the practice in order to stay with it; you may not want it and you may not be able to afford it. The dilemma is that you will be asked to agree to this term even before you have worked in the practice.

The agreement may force you to purchase the practice if the senior physician becomes totally and/or permanently disabled from practice and you elect to practice in the area. Try to retain the *option* of purchasing the practice in these situations, rather than the *obligation*.

Purchasing the practice assets means buying the equipment, medical, and clerical supplies and inventories; possibly purchasing the right to use the senior physician's name for a limited period of time; buying out the lease (where permissible); and *sometimes* purchasing the practice goodwill.

If this death or disability buy-out clause is a term in your offer, be sure to have your attorney review it in your contract. Also evaluate if you can realistically afford the price of the practice.

Buying Into the Practice (Co-Ownership)

Is an equity position in a practice important to you? If so, discuss whether the possibility of co-ownership exists. If equity is an option, know the owners' timetable for this.

Explore and clarify what (stock or partnership) co-ownership means in this practice. Usually it means gaining some ability to vote on corporate matters, sharing in financial risks and rewards (including liabilities), and generally having a vote on, or at least a voice in, management issues. When you become an owner in a practice, the biggest benefit is often a change in how you are compensated. Usually all owners have the same compensation system; for example, they all get paid the same percentage of their production or they all pay equal overhead from their production. Becoming an owner most often means getting an increase in your compensation, but losing any guaranteed income.

Becoming an owner in the practice generally assumes you will be working full time. Should you be considering working part-time and raising a family, then an equity position may not necessarily be an arrangement you might strive for. In any event, outlining in the employment contract the buy-in arrangements, the criteria for a buy-in, the basis upon which the cost to buy-in will be assessed, and the timing of the transaction are all very important factors. Once you've spent months or years in the practice without these conditions enumerated in your employment agreement, they will all be much more difficult to negotiate after you have helped build a more successful—and more valuable—practice.

Evaluation Criteria for Co-Ownership

If co-ownership is not automatic after some number of years, and if it is based on specific criteria, then the criteria against which you will be judged should be stated in your agreement. For example, typical co-ownership criteria include at least the following:

- The *commitment* of your time and energy to contribute to the practice success
- Your *productivity,* efficiency, and contribution to the bottom line
- Your *acceptance* of the practice burdens and responsibilities, as an ongoing matter
- Your *interest* in the practice from an entrepreneurial standpoint
- A clearly demonstrated *ability* for you to work together with the other physicians and the staff
- Your becoming and remaining *board certified* in your specialty
- Often there may also be a *minimum number of years* (2–5) that you must be continuously employed by the practice

Valuing a Practice

It is true in any sale that the transaction will only happen if a willing seller and a willing buyer can agree on a price and terms. If there is no agreement, the item doesn't get sold. The same is true for purchasing an interest in a medical practice—you will only become an owner if you and the seller can agree on price and terms. There are a number of ways that the price and terms of a practice are established.

Subjective Value Sometimes the selling doctor will have a figure in mind that he or she wants to get for selling a portion of the practice. That figure may come from a friend's practice that was sold for the same amount or a simple formula heard at a seminar (eg, "practices are worth two times their annual revenues"), or it may be related to some financial need the doctor has, such as debt that needs to be retired. In these cases, the figure the selling doctor has in mind may or may not be close to the real value of the practice.

Historical Value If there are several doctors in the practice who have become co-owners, the method under which they bought into the practice will usually be used for new owners. Sometimes practices will figure the value of the practice at a given point in time and then annually adjust that value by a vote of the owners, without going through the formal process of reappraisal.

Net Asset Value The simplest conceptual way of valuing a practice is to appraise the value of all of the tangible assets (eg, ophthalmic equipment and supplies, furnishings, office equipment and supplies, and inventory) and all of the intangible assets (eg, patient flow and goodwill, practice name and reputation, location, and logo). The value of account receivables also needs to be factored into the value of the practice. The tangible assets are relatively easy to appraise; used equipment brokers can determine the value of your ophthalmic equipment and furniture brokers can appraise your furnishings. The difficulty is in determining the value of the intangible assets. How much is it worth to a practice to be on the ground floor of a busy medical office building? How much value is there in the flow of patients that has been established in the practice? The patient flow question is answered in a practice appraisal by assigning a value to all of the active charts. In other words, an appraiser might count all of the charts and multiply that number by $4 to arrive at a value for the patient flow. However, the question when this approach is taken is always: Why was $4 per chart the figure used? Why not $6 or $2? There is no established standard for the value of an ophthalmology chart, so valuing patient flow based on a per-chart figure that an appraiser randomly assigns is not a defensible way to approach the question of the value of a practice. Because intangible assets are so difficult to quantify in any objective way, the net asset value method is not an appropriate method for valuing most ophthalmology practices except as noted in the next section.

Excess Earnings Value The real value in an ophthalmology practice is in the earnings that the practice generates in excess of its expenses. Another way to look at this is to estimate the earnings that a practice would generate if someone bought it as an investment and replaced the selling doctor with an ophthalmologist who could do the same work. For example, in a practice where the owner makes $250,000 per year and the new owner could hire a replacement doctor for $150,000 per year, the owner would have excess earnings of $100,000 per year. An investor who bought the practice and hired the replacement doctor would earn $100,000 per year on the investment, so how much would the investor be willing to invest to earn that $100,000 per year? (Ignore for the purposes of this illustration the laws in many states that prevent non-MDs from owning practices.)

Since return is always related to risk—in other words, if an investment has greater risk, a greater return is expected—the amount we would pay today (the "present value") of a cash flow of $100,000 per year is less as the risk becomes greater.

Here is an illustration of that concept. For example, the federal government may pay 4% on its treasury securities, a figure that is barely above the inflation rate, which in the last decade or so has hovered around 3%. So if the United States Treasury will pay a cash flow of $200 per year for 10 years ($2,000 total), an investor would be willing to invest maybe $1,600 today to receive that stream of cash flow. On the other hand, corporations pay higher interest rates because there is more risk they will not be able to pay the money back. Investors might only pay $800 today for those cash flows, because the risk that they might not receive the promised payments is much higher for a company than for the government.

Ophthalmology practices are personal service businesses that carry even higher risk. The risks are relatively high that the practice may experience adverse effects such as financial struggles, reduced reimbursement rates, or death or departure of a key physician. Consequently, the rate an investor requires for an investment in the practice is also high. When one looks at valuing future cash flows, one does not add interest to them, but instead discounts those sums every year into the future that they occur. So, the higher the "discount rate" the lower the value of those cash flows.

Based on research and writing that has been done on the various levels of discount rates for many types of businesses, the typical risk-based discount rate for medical practices is in the range of 25%–45%, and where a particular practice falls in that range depends on its own specific risk profile. To get the rate used in determining the value of the cash flows in a practice, the risk-based rate is added to the risk-free rate (the rate the U.S. government pays) to arrive at a "capitalization rate." That rate is then used in the following formula to determine the value of the excess earnings: $V = EE/(d - g)$, where V is the value of the practice, EE is the annual excess earnings of the practice, d is the discount rate as defined above, and g is the average annual growth rate of the excess earnings in the practice. See Table 3-1 for a specific example of this calculation.

Please note that this value includes all of the assets of the practice, since they are used in creating the excess cash flow. Any liabilities and debts of the practice would be subtracted from this figure to arrive at the net value of the practice. In the case illustrated in Table 3-1, if you were going to buy into the practice as a 10% owner, it would cost you $33,333 assuming that was the agreed-upon amount. If you bought in at 50%, it

Table 3-1 Excess Earnings Value Illustration

Owner earnings	$250,000
Replacement doctor costs	$150,000
Excess earnings	$100,000
Discount rate	40%
Growth rate	10%
Formula	$100,000/(40% − 10%) or $100,000/30%
Value	$333,333

would cost $166,667. Most often, these payments are spread over 3–7 years, with the practice acting as a bank in loaning the money to you, although in some cases you may have to go to a bank or credit union and borrow the money if you do not have personal funds sufficient to cover the amount.

Alternate Method for Buying Into a Practice

In some situations a practice ownership purchase is accomplished without valuing the practice directly. For example, you might encounter a situation where your buy-in results from your taking less than your full share of compensation as a partner. Table 3-2 gives one example of this method.

In this example, during your first year of partnership you would receive 60% of what you would have received as a partner, in the second year 70%, and so on. In this method, as in any other, coming to a final agreement with the seller of ownership in the practice depends on the ability of both parties to agree on the terms.

Note that some very large practices (30–100 physicians) find that their practices are valued at such a high price, and they add doctors so often, that it is impractical to appraise the practice every time a doctor qualifies for ownership. In addition, because of their high value, a young doctor would be hard-pressed to be able to purchase an equal share of the practice. In these cases, the practice institutes what amounts to a membership fee that is charged to new doctors. The new partner pays $10,000 or $15,000 to obtain the benefits of ownership, which are usually limited to a more permanent position and some eventual input into the operations of the practice. As owners leave the practice, their shares in the corporation are bought back from them for the same amount as the purchase price.

There are implications of buying in with this approach and how it affects the taxation of net income when you are eventually bought out. Also, buying in through reduced compensation is in effect done with before-tax dollars while writing a check to the practice is with after-tax dollars. The IRS has guidelines for these transactions, including the tax-basis for stock in such transactions, so you should review these issues with a certified public accountant and with a tax attorney.

Income Division Among Owners

How the owners of a practice divide income among themselves dramatically affects your perception of whether a given value for the practice is reasonable. Income division methods affect how much you will make as a partner as well as how the doctors in the practice

---

Table 3-2 Alternate Method Model

Income Entitlement for Ownership, by Year	Income Share
Year 1	60%
Year 2	70%
Year 3	80%
Year 4	90%
Year 5	100%

interact with each other. Practices use five basic methods to divide owner income: equal pay, equal overhead, equal percentage of overhead, equal resources, and profit sharing.

Before you buy ownership in a practice, you need to understand in detail how income will be divided among owners, because misunderstandings in this area can be very detrimental to the relationship between co-owners. Keep in mind that if you are going to become a co-owner with a solo doctor who has never had a partner, he or she may never have thought much about how to split up the income, and it may take some study to come to a conclusion as to which way is best for that situation.

Equal Pay In this method, each owner receives the same compensation, regardless of his or her individual production. This method works well if all partners have similar work habits and production (and work an equal number of days), but usually causes problems when work habits and production are dissimilar.

Equal Overhead Under this system, each partner is responsible for an equal dollar amount of overhead. For example, if overhead is $1,000,000 and there are two partners, each partner would be responsible for paying $500,000 in overhead; any collections over that amount would be income to the partner. This method provides an incentive to produce as much as possible, but creates difficulties for young partners who are growing their practices and senior partners who want to slow down because they have to pay the same overhead as those who are in the prime of their practices.

Equal Percentage of Overhead This arrangement calculates the overhead percentage for the entire practice and then charges that same percentage of collections to each partner. For example, if the overhead percentage is 60%, and one partner produces $1,000,000 in collections, that partner would be charged $600,000 in overhead. If the other partner produces $500,000 in collections, they would pay $300,000 in overhead. This is the most commonly used compensation method, and it allows for growing into a practice and for slowing down at the end of a career. Sometimes the high producer in this system, however, feels like he or she is bearing a disproportionate share of the overhead.

Equal Resources Some practices calculate how much of the practice resources each owner/physician uses and then deduct that amount from the doctor's collections. For example, if one doctor uses four techs and the other uses two, the doctor using more tech time would be charged more. The same type of calculation would be made for rent (percentage of rooms used), billing staff (number of claims filed), and so on. This might be the fairest way of splitting expenses, but it does require significant accounting resources to track and allocate each category of expense, and it often leads to ongoing divisiveness among the partners regarding the most appropriate ways of assigning costs.

Profit Sharing In this method, each doctor receives a salary and then any owner compensation remaining is split based on the percentage of ownership. This method is almost never used as the sole method of compensation division for ophthalmology practices, but it is often used if there is income remaining at the end of a year that has not been distributed in the usual way.

Buy-Ins and Payouts—Structuring the Arrangement

Reviewing this section will help you understand what you need to know and do to have your contract facilitate the buy-in process. This section will also help you better understand what the seller-physician is thinking about when he or she is ready to retire from, or have partners in, the practice.

Accounts Receivable Unpaid customer invoices, or accounts receivable (A/R), may be handled separately from the value of the practice in a purchase, depending on the situation the young doctor has been in before becoming an owner. If the practice has taken on the risk of adding the new doctor by guaranteeing him or her a salary, then the A/R rightfully belong to the practice. If the new doctor has been paid a percentage of his or her production (with or without a base draw against those earnings) and that percentage is all the practice has paid over the course of the employment contract, then the young doctor has *earned* his or her A/R and should not be expected to pay for them separately. The following example helps illustrate this concept:

1. A young doctor has a contract that pays her 35% of whatever is collected from her professional services.
2. Since collections lag the dates of services by several months, especially in the early months, the practice gives her a draw against earnings of $8000 per month so that she can pay her bills.
3. At the end of each quarter, reconciliation is made and any remaining compensation is paid to the new doctor in the form of a bonus.
4. At the end of the first quarter, the practice has collected $20,000 on the work of the new doctor and has paid out $24,000 in compensation. The compensation the doctor earned for that quarter is $7000 (35% of $20,000). That amount subtracted from the draw she received for that quarter leaves her in a negative position of $17,000. The doctor owes the practice $17,000, but no check is written—the amount is just carried over to the next quarter.
5. In the second quarter, the doctor's collections are $60,000, so her compensation is $21,000, but her draw has paid $24,000, so she is in a negative position by another $3000, or $20,000 total.
6. In the third quarter, her collections are $90,000, so compensation is $31,500 (35% of $90,000.) Her draw was $24,000 again, so the bonus is $7500.
7. However, she owes the practice $20,000, so a bonus is not paid, but rather the bonus amount is subtracted from the debt, leaving $12,500 in remaining liability.
8. In the fourth quarter, her collections are $120,000 and her compensation is $42,000. Subtracting the draw leaves a bonus payable of $18,000. From that amount, the practice subtracts the $12,500 in remaining debt and the bonus check is $5500.

At this point in the example, the practice has paid the new doctor exactly 35% of what she has produced in collections and the liability and expense it undertook in employing the doctor has been repaid in full. The doctor has earned her A/R and would not have to buy them separately as she buys into the rest of the practice. It is common, however, for practice operating agreements to require at least 1 year's notice if an owner is going to leave the practice through retirement or relocation. If proper notice is given, then the doctor would receive her A/R as the money is collected (less 5%–15% as a collection fee or in a lump sum adjusted for the historic collection ratio). If less notice is given, then the A/R would revert to the practice so that it can pay the costs incurred in recruiting a new doctor.

Payouts When you as a co-owner leave a practice, you might receive two sums of money, depending on your practice agreement:

- A buy-out of your practice ownership or equity
- A buy-out of your A/R

As mentioned in the preceding text, the A/R amounts are usually collected over time and paid out to you minus a collection fee. The practice ownership is usually valued at the time of your leaving and that sum may be paid to you by a new partner as his or her way of buying into the practice, or by the practice as a whole. Most often, the amount is spread over 3–7 years to lessen the burden on practice cash flow.

Payouts may be structured in one of two ways: *deferred compensation* and *stock or equity redemption*. In most cases, a payout will combine these methods. In deferred compensation, the payout is characterized as compensation, which is deductible to the medical practice and taxable as ordinary income to the departing physician. In stock or equity redemption, this portion of the payout is not deductible to the medical practice and is taxable as a long-term capital gain to the departing physician.

Other Contract Terms

Table 3-3 summarizes typical contract terms. Here are some of the other terms you may see in an employment contract, a buy/sell agreement, or a practice operating agreement:

- *Complete understanding:* In an increasing number of contracts, only the terms written in the contract control the terms of the arrangements; no other terms apply. These are called *merger* (or *integration*) *clauses*. Therefore, you may not rely on a "side letter," a verbal assurance, or any other understanding not made part of the final contract.
- *Assignment:* With all the mergers and acquisitions in the health care field, you may find that your contract may be assigned to a new party whom you do not want to join. Therefore, your contract should be modified to state that it shall become void if, for example, more than half of the practice shareholders change, or if the practice assets or stock are sold. Many practices, for apparent reasons, may not concede this issue.

Table 3-3 Typical Contract Terms

Contract Area	Example
Contract term	2–3 years employment
Termination	60–90 days written notice "at will"
Compensation scale	Base pay, 10%–20% increase/year and/or bonus incentive
Business expenses	Professional malpractice insurance Society dues and subscriptions Hospital staff fees Travel, CME, board costs up to a negotiated limit Portable phones, pagers, computers, and other business equipment, as necessary
Fringe benefits	Health and major medical for physician and family Group term life insurance to $50,000 Payment or allowance for disability premiums Retirement plan contributions
Vacation	3–4 weeks, increasing 1 week/year until parity
Sick pay	6–15 days/year
Restrictive covenants	Noncompete, variable Nonsolicitation, variable
Co-ownership	Addressed, but variable
Assignment of contract	Becomes void if percentage of shareholders changes or practice assets are sold, variable

- *Penalty for failure of performance:* An increasing number of contracts state that once you sign on, if you fail to work for the practice for at least 3 months (or thereabouts), you must pay the practice agreed liquidated damages of $10,000–$20,000. These clauses are more common if the practice purchased equipment because of your employment, used a recruiter to find you, invested significantly in marketing your services, or paid you a signing bonus.

See the box "Pointers About Contracts" for some basic do's and don'ts when it comes to reviewing your contract.

A Second Opinion

Where contracts are concerned, seek good professional advice early on. Ideally, that advice comes from a health care attorney or health care consultant who is familiar with the contracting process and aware of the fundamentally different areas of medicine and types of practices, styles of medical groups, and how these variables affect the offer you receive.

Use someone whom you trust or who is recommended to you, but be sure that professional has the expertise you need in the physician-contracting area. Expect to pay $150–$350 per hour for this expertise, but do not buy more talent than you need. You may want to personally try to negotiate the contract, with your advisor available to coach you on trade-offs, good arguments for your case, and the actual industry norms. Be sure

Pointers About Contracts

- When in doubt about the meaning or the intent of a term in an agreement, ask. As needed, have that clause revised.
- Never sign a contract with ambiguous language or based on verbal assurances that are contrary to the stated contract language.
- Deal directly with the practice representative to discuss the contract terms. You and the practice representative should agree on the issues and direct the respective attorney to create the appropriate documents. Do not just have your lawyer talk to the practice lawyer. Avoid negotiating with the practice's lawyer. He or she may be a better negotiator than you, and the attorney's job is to protect the practice.
- Have a lawyer or consultant familiar with these types of contracts review your arrangements to help determine if your contract is fair, reasonable, complete, and fully legal.
- Pay attention to the practice's negotiating style. Are they being reasonable or heavy-handed? Does this negotiation lead you to believe that problems may develop? Is there information that the practice has not fully disclosed?
- Understand the trend toward more practices moving to a fixed-salary arrangement.

that your advisor has no conflict of interest in representing you and that he or she has the experience you need.

Next Steps

Whether you sign a contract with an employer or decide to set up your own practice, your attention to the business issues involved strongly contributes to an efficient, successful practice. Even though higher-level administrators may handle the complexities of managing the business, you need to understand what is involved. Chapters 4 through 12 lay out business basics for you.

Appendix I features practice management resources that include descriptions of products and services from the American Academy of Ophthalmology and the American Academy of Ophthalmic Executives, suggested reading, and sample materials.

CHAPTER 4

Financial Management and Business Performance

While many doctors would like to simply practice medicine without dealing with the financial aspects of modern medical practice, a doctor in private practice needs to understand at least the basics of financial management. Ophthalmology is a clinically demanding profession, and the business aspects of practice are equally demanding. A lack of attention to the details of the financial side of your practice can lead to disaster and may prevent you from practicing in the way you would prefer. In introducing you to the principles and intricacies of financial management and business performance, this chapter helps you prepare for an aspect of practice that will impact your success for the duration of your medical career (Figure 4-1). See the box "A Tale of Financial Irresponsibility" for a scenario to set you on your way.

The Basics of Accounting and Budgeting

Two basic methods of accounting are accrual basis and cash basis. In accrual basis accounting, revenues are recognized when the work that generates them is done, and expenses are recognized when they are incurred, whether or not they have been paid at that time. In cash basis accounting, funds are added to your bank account and financial statements when they are deposited in the bank, and expenses are subtracted from your records when a check is written.

Most small- to medium-sized ophthalmology practices use the cash basis of accounting because it is simpler to administer. However, the accrual basis is generally more accurate and harder to manipulate. For example, a practice using the cash basis of accounting can hold checks at the end of the year and not deposit them in the bank, thereby reducing their revenues for that year and postponing taxes due on those revenues. Under the accrual method of accounting, there would be no incentive to postpone depositing checks, since that revenue would have been accounted for when the work was performed.

Using the Balance Sheet as a Financial Management Tool

There are two key financial reports that every business should monitor, including ophthalmology practices: the *balance sheet* (discussed in this section) and the *income statement* (discussed in the next section). The balance sheet is a summary of the values of all

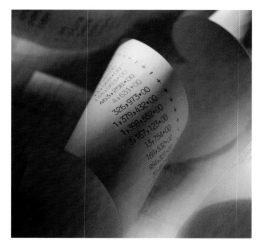

Figure 4-1 A basic understanding of the intricacies of financial management helps you prepare for an aspect of practice that will impact your success throughout your medical career.

of the practice assets, liabilities, and equity. In a balance sheet, the sum of the value of the assets must always equal the sum of the liabilities plus the equity. Think about it in this way: If you own a car (asset) that is worth $20,000, and you owe the bank $15,000 on its loan (liability), you have $5000 in equity in the car. In other words, if you sold the car for $20,000, you would have to pay the bank $15,000 to clear the loan, and you would be left with $5000 from the transaction.

Assets Listed on the Balance Sheet

A balance sheet typically lists three types of assets: current, long term, and other.

Current assets are easily turned into cash and are usually used within a year. Examples of assets in this category are cash, supplies, checking and savings accounts, and liquid investments such as stock or bond portfolios. Money owed to the practice that will be paid within a year can be included in current assets, but usually accounts receivable are not included in ophthalmology practice balance sheets, since it is difficult to know their true value after the contractual write-offs and how much of the remainder is collectable.

Long-term assets are items that last more than a year, such as equipment, furnishings, and buildings. Long-term assets are depreciated each year, meaning that the IRS allows you to write off a portion of their purchase price each year as a deduction from your revenues, thereby allowing you to save funds for their replacement. For example, you might purchase a slit lamp for $14,000 and deduct $2000 each year from your revenues for 7 years, until the slit lamp is entirely depreciated. Although you may have written off the entire amount, so that the equipment no longer affects the balance of your assets on your balance sheet, you may still use the asset for many years. For this reason, the value of your assets on the balance sheet, especially after years in practice, will not reflect their true market value, which is what you could sell them for on the open market. The IRS

A Tale of Financial Irresponsibility

"How much money do we have in the bank?"
The question was directed to the office manager by the sole owner of the practice, an ophthalmologist who had been in practice eight years. The manager thought about how nice it was to have a practice that was doing well finally, after many years of uneven growth and lots of struggles. She quickly checked the balance on her computer and gave the verdict: "A little over $50,000 as of this morning's deposit."

"Well, write me out a check for $50,000 because I need to put a down payment on the cabin I am buying up by the lake. Thanks!" The office manager was so shocked, she couldn't even manage a response. How would she make payroll in three days if all the cash was taken out of the bank? Was he really serious? Didn't he understand all of the demands on the practice for payments? She quickly recovered, and chased him down the hallway, took him into an empty exam lane, and tried to explain why it would be very unwise to take all of the money out of the bank account. The doctor seemed surprised that she would deny him his money, but he finally relented and settled for half the amount.

has rules for the depreciation length for various types of long-term assets—some may be written off over 3 years, some 5 years, others 7 years. Leasehold improvements and other buildings may have long depreciation periods such as 30+ years in some cases. Your accountant will set up depreciation tables for all of your depreciable assets so it is important that he or she know purchase dates and purchase prices for all of your long-term assets. Other assets include the costs incurred in organizing a practice, goodwill acquired in the purchase of another practice, intangible assets such as trademarks and copyrights, and so on.

Liabilities and Equity

A balance sheet lists two types of liabilities: current and long term. Current liabilities include accounts and notes payable and other debt payments due within 1 year. Long-term liabilities include notes payable, loans payable, and any other liabilities with a term of greater than 1 year.

The balance sheet also has two types of equity: paid-in capital and retained earnings. Paid-in capital is money that has been invested in the business. Retained earnings are profits not withdrawn from the business.

On the balance sheet, three areas are key indicators of practice health:

- If current liabilities exceed current assets, the practice may be in danger of defaulting on accounts payable. Note that because there are usually accounts receivable that are regularly turned over for collection but are typically not included on the balance sheet, you may see current liabilities exceeding current assets and yet the practice may be financially solid.
- If liabilities unexpectedly grow, the practice is taking on more debt. The cost of interest to service excessive debt can adversely affect the financial health of a practice, especially in times when revenue growth slows.

- Shrinking equity is also a possible cause for concern on the balance sheet. However, a stable practice may have shrinking equity in times when assets are being depreciated and no earnings are being retained in the business.

Figure 4-2 shows an example of a simple balance sheet for an ophthalmology practice.

Understanding the Income Statement

While your balance sheet gives you a good idea of the level of assets, liabilities, and equity in your practice, the income statement is your guide to your practice's revenues and expenses. The income statement (also called a *profit and loss statement*) lists the collections in the practice and basic categories for practice expenses for a specific period.

The most helpful analysis on the income statement is found by calculating ratios for specific expenses. For example, by dividing your staff payroll expenses into your total revenues you can calculate a staff payroll ratio. Likewise, by dividing your total practice expenses (not including owner income or benefits) into your total collections you can figure your overhead ratio. See the section on benchmarking later in this section for more information on other financial ratios.

One of the most important uses for the income statement is in comparing any current year's financial results to previous years. Watching your expense levels and ratios

---

Balance Sheet
Central Ophthalmology Practice
As of December 31, Year 2

Current Assets:		
Cash	25,261	
Securities	31,222	
Supplies	2,310	
Optical Inventory	21,989	
Total Current Assets:		80,782
Long Term Assets:		
Equipment	214,675	
Furnishings	45,671	
Leasehold Improvements	18,011	
Total Long Term Assets:	278,357	
Less Accumulated Depreciation:	(128,332)	
Net Long Term Assets:		150,025
Total Assets:		**230,807**
Current Liabilities:	1,255	
Long Term Liabilities:	53,293	
Total Liabilities		54,548
Equity:		
Paid in Capital	1,000	
Retained Earnings	175,259	
Total Equity		176,259
Total Liabilities and Equity:		**230,807**

Figure 4-2 Sample balance sheet.

year after year or quarter by quarter will alert you to dangerous increases in expenses, reductions in collections, and sometimes even theft from the practice. Some expenses typically grow each year. For example, most employees want a pay raise annually, so your payroll expenses will increase each year. Most office leases include escalator clauses that increase your rent each year, most often by a percentage equal to the change in the Consumer Price Index. For these reasons it is very important for practices to find ways to increase their collections year after year.

Figure 4-3 is an example of a simple income statement for an ophthalmology practice. Note how the report calculates the ratio of each expense to the total revenue for each year and shows the change in revenues and expenses from the first to the second year.

Many practices develop separate income statements for different departments such as optical, refractive surgery, contact lenses, or ambulatory surgery center. Each different type of business or department must be compared to itself on a year-to-year basis.

Fixed vs Variable Expenses

You will find two types of expenses in your practice: fixed and variable. Fixed expenses do not vary with changes in your collections. For example, your rent will be the same regardless of how much money you collect. One of the basics of practice financial health is to make sure that the sum of your collections exceeds the sum of all fixed practice

	Income Statement Central Ophthalmology Practice				
	Year 1	Yr 1 Ratio	Year 2	Yr 2 Ratio	Change
Total Revenue	1,504,062	100.0%	1,601,935	100.0%	97,873
Expenses					
Advertising & Promo	9,429	0.6%	10,580	0.7%	1,151
Automobile Expense	5,123	0.3%	5,678	0.4%	555
Bank Charges	9,544	0.6%	11,135	0.7%	1,591
Contact Lens	25,214	1.7%	31,120	1.9%	5,905
Depreciation	37,859	2.5%	22,892	1.4%	(14,967)
Facility Expenses	22,790	1.5%	25,318	1.6%	2,528
Insurance	62,018	4.1%	81,548	5.1%	19,530
Legal & Accounting	3,900	0.3%	4,200	0.3%	300
Medical Expenses	35,375	2.4%	40,596	2.5%	5,221
Office Expenses	22,086	1.5%	31,958	2.0%	9,872
Optical Expenses	247,742	16.5%	241,413	15.1%	(6,330)
Personnel Expenses	497,497	33.1%	522,606	32.6%	25,109
Prof. Dues/Educ.	2,040	0.1%	4,929	0.3%	2,889
Rent Expense	58,095	3.9%	63,722	4.0%	5,627
Taxes & Licenses	2,313	0.2%	2,351	0.1%	38
Telephone Expense	5,772	0.4%	6,480	0.4%	708
Total Expenses:	1,046,798	69.6%	1,106,525	69.1%	59,728
Owner Income	457,265	30.4%	495,410	30.9%	38,145

Figure 4-3 Sample income statement.

expenses. Variable expenses vary with changes in collections. An example of a variable expense is the cost of optical goods sold. The key to managing variable expenses is to price goods and services so that the variable expenses are covered and there is something left over to help pay the fixed expenses that are required to provide those goods or services. Staff payroll is generally considered a fixed expense, because it doesn't automatically vary with the volume of revenues in the practice. Some practices vary payroll expenses by having some staff members work part time or on an on-call basis. However, in most cases it is difficult to retain employees if they cannot depend on some level of regular income.

The balance sheet and the income statement are calculated together at the end of each tax year (and sometimes more often, depending on your needs). The figures in the balance sheet affect the income statement and vice versa. For example, the depreciation for a fiscal year shows up on the income statement and adds to accumulated depreciation on the balance sheet. Your accountant will reconcile your financial statements as part of preparing your tax returns each year.

Understanding the Chart of Accounts

The chart of accounts is simply a list of numbers that identify each category of expense in your practice by department. Your accountant will help establish a chart of accounts that provides for allocation of expenses for tax purposes and cost accounting.

As an example, assume that the account number established for medical supplies is 105. A check is written to XYZ Ophthalmic Supply Company for eye drops. The check should be made out to XYZ Ophthalmic Supply Company in the proper amount, and the account number 105 should be noted on the check stub. This number tells the accountant that the check to XYZ was for medical supplies. For internal use, the invoice numbers that are paid should also be listed on the stub.

Correctly allocating expenses is essential to efficient practice operations. For accuracy, the person writing the checks—not the accountant—should be responsible for determining the account number to put on the check stub. The accountant may not know what supplies XYZ Company sells. Keep a copy of the chart of accounts available for ready reference.

Managing Accounts Payable

The accounts payment process works best if bills are paid only once each month. Unless a substantial discount is offered for early payment, pay bills closer to 30 days from the date of purchase. This practice keeps the money in the bank working for you as long as possible, and not in the vendor's bank earning interest.

In general, it is best to pay bills from invoices, not from vendor statements. Vendors seldom have the same billing cycle you have. If payments are made from a statement, an invoice may mistakenly be paid twice. Most vendors will allow you to determine your invoice date.

At the same time each month, follow the routine for paying bills shown in the box "The Payment Process." Establishing a workable accounts payable system at the start of your practice is critical. Accurate tracking of supply costs reduces overspending and panic buying, provides information needed for budgeting and forecasting, and gives the accountant the information necessary to prepare financial statements and tax returns.

The Payment Process

1. Collect all the invoices that have been received from a vendor in the previous 30 days. Make sure that the person receiving the goods has initialed the invoice to show that all goods ordered were received and in the proper quantities. Total the invoices and write a check for this amount.
2. Write every invoice number that is being paid and the amount on the check stub. Do not forget to put the chart of accounts number on the check and the check stub.
3. Staple the invoices together, mark them paid, and write the date and check number on them.
4. File the paid invoices in the vendor folder for that company. Keep only the invoices for the current year in the folder. At the end of each year, the invoices should be filed with other accounting papers for that year.

Managing and Tracking Cash Flow

There is a saying in finance that "cash is king." Although that may be debatable in the investment field, having enough cash on hand to pay your bills and obligations is absolutely critical to the smooth operation of any practice. One of the most disconcerting events for any practice is finding that its cash in the bank is not enough to cover its immediate needs. While some accounts payable can be temporarily postponed to conserve cash, some obligations have fixed due dates that are inflexible such as payroll, taxes, or rent. Missing a payroll date can result in reduced morale among employees, increased turnover, and financial distress for the practice.

Highly profitable practices with healthy cash flow may feel less pressure to project and manage cash flow, because the high profits enable the owners of the practice to work within the shifting flow of collections and expenses. On the other hand, even strong, healthy practices can have a cash flow crisis if circumstances conspire to limit collections or dramatically increase collections.

Here are the key steps in managing your cash flow:

1. Collect your money as soon as possible. Make reasonable effort to ensure patient co-payments and deductibles are paid on the day of service whenever possible. A reasonable deposit may be required for optical orders for new patients to the practice, with the balance due upon delivery of the product. Allow established patients with a good patient record more flexibility. Make sure insurance billing is done promptly, and that denied claims are corrected quickly and re-sent immediately.
2. Make payments to vendors as noted earlier in this section. Know what discounts are available for timely payment and meet those timelines.
3. Once you have a track record of collections per month, use those figures to project your probable receipts at least 3 months ahead. Keep in mind that time away from the office usually reduces collections 1 to 3 months later, so take vacation and CME time off into account when making projections.
4. Project collections for each month separately, and compare to the expected expenses for that month. Some expenses (eg, rent, equipment leases) are the same

each month, but others vary by the number of workdays (eg, staff payroll) or are annual or quarterly payments that occur in specific months (professional liability insurance).

5. Shortfalls in net revenues (expected revenues less expected expenses, including your own needed income) can be made up from excess revenues in previous months, by reductions in or postponement of expenses, by increases in revenues or collection activity, or by borrowing money.

6. Some expenses may be due annually. You may want to divide the anticipated expense into monthly amounts and deposit that amount each month into a separate money market account to have the ready cash for that larger annual payment.

Budgeting

Budgeting is related to the process of managing cash flow, but also includes the process of managing specific budget categories. Although almost everyone thinks budgets are a good idea, budgets require some time to set up and track, and some discipline to use properly. Many practices skip this tool, often to their detriment.

A simple process for setting up and using budgets is as follows:

1. Use your income statement as a basis for revenues and expenses. If you are starting a new practice, you will need to estimate what revenues will be. Expenses are easier to predict, as you will know what your rent, staff payroll, utilities, phone service, and so on will cost each month.

2. Adjust revenues to reflect your best estimates for the upcoming period, typically a year.

3. Adjust each expense category to reflect your best estimates. For example, if your phone directory ad starts in March, and costs $1000 per month, you would budget $9000 for that item for the calendar year. If your rent increases by $500 in June, you will need to include the higher figure in your budget once the increase begins.

4. Some expenses vary according to revenues, and can be projected as a percent of expected revenues. For example, if your cost of goods sold (frames + lenses) for glasses runs about 38% of your optical collections, and if your optical collections are expected to increase from $200,000 to $300,000 this year, you would expect that frames and lenses would be budgeted at $114,000 this year, up from $76,000 last year.

5. Each month create a report that compares your expenditures for each major category (revenues and expenses) to the projected amount for that month and for the total amount for the year to date.

Tracking budgets in this way allows you to make mid-course corrections before unpleasant surprises cause major financial discomfort. Budgets also help instill fiscal discipline, helping you plan for major expenses and purchases rather than incurring those costs on whims. Budgets are particularly helpful in group practices where the absence of agreed-upon budgets between the partners in a practice can result in discord regarding unplanned expenses or purchases. Budgets can help tremendously in delegating responsibility and accountability to managers and supervisors because they help managers and supervisors have an incentive to maximize the productivity of their respective departments. For example, a front desk supervisor who is given a payroll budget is more likely to work on optimizing the staff schedule to stay within the budget than if he or she has no budgetary guideline.

However, budgets should be guidelines, not laws. A clear and present opportunity for increasing revenues and net income may need to be undertaken for the good of the practice even if not immediately contemplated in the budget.

Benchmarks of Business Performance

Most ophthalmologists like to know how their practice is doing financially or in terms of patient flow compared to other ophthalmology practices. The process of comparing key measures of practice health to other practices has been termed *benchmarking*. Benchmark figures can be useful if they help a practice understand its current structure and help the practice strive for better performance. On the other hand, benchmarks can be harmful if used inappropriately. For example, when told that his practice's staff payroll ratio was a little high, one doctor thought he would just fire somebody to bring the ratio back into line with national averages. In that particular case, any loss of personnel was likely to put so much pressure on the remaining staff members that additional, unwanted defections were almost inevitable.

The best use of benchmarks is to track your practice's own figures over time and use those comparisons as a springboard to improvement. For example, if your revenues are $400,000 and your staff payroll is $140,000, your staff payroll ratio (percentage of collections spent on staff compensation) would be 35%, which is higher than average for an ophthalmology practice. If you wanted to have a staff payroll ratio of 25%, you could reduce staff hours by about 30% to reach that ratio, but that is often difficult, and reducing hours too much can result in reduced production, reduced collections efforts, loss of personnel, and so on. You could reduce the number of employees, but you would need to save about $40,000 in payroll, so that may mean eliminating two employees, depending on their pay rates.

Those approaches may be necessary in some cases, especially if the practice is in financial trouble. However, increasing revenues will have the same effect and will have the additional benefit of increasing net income—the amount of money available for the owner(s) to take out of the practice.

National benchmarking figures change over time. Fifteen years ago, many ophthalmology practices had overhead ratios of 50% of revenues, but that figure is rare these days, and the average is now a little above 60%. Tables 4-1, 4-2, and 4-3 show a range of benchmark calculations for revenue, patient flow, and relative value, with the best-of-class practices at the higher ends of the ranges. Few practices track all of these benchmarks; it is usually best to choose five or six that are most important to your practice and pay careful attention to those, especially tracking how they change in your practice over time.

Keep in mind that benchmarks differ among practice types. For example, a pure cataract referral practice may have an overhead of 40%, where a comprehensive group ophthalmology practice with an optical dispensary and contact lens service may be 65%–

Table 4-1 Revenue Calculations

The calculation of the following benchmarks use figures from your income statement, plus the number of full time equivalent (FTE) staff and doctors (FTE = 40 hours/week).

Benchmark	Range	Calculation
Overhead ratio (% overhead)	35%–70%	Total practice-related expenses (not including physician-owner income) divided by total net collections (collections less refunds)
Profit ratio	30%–65%	Total physician income divided by total net collections
Staff payroll ratio	18%–28%	Total staff payroll expenses divided by total net collections
Occupancy expense ratio	4%–10%	Rent or mortgage payment divided by total net collections
Collections per FTE staff member	$100,000 or more	Total net collections divided by FTE staff member
Collections per FTE physician	At least $300,000	Total net collections divided by FTE physicians

Table 4-2 Patient Flow Calculations

Most practice management computer systems provide the information needed to calculate the following ratios, although the number of doctor hours usually must be figured separately.

Benchmark	Range	Calculation
New patient ratio	9%–18%	Total number of new patients divided by total patients seen
Cataract surgery yield	20–30 for practice with typical 65+ age distribution of 40%	Total number of patient visits divided by the number of cataract surgeries performed
Refractive surgery yield	Too variable for an average benchmark	Total number of patients seen divided by the number of refractive surgeries performed
Average collections per patient visit	At least $95 for a general ophthalmology practice; more for retina or practices with high surgical volume	Total net collections divided by total patient visits
Number of patients seen per doctor hour	4–10	Total patient visits divided by total doctor hours spent seeing patients

Table 4-3 Relative Value Calculations

The following benchmarks use practice management reports and income statements to generate ratios based on the resource-based relative value units (RVUs) published by the Centers for Medicare and Medicaid Services. These require generation of a practice management report that lists all current procedural terminology (CPT) codes billed in a given time period. Those codes then must be converted to RVUs by multiplying the RVU value for each code by the number of times that code was billed and then summing all of the RVUs to yield a total number of RVUs generated for the time period. That figure ("Total RVUs") is then used in these calculations.

Benchmark	Range	Calculation
Average collections per RVU	Medicare pays about $38 per RVU; most insurance companies pay more	Total net collections divided by total RVUs
Average expenses per RVU	Varies widely	Total net practice expenses (not including physician income) divided by total RVUs
RVUs per FTE physician	At least 7500 per year	Total RVUs divided by total FTE physicians
RVUs per FTE staff member	At least 2500 per year	Total RVUs divided by FTE staff members

70%. While benchmarking can provide a basis for comparison and ultimately direction for improving business performance, it is imperative that you use benchmarks from practices similar to your own.

Organization for Smoother Operations

The preceding sections introduced you to the basics of financial management and how to use benchmarks to track your practice's own figures over time. Now you are on to some practical steps: organizing the purchase of supplies, pulling together your pool of financial and legal advisors, setting policies and procedures for office staff, and determining how to schedule patients efficiently.

Purchasing Supplies

In a medical practice just starting up, an organized purchasing system helps ensure profitability of the practice. The first step is to centralize the ordering process. Assign one person to be responsible for ordering supplies. Having one person in charge (usually the office manager or office assistant) eliminates duplicate orders, adds objectivity, and prevents having sales representatives talk to more than one person. The employee in charge of purchasing becomes familiar with supplies and prices and thus can shop around for the best prices (Figure 4-4). Centralized ordering also allows the purchaser to establish the quantity of each supply used over a given time (eg, monthly). These usage guidelines allow development of an inventory process that will reduce unnecessary inventory and minimize the tendency to place panic orders that increase expenses.

Develop a form with the most common orders listed. Each employee who needs supplies or uses the last of the current inventory can list the item in the order book. The office manager will order supplies based on what is written on the form. The box "Tips for Purchasing Supplies" describes ways to help minimize the cost of supplies, such as using the Academy's SimplifEye buyer's program.

Selecting Financial and Legal Advisors

To ensure that the practice is positioned for the best tax advantages and flexibility, you will need to engage an experienced accountant. In addition, every practice and every physician will need legal advice at various times.

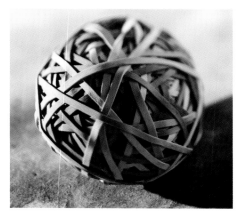

Figure 4-4 Organizing a system for purchasing supplies—whether for the office or patient care—is a practical step that contributes to smooth operations.

Tips for Purchasing Supplies

- Create vendor files by company name and file all invoices and statements in chronological order. File the folders in alphabetical order.
- Be familiar with price breaks for regularly used items so that they can be ordered in quantities that provide the best price.
- Purchase office supplies at local office supply discount stores instead of ordering by telephone from an office supply business. This can save the practice up to 50% on some items.
- Every 6 months, check the prices on standard items and compare vendor prices. Ask for competitive bids from three different vendors.
- Ask for a 45-day payment window.
- Be aware of items being put on backorder. Never accept payment responsibility unless the order is received.
- Participate in the Academy's buyers' group program called SimplifEye. Members save 15%–35% off list prices of Henry Schein, Inc. Discounts apply on purchases of pharmaceuticals, disposables, and major equipment. This service is free to members and no minimum purchasing requirements or contracts are involved. It's simple, and effective.
- Negotiate for better prices with all of your vendors.

Accounting Professionals

Along with the attorney, an accountant should be consulted before setting up your legal structure because the legal structure can affect tax advantages and flexibility. The accountant assists with setting up accounting processes as well as establishing the internal controls for tracking cash flow, profit and loss statements, payroll withholdings, quarterly taxes, and operating budget. The person providing accounting advice does not necessarily have to be a certified public accountant (CPA). Nonetheless, selecting the right accountant should be considered on the basis of technical knowledge and experience in health care and the ability to meet your needs. The following descriptions will help differentiate between the various types of accounting services.

Certified Public Accountant A CPA has successfully passed rigorous certification requirements. As with other certified professionals, CPAs must comply with mandated regulations. A CPA generally charges by the hour and his or her services are typically more expensive than other accounting services. Finding a CPA who is experienced in operations of medical practices will be well worth the extra investment. CPAs are typically used to prepare tax returns, assist in tax planning, and offer financial advice. Using your CPA to write your checks and handle your bank accounts can be very expensive, though, unless the CPA's firm also provides less costly bookkeeping services.

Bookkeeping Services Bookkeeping services generally provide some of the same types of services as that of a CPA, but they may be limited in how much tax planning and/or business advice they can provide. Bookkeeping services most often handle the day-to-day tasks of writing checks, preparing financial reports, and balancing bank accounts. Carefully check references and the reputation of bookkeeping firms that you are considering and, more significantly, verify that they are experienced in operations of medical practices.

Accounts Payable/Payroll Employee This person is an employee of your practice who writes checks, balances the bank accounts, prepares financial reports, and handles payroll. Often, your office manager or billing supervisor may be responsible for these tasks in addition to their other responsibilities.

Responsibilities of Your Financial Advisor(s)

Whether you choose to use a CPA, a bookkeeping firm, your own employee, or some combination of these entities to handle your financial needs, the basic tasks involved are the same. Your financial advisors have a wide range of responsibilities, including the following:

- Establishing budgets and financial forecasting
- Periodically reviewing the financial performance of the practice, including monthly or quarterly preparation of financial statements
- Performing routine audits, and checks and balances
- Reconciling bank statements, bank deposits, credit card transactions, and accounts payable
- Offering knowledge and consultative reviews of IRS laws and penalties

- Advising on 401(k) contributions, real estate, investing, and financial planning
- Preparing payroll and submitting payroll taxes
- Holding regular meetings to discuss the performance of the practice and to recommend improvements where needed

The initial start-up phase of the practice involves the services of advisors such as brokers, real estate agents, and lenders. A local bank can also be a resource for options on establishing a line of credit. Most lenders require a business plan or pro forma financial statement for the business.

Legal Assistance

Just as you would never consult a cardiologist for help with an ankle sprain, take care to match your needs with the appropriate specialty within the legal profession.

Unlike medicine, however, where each specialty has a specific and clear title, lawyers become "specialists" more often by their on-the-job experiences than by specialized education. In addition, many attorneys are generalists who tackle a wide variety of legal issues and projects, so it is sometimes difficult to find an attorney with deep experience in your specific area of need.

Medical practices deal with three types of attorneys primarily: general business attorneys, health care law specialists, and malpractice specialists.

General Business Attorneys These lawyers help you with office and equipment leases, employment contracts, partnership or corporate operating agreements, and other general business issues. It is always best—and the most efficient use of your time—to use an attorney who has some familiarity with medical practices, even in seemingly straightforward transactions such as office space leases, because medical practices have needs that differ from those of an insurance office or a stock broker. An attorney who understands ophthalmology is even better, although in some locations finding that person may be an elusive goal.

Health Care Law Specialists Because so many laws and regulations regarding health care have been put on the books in the last couple of decades, some attorneys have found a niche by specializing in the federal and state laws that pertain to health care. Fraud and abuse statutes, the Stark II group practice regulations, and state laws regarding practice ownership, fees for referrals, and certificate-of-need processes are often difficult to apply and require review by a specialist in health care law.

Consider this scenario as you select the best attorney for your particular issues and need: A retinal specialist wanted to enter into a deal he had agreed to with a general practice that needed his part-time services. It was not until his *second* legal consultation—with a health care attorney—that he discovered his proposed deal was illegal. This second legal opinion surprised him because his own attorney, a general business lawyer who had helped him on some real estate purchases, did not see anything wrong with it. The health care attorney assisted the parties in restructuring the deal to avoid problems with Medicare regulations. Since many of the laws that apply to doctors and hospitals are very different from those that apply to businesses in general, an attorney who does not specialize in health care law is not in a good position to advise you on some of the more complicated regulations.

Malpractice Specialists If you are faced with a professional liability action, your malpractice insurance company will take a leading role in defending you, and it will have its own attorneys who specialize in malpractice defense. Keep in mind that lawyers always represent and work on behalf of their clients, and even though a malpractice carrier's attorney is defending your actions, his or her client is the insurer, so it is often advisable to also have your own malpractice attorney to assist in that defense and to make sure your interests are represented.

Attorneys' Conflict of Interest

Conflict of interest rules that the legal profession abides by may dictate that a local attorney cannot represent you if he or she also represents one of your competitors, especially if issues exist that might be in conflict between the two parties. If your attorney draws up an employment agreement for a potential new associate, be sure to encourage that new doctor to get the document independently reviewed by his or her own legal counsel; likewise, if you are the new doctor make sure that you engage an attorney to review contracts on your behalf.

Setting Policies and Procedures

For a myriad of reasons, every practice must have policies and procedures in place. Some of the important reasons are related to efficiency, structure, and liability. Many of the ways your practice does things will change as the staff grows and the practice builds its patient base. Written policies and procedures are essential for training and holding the staff accountable for the delivery of quality patient care. They also will accelerate the learning curve for new employees, especially when there was no overlap between the new employee and the departed employee.

Preparing written policies is a good exercise in thinking through the processes and examining their validity and accuracy. A policies and procedures manual should be prepared with greater detail and bound separately from the employee handbook, which is discussed in Chapter 9. Each employee should sign a form that will be maintained in the employee's personnel file acknowledging that the policies and procedures have been read. The box "The Policies and Procedures Manual" describes what such a manual should accomplish. For other policies and procedures to consider, also see "Identifying and Remedying the Risks" in Chapter 7.

The physician will likely assume responsibility for the preparation of the policies and procedures manual in the early stages of a practice. How each policy or procedure will be carried out or conducted should be defined. After the initial office set-up phase, this task can be turned over to the administrative staff for updates and maintenance.

Scheduling Patients

Inefficient patient scheduling can significantly impede the progress of your day. There are many effective methods from which to choose, and you can experiment with different appointment schedules to learn what works best for the practice.

The Policies and Procedures Manual

- Provides step-by-step guidelines for completion of each task in the office.
- Identifies key personnel to use as resources for each task.
- Includes samples of forms to be used.
- Lists frequently called telephone numbers.
- Advises about miscellaneous office matters (eg, location of keys, how to reorder forms).
- Addresses the following functions with specific policies and instructions:

Communicating clinic and surgery charges	Scheduling patient appointments
Purchasing protocols	Closing and reconciling day's activities
Office collections routine	Cleaning equipment
Releasing patient records prerequisites	Working up a patient
Billing policies follow up	Scheduling ancillary tests
Registering a patient	Handling test and laboratory results (eg, notifying the patient)
Setting up a patient's file	
Completing a superbill	

Here are some samples of methods practices use in scheduling patients:

- *Typical method:* One patient is scheduled every 15 minutes regardless of whether the patient requires a full exam or just a follow up. This method is often driven by appointment scheduling software that defaults to one type of appointment time slot. Since this method results in very inefficient scheduling, it is almost always modified by staff members to better fit patient and practice needs.
- *Wave method:* Three patients are scheduled to arrive on the hour and half hour, based on the concept that one patient will always be early, another on time, and the third 5–10 minutes late.
- *Need method:* Patients for follow-up visits or short exams are scheduled for shorter time periods, while new patients and cataract or refractive surgery evaluations are given more time and are scheduled at specific times such as the first and last patient each morning and each afternoon.
- *Open access:* Patients are seen on the day they call, with designated time slots for types of visits. This method is rarely used in developed ophthalmology practices, although it is sometimes used in other specialties such as family practice.

Whatever method is used, take note of the receptionist's demeanor and whether the receptionist asks permission before putting a patient on hold. Such courtesies help reinforce the patient's goodwill toward your practice. Let the office staff know that it is imperative patients wait no longer than 15 minutes in the reception area without the physician being made aware of the situation. The staff should also be responsible for keeping the patients informed of any delays. Patients usually do not mind waiting an extra few minutes if they are regularly updated and given the opportunity to reschedule.

Managing Patient Flow

Your own responsibility for maintaining a prompt appointment schedule cannot be overstated. Excess waiting time is still the number one complaint of most patients. Patient satisfaction is crucial in today's competitive health care market, and being on time goes a long way toward achieving patient satisfaction. (See "Developing Patient Satisfaction" in Chapter 10.)

Consider the pointers in the box "Tips for Efficient Scheduling" when addressing scheduling issues. These tips will improve access and increase efficiencies, benefiting you and your patients. Ensure that your staff has this information available to them through your policies and procedures manual.

The following are some of the procedures often used to manage patient flow:

- Ask patients calling to cancel appointments why they are canceling and if and when they would like to reschedule. The ophthalmologist should review charts for established patients who do not reschedule. If medical necessity requires a follow-up visit, it may be appropriate to send a certified letter to the patient.
- Be sure to document their cancellation and your response in their chart and in the appointment book.
- Call patients scheduled later in the week who might like to come in earlier.
- Script instructions or statements to callers who have previously been no shows.
- Have a policy and procedure for working in patients who are more than a specific number of minutes late or patients who do not have an appointment but would like to, or need to, drop in.
- Have a policy and procedure for handling a situation in which another family member hopes to be seen in an appointment time reserved for just one.
- Have a policy for patients arriving early.
- Have a policy and procedure for interacting with pharmaceutical sales representatives who arrive without an appointment.

Tips for Efficient Scheduling

- Arrange office hours to fit community needs. Consider seeing patients during evening hours two or three times a week or Saturday mornings.

- Use an appointment scheduler customized according to physician preferences. In a partnership or group, scheduling preferences may vary by physician. Provide for evening and weekend coverage and vacations.

- Establish an office policy for screening telephone calls. Be sure to set aside specific times for callbacks.

- When an emergency results in a delay, explain the situation to waiting patients; give them a choice of waiting or rescheduling. Contact patients who are not yet in the office.

- When a patient requests an appointment time that is already filled, offer at least two other times that are available. Chances are the patient will choose one of the other times being offered.

- Identify more lengthy appointment types, and "high risk, no show" patients (ie, new patients) and send them written or oral reminders. Mailing new patients a "Welcome to the Practice" letter or brochure along with the new patient information forms to fill out prior to coming to the office is an excellent way of reducing new patient "no shows" while making the patient registration process much smoother.

- Avoid canceling patient days if at all possible. If canceling an appointment is unavoidable, notify the patient as soon as possible.

- If the physician makes visits to referring physicians, nursing homes or other institutions, schedule these trips realistically so they do not conflict with office hours.

- Do not overcrowd the schedule. Allow two or three times during the day for catching up, work-ins, or emergencies. Some busy practices set aside specific appointment slots for new patients who may find another eye doctor if they aren't seen within a reasonable number of days.

- For slow days, keep a stand-by list available of patients who can be called in on short notice in case of cancellations.

CHAPTER 5

Payment for Services

Delivering high-quality patient care and service starts your practice on the road to success. Doing a good job collecting from patients and third-party payors keeps it on track. Have good billing and collection protocols in place and a well-trained staff to carry them out. An experienced health care consultant can help the practice get off to a good start.

Consider this real-life example of what can happen when you are starting out, if you are not careful. A young doctor had been working for a solo practitioner for less than a year when he found out that his employer was having financial difficulties. In fact, his employer's home electricity service had been cut off for lack of payment. Although he enjoyed the practice, the young doctor wanted help finding another job because he feared that his paycheck would bounce. Clearly, the practice was suffering financially for a lack of collecting money owed to the practice by insurance companies and patients. The solution is obvious: Put systems into place that will allow the practice to collect the money that it is owed so that its bills can be paid.

The Fee Schedule

The first key step in making sure your practice is compensated appropriately is to establish a fee schedule for your services. Although federal law prohibits calling other practices and asking their fees as a method for establishing your own fee schedule, there are various accepted methods for establishing and reviewing fees in a medical office, including the following:

- Refer to publications such as the *Physicians Fee and Coding Guide* (updated annually) available in most medical bookstores.
- Use the resource-based relative value scale (RBRVS) compiled by the Centers for Medicare and Medicaid Services (CMS).

Resource-Based Relative Value Scale

The Medicare fee schedule has been based on the RBRVS system since 1992. Most indemnity insurers and managed care organizations are beginning to base their reimbursement on this system as well.

RBRVS at a Glance

The RBRVS is used to determine allowable reimbursement amounts and global days for surgery for Medicare Part B physician services. Medicare Part B medical insurance helps pay for doctors' services, outpatient hospital care, and other medical services that are not covered by Part A hospital insurance. In the development of the RBRVS system, CMS (then the Health Care Financing Administration, or HCFA) assigned a relative value unit (RVU) to more than 7000 current procedural terminology (CPT) codes. (For the complete and comprehensive history of RBRVS, visit www.RBRVS.com. The web site provides free downloads, such as RBRVS spreadsheets, formulas, and published Medicare data. Also see "Case Study 1: Reimbursement" in Chapter 21.)

Each RVU has three components that, when added together, equal the total RVU: work RVU, overhead RVU, and malpractice RVU.

Recognizing that the cost of practicing medicine varies in different parts of the country, CMS, then HCFA, assigned a geographic practice cost index (GPCI) to each component of the RVU for each CPT code. To arrive at the Medicare allowable amount for a given location, each RVU component is multiplied by its corresponding GCPI; the sum of those three figures is multiplied by a "conversion factor" that converts the RVUs into a dollar figure. The conversion factor changes each year depending on CMS formulas and legislative decrees. The 2005 conversion factor is likely to be $37.8975, barring any additional legislative changes. If the 2006 conversion factor increases by 1.5% over 2005, that figure will be about $38.4660. Figure 5-1 displays the complete RBRVS formula; Figure 5-2 shows an example of how the formula works in practice. (Also see "The Bottom Line" later in this chapter for further drill-down into this example.)

Setting Your Fees

When developing a fee schedule(s) there are many factors to consider. CMS, in collaboration with specialty societies (including the American Academy of Ophthalmology) has determined and continues to re-evaluate the RVUs for each CPT code. While Medicare establishes their fee schedule with RVUs, geographic region indicator, and the annual conversion factor, not all commercial payors follow this formula. So establishing your fees on the RBRVS system is only one method of establishing your fees. The Medicare fee schedule is published annually online on the CMS web site (www.cms.hhs.gov).

Commercial Contracts and RBRVS Most commercial payors use a different conversion factor to arrive at their allowable RVU amounts. Some health plans designate different conversion factors for exams and surgical vs nonsurgical services. If you can determine the conversion factor(s) for the plans for which you are a participating provider, it is relatively easy to make sure your fees are appropriate by using a conversion factor that

---

[(Work RVU X Work GPCI) + (Overhead RVU X Overhead GPCI) +

(Malpractice RVU X Malpractice GPCI)] X the conversion factor = Total Allowable Amount

Figure 5-1 The complete RBRVS formula.

Calculation of Medicare Allowable Amount

CPT 66984 - Cataract Surgery With Insertion of IOL

Dallas, TX Region

	RVU	X	GCPI	= Total
Work	10.21		1.010	10.3121
Practice Expense	7.63		1.065	8.12595
Malpractice Expense	0.49		0.996	0.48804
			Sum of Totals	18.92609
				X
			Conversion Factor	$37.3374
			Allowable Amount	$ 706.65

Figure 5-2 Sample calculation of Medicare allowable amount. All physicians in a given geographical area are reimbursed the same amount for a CPT code regardless of specialty.

is higher than the insurance companies'. You can contact the provider relations department for your plan and request a copy of their fee schedule. Many plans have several carve-out plans as well and you should obtain those fee schedules too. A carve-out plan is a specialized plan. It provides coverage on selected individuals by "carving out" all or a portion of their coverage under an employer-sponsored group plan.

Multiple Fee Schedules Note that you may have more than one fee schedule. The rule is that you cannot charge your Medicare patients a higher amount than your usual and customary charge.

The Bottom Line Using the data shown in Figure 5-2, how would you determine your fee for the same service? Let's say the Medicare allowable for participating physicians in your state is $706.65, and the BlueCross/BlueShield allowable for participating physicians is $864.92. You will want to set your fee at an amount that will be higher than each of these allowed amounts. By setting your standard fee at $1060 you are making sure your charged amounts exceed the allowed amounts while still being competitive in the area.

Cost of Providing a Service vs Practice Fees However the fees are set, the practice cannot afford to deliver a service for a fee that is less than the cost of providing the service.

It is a fact that CMS took the cost of providing a service into account when it established the overhead RVU for each service. However, the CMS perspective of a reasonable profit margin may differ from a physician's perspective, and it may not consider all the expenses in managing a medical practice. To maintain a practice that affords a reasonable profit/salary margin after the bills are paid, keep in mind the cost of supplies and other operating expenses. In time, expenses—with the exception of some variables—should be somewhat predictable.

One way of estimating how much it costs your practice to provide a service is to use RVUs. To do so, follow these steps:

1. Calculate the total number of RVUs produced by your practice in a given time period, typically a year. To do this, list every code you billed and how often you billed it, and then multiply the number of each code done by its RVUs. For this example, assume that you use 7500 RVUs produced in a year.
2. Divide the number of RVUs produced (7500 in this example) into the total costs of operating your practice to figure the cost per RVU. Do not include in the costs any income, benefits, retirement or personal business expenses (eg, CME courses) paid to or on behalf of the owners of the practice. For this example, imagine that you have $150,000 in practice expenses. You would divide that figure by 7500 RVUs to arrive at a cost per RVU of $20.
3. Then multiply your cost per RVU by the RVUs in any code to figure the approximate cost of providing that service. For example, using the $20 per RVU calculation, a cataract surgery as noted in Figure 5-2 would be 18.92609 RVUs. That figure multiplied by the $20 per RVU figure means that it costs the practice approximately $378.52 to perform a cataract surgery, not including any income to the doctor.

By comparing your costs for common CPT codes to the fees offered by health insurers and vision plans, you can decide whether the fee schedules are sufficient for your practice.

Practice Fees vs "Allowable" Fee Schedules Most insurance plans have an "allowable" fee for every CPT code you bill. This fee is the total amount the plan allows you to collect—typically the plan pays part of the fee, and the patient pays another part. (Some patients must pay 100% of the plan's allowable amounts up to their annual deductible.) In most cases, your contracts with the insurance plans prevent you from billing the patient more than the plan allows you to, although if you are not a paneled physician with a plan you may be able to bill the patients the entire amount and then let them collect what's due from their insurance company.

Be careful to understand the requirements of any contracts you sign with insurance companies. For example, most contracts with BlueCross/BlueShield (BCBS) plans in a particular state require that you treat all other BCBS plans the same as the one you are contracted with. So, if you are contracted with BCBS in Idaho and someone who is a member of BCBS in Iowa is cared for in your practice, you have to accept Idaho's allowable as payment in full, even if the Iowa plan would pay more.

It is best to get the fee schedules from all of the plans that you are contracted with, and then to make sure your fees are set at least as high as the best allowable amount from any of those plans for each CPT code.

Reviewing your fees at least once a year is mandatory if you are to keep on top of changes in fee schedules. Also review your fees if either of the two following events occurs:

- You receive a notice of changes in a contracted plan's fee schedule.
- You receive a check from a contracted insurance company that has the allowable equal to your charge. In this case, the actual allowable is probably greater than your charge for that CPT code and you may consider raising your fee.

Write-Offs Insurance plan contracts require that you "write-off" any amounts that you charge in excess of their allowable fee amounts. For example, if your charge for cataract surgery is $1060 and the insurance allowed amount is $900, the transaction would look like this:

1. You collect a co-pay from the patient of $15 on the day of service, and that amount is entered into the computer system's payment screen for that patient.
2. You send a claim to the insurance company for $1060 for code 66984.
3. The insurance company sends you a check with an Explanation of Benefits (EOB) form. The check is for $885 (the allowable less the $15 co-payment) and the EOB indicates that you must write-off $160, which is the difference between your $1060 fee and the $900 allowable.
4. Your billing clerk then enters the insurance payment of $885 and then credits the additional $160 as a contractual write-off. The total of $15 patient payment, $885 insurance payment, and $160 credit posted against the original $1060 charge clears the account to a zero balance.

Coding and Billing

The CPT codes referred to here are published annually by the American Medical Association and must be used for virtually all of your insurance billing. The CPT code manual also gives descriptions of what each code entails and includes modifiers that are used to clarify special billing situations. Every practice needs to obtain the CPT code manual each year and to carefully follow its guidelines when billing insurance companies.

Resources The American Academy of Ophthalmology and the American Academy of Ophthalmic Executives provide a number of publications and resources related to coding. See Appendix I for more information. To find a copy of the Medicare RVU values for each CPT code, along with Medicare days included in postoperative care for each surgery code, visit the CMS web site (www.cms.hhs.gov).

Your Payment Policies

Your practice must have a policy and specific processes for billing and collecting from insurance companies. Many practices have found themselves in serious financial trouble because they did not have a good process for getting paid by insurance companies.

Because it can take 1–3 months for a health plan to pay you, problems that delay payments can turn serious quickly. For example, if you experienced a computer problem on March 1 that prevented your electronic claims from being sent out, you might not know you had a problem for a month, when the lack of payments for those claims would be noticed. If it takes a week to fix the problem, and then you re-bill the claims, it can be May 1 or later before you begin receiving payments. Now, usually you receive confirmation that your electronic claims have been received (in the form of an electronic report) so you should know before a month goes by that your claims have not been received for processing. In some instances problems within the billing staff have caused claims to be delayed and the physician did not realize there was a crisis until the checkbook was empty.

Table 5-1 lists 21 basic checkpoints that every practice must take to make sure their billing is handled correctly and efficiently. The table also includes some ways to measure your success in each step. The "Measurement" column is for including the measurement for your practice. The "Score" column is used to indicate where your practice meets the standard and where extra work is needed. Most practices do not constantly measure every one of these steps, but you should choose several that are most important to your practice and make sure you are measuring up in those areas.

During the early stages of a practice startup—before bad habits have a chance to develop—institute a payment policy. See Appendix I for an example of procedures that have been set up for handling insurance and patient collections at a practice.

Interfacing with Insurance Companies

About 80%–90% of your patients are covered by some form of insurance. An efficient computer system simplifies claims processing, yet there are still obstacles to overcome in order to collect reimbursements. The more you know about how insurance companies work, the more successful you will be in collecting.

Understanding the Plans Available

Following is basic information on various types of plans and an overview of how they will affect your ability to collect your charges.

Indemnity Plans

The traditional insurance companies are known as *indemnity* or *commercial* insurance plans. Sometimes called *80/20 plans*, their marketing materials typically state that they pay 80% of the patient's medical bill, and the patient only pays the remaining 20% after an annual deductible is met. This type of advertising can be misleading to patients, because these companies base the 80% they pay on what they term a *usual and customary reimbursement*, or UCR (see the box "Example of 80/20 Plan in Action"). The insurance company's UCR for a particular service is seldom, if ever, the same as your fee for that same service. Insurance companies generally do not explain how they establish their usual and customary fees.

Table 5-1 Checkpoints for Accurate Billing

Area	Standard	Measurement	Score
1. Initial patient phone call	98%+ complete information		
2. Form completion	98%+ of forms complete		
3. Patient data entry	1% or less denied claims due to data entry		
4. Insurance card copying	95%+ cards copied or verified		
5. Insurance verification; pre-authorization; referrals	2% or less of denied claims		
6. Procedure coding	96% claims are coded properly		
7. Charge entry	24 hours or less between service and charge entry		
8. Charge entry verification	99% accurate entry of charges		
9. Patient date of service collections	95% of co-pays collected on date of service		
10. Claims submission	24 hours or less between service and claims submission		
11. End of day close	100% balance at end of each day		
12. Payment entry and deposits	Checks and cash deposited daily		
13. Patient billing	Patient statements sent at least monthly		
14. Denial tracking	3% or less of total claims denied		
15. Insurance follow up	10–20% of billing staff time spent on follow up		
16. Patient account follow up	80% of patient statements paid within one month		
17. Month and year-end close	Done each month and at year end		
18. Monthly Reports	Owners receive a clear one-page summary monthly		
19. Fee Schedule	Update fee schedule annually		
20. Insurance Contract Review	Annual contract reviews for appropriate payment levels		
21. Compliance Plan	Charts sampled for each provider at least quarterly		

Managed Care Plans

New physicians entering the marketplace have an advantage in that they grew up with the managed care concept. Physicians that have been in private practice for many years have had to learn a new payment process and modify the way they view patient care.

Several types of plans are offered in most areas, and most insurers sell some type of managed care plans that generally pay the provider on a discounted fee for service or a capitated basis.

Discounted Fee-for-Service Plans In a discounted fee-for-service plan, the payor/insurance plan negotiates with the physician for a discount off the regular fee for a particular

Example of 80/20 Plan in Action

You charge a patient $1500 for a trabeculectomy surgery. The indemnity insurance plan says the usual and customary fee is $1200, so they pay 80% of $1200 ($960), not 80% of $1500. The patient then is responsible for paying $540 to the physician instead of the $240 (or 20% of $1200) he expected to pay. The patient receives an Explanation of Benefits (EOB) form that states "Your physician's fee is higher than the usual and customary fee for this procedure. The usual and customary fee for this procedure is $1200, so we are reimbursing 80% of $1200." Without an understanding of how the insurance company pays for a particular procedure, or how this fee is calculated, the patient is likely to be annoyed with you.

Here's what you can do: Conduct some patient education before performing a service or surgical procedure. Explain to the patient that the fee for the service may not be the same as the insurance company's reimbursement. Also explain that your fees are set so that you can provide a high-quality service, pay your expenses, and remain competitive in the marketplace. Open communications help keep patients happy and set successful physicians apart from their peers.

service in exchange for the promise of a potential increase in patients. Generally, the physician receives no guarantee in the number of patients he or she will receive from the plan. These plans are typically called preferred provider organizations (PPOs), health maintenance organizations (HMOs), or point-of-service (POS) plans.

Most PPOs involve an insurance company contracting with certain providers who agree to accept the plan's reimbursement rates, rules and regulations. Patients may only be covered for medical services if they use the providers on the health plan's panel, so there is usually a big incentive for patients to avoid nonpanel providers.

HMOs are similar to PPOs in most respects, and in some states the only difference between the two may be what they call themselves. However, some HMOs use a "staff model" approach in which they hire most of the doctors they need as employees, build their own office buildings and hospitals, and control most of the provision of services for their members. On occasion, a staff model HMO may contract with a local ophthalmologist to provide services to its members. Such an arrangement is usually temporary; as soon as the volume of patients warrants the HMO typically hires its own ophthalmologist because that is viewed as being a less expensive way of providing eye care to its members.

A POS plan looks like a PPO or HMO, with a list of contracted doctors, but also has the option for patients to seek care outside the plan panel. In most cases, if a patient sees a doctor who is not on the panel, the health plan's reimbursement is less and the patient pays a larger share of the cost.

Capitated Plans In a capitated arrangement, the physician agrees to provide a specified list of services to each patient assigned to the practice for a set dollar amount each month (eg, per member per month). The insurer pays the physician this specified amount whether or not the physician sees the patient in the office. The amount may range from 25¢ per patient per month for very limited ophthalmic services provided to a young patient base to $10 per patient per month for a full range of services provided to senior patients. Capitated plans are often called *risk-sharing arrangements,* although in some cases nearly all of the risk for the patient's care is shifted to the physician.

Here's an example of a capitated plan: A physician has 1000 patients assigned to her practice for which the insurer pays a capitated fee of $1 per member/per month (pm/pm), or a total of $1000. If the physician sees 20 of these patients in a month and these patients require a total of $1800 worth of services, she has come up $800 short of what she would have collected had the patients been seen on a fee-for-service basis. However, if the physician sees only 5 of the 100 patients in a month and their services total $200, she has made $800 more than she would have under fee for service. Seeing the risk involved in this arrangement is fairly obvious.

Medicare

Medicare is the government's health plan for people in three categories:

- Virtually everyone over 65 years of age
- Some people under 65 who have disabilities
- People with end stage renal disease

Medicare is administered by the Centers for Medicare and Medicaid Services (CMS), which is part of the Department of Health and Human Services of the federal government.

Typically about 60% of a general ophthalmologist's practice includes patients with Medicare coverage. Medicare is considered to be among the lowest-reimbursing health plans in most parts of the country, although in some areas managed care plans reimburse significantly lower than Medicare. Medicare Part B benefits pay physicians for their services, while Part A pays hospitalization costs. Most Medicare recipients get Part A coverage at no charge to them but have to pay a small monthly fee for Part B coverage, so it is possible you could see a patient who only has Part A coverage.

Medicare operates as an indemnity insurer, paying 80% of allowed charges while the patient is responsible for the remaining 20% plus an annual deductible, which, for example, was $100 in 2004. For this reason, many Medicare patients have secondary insurance (sometimes called *Medigap insurance*) that pays some or all of their portion of the allowable amount. If a patient has a secondary insurance, you need to bill Medicare first, then submit a claim for the balance to the secondary carrier and include the Explanation of Medicare Benefits (EOMB) form with the claim to show the secondary insurer what Medicare allowed and paid. In some cases, Medicare can now forward the claim on to the secondary insurer electronically so your practice does not have to bill both entities. Once both Medicare and the secondary carrier have paid, you may need to bill the patient if a portion of the allowable amount remains outstanding. You must make a good faith effort to collect deductibles and co-payments from Medicare patients; failure to do so routinely can result in adverse consequences from the Medicare program.

Medicare does not actually pay doctors directly, but Medicare claims processing is contracted to various insurance companies (called *Medicare carriers*) who each have a particular region of the country assigned to them. If you see patients in two different states, you may have to file claims with two different Medicare carriers and deal with both carriers in the event of claim appeals and so on.

Medicare has set certain payment policies that all carriers are expected to follow, called *national coverage determinations* (NCDs). Medicare allows the carriers some latitude in other policies, and the carriers publish *local coverage determinations* (LCD) to educate providers and patients on those policies. LCDs must not contradict or conflict with NCDs, but they can be more specific or cover areas not yet published in an NCD. Most Medicare carriers have their own web sites where you can access LCDs. To research both national and local coverage determinations for specific codes, visit the CMS web site (www.cms.hhs.gov).

Doctors have three options when working with the Medicare program:

- You can "accept assignment," which means you agree to accept Medicare's allowable amount as full payment for your services. If you agree to always accept assignment on every claim, you become a "participating" provider with Medicare by signing a participating agreement.
- You can be a Medicare provider but not accept assignment, which means that you can collect up to 115% of the Medicare allowable amount. In this case Medicare reduces the allowable by 5%, so your limiting charge that you can collect is 115% of 95% of the normal allowable, or 109.25% of the usual allowable. Medicare then pays 80% of the reduced allowable and you can bill the patient for the remaining amount. For example, if the Medicare allowable for a CPT code is $100, and you charge $150 but do not accept assignment, Medicare allows you to collect $109.25—$76 from Medicare (80% of the $95 reduced allowable) plus $33.25 from the patient. You can accept assignment on a case-by-case basis unless you are a participating provider.
- You can opt out of the Medicare system entirely and charge patients whatever you decide. In this case the patient signs a private contract with you and gives up any Medicare benefits for care that you provide. You must officially notify Medicare of your decision to opt out, and you must remain out of the system for at least 2 years. Opting out of Medicare is not a good option for most ophthalmologists unless you provide exclusively cosmetic or refractive surgery.

Medicaid

Medicaid is a federal and state program for low-income families and individuals. It is federally mandated and state-run, so there is considerable difference in reimbursement levels from state to state. In general, Medicaid (called *Medi-Cal* in California) pays the lowest reimbursements of any third-party payor. In some cases, patients may have both Medicare and Medicaid ("Medimedi" coverage) and in those situations Medicaid may pay a portion of the patient's responsibility.

Workers' Compensation Insurance

All employers must provide workers' compensation insurance to cover the medical and disability expenses incurred by the worker from a job-related injury. Many states administer workers' compensation insurance billing directly. In these states, the physician sends the claims directly to the state's agency. Other states require employers to contract with an insurance company for payment of work-related claims. In either case, legislation predetermines the benefits and payments, based upon the state and the company. Request a packet of information from your State Workers' Compensation Board in preparation for accepting patients with work-related injuries and before processing claims.

When accepting a patient for a work-related injury, follow these guidelines in order to receive reimbursement for your services:

- Before providing services to the patient, get authorization for treatment from the employer.
- Try to get a written request for treatment from the employer.
- If a written request is not possible, call the employer for authorization. Use a simple telephone consent form to record the authorization.
- The employer must notify the insurance company of the injury. Without a "first report of injury" notification, reimbursement will be delayed.
- Treat workers' compensation claims as any insurance claim, filed in the unpaid claim file, and routinely followed up.
- The first claim form should reach the insurance company within 10 days of first treatment, even if treatment is not completed.
- Physicians cannot bill patients for treatment of work-related injuries.

Self-Payers

Every practice has some patients who pay for care themselves. In some cases they may not be insured; in others they may have a high deductible so your care is their financial responsibility unless the amount exceeds their deductible. Many plans, including Medicare, do not pay for routine eye exams, glasses or contact lenses, so patients must pay for those services themselves.

It is important that self-payers be apprised of (1) the cost of services before those services are provided and (2) the need to pay on the date of service for services rendered. It is appropriate to refuse to provide care if a patient is not willing or able to pay for your services, although you may decide to do some pro bono work for indigent patients. Patients who arrive on an emergency basis should receive care without waiting to verify their ability to pay.

Refractive surgery and cosmetic patients are very often 100% self-payers, and their payments should be collected before services are provided. You will find it helpful to accept credit card payments for these patients, and it is usually a good idea to provide access to local banks or other companies that finance medical procedures. In no case should your practice finance elective surgeries unless you own a bank.

Filing Insurance and Following Up on Claims

Insurance claims processing consumes a large portion of administrative time. Setting up workable policies and systems initially helps assure that insurance reimbursement provides a steady flow of cash into the practice.

Most medical management software can print the CMS-1500 insurance form used for filing a claim with Medicare, Medicaid, and insurance companies (see a sample of the front of this form in Appendix I). Automation simplifies the filing process and allows the practice to submit claims daily, if desired. However, the claim filing process is only one small part of the reimbursement process. Monitoring the filed claims and assuring that insurers are paying them quickly requires much more effort.

Develop a claim filing protocol similar to the following example to streamline this process:

- File claims at least twice weekly; daily is preferable.
- Check all claims for accuracy and completeness of information before mailing. Most insurance companies promise a 30-day turnaround time for payments if they receive a clean claim. Some states have enacted legislation requiring payors to pay claims within a certain time frame and to pay interest on late claims. Be aware of the laws in your state and report any violations to the proper authorities.
- Print out daily a claims pending report; call the insurance carrier on all claims that they have not paid within 30 days of the filing date. If your computer cannot generate this report, enter filed claims on an insurance log. Enter the date, the patient's name, the insurance company, and the amount filed on the log sheet. Check the log sheets every day to determine which claims have not been paid in 30 days and follow up by telephone.
- Call the insurance companies to ask about an unpaid claim. Calling is more effective than simply resubmitting the claim. If the insurance company says it has not received the claim, then it must be resubmitted. Some health plans now allow you to check the status of claims on the Internet, and you may find this is faster than calling on past due claims. However, you may still have to call on some claims if the web site does not give you enough information to know how to correct and re-file the claim.
- Print out an aged accounts analysis by payor each month to learn which companies pay on time and which ones habitually exceed a 30-day turnaround time. (This is not a standard report on every system. It is worthwhile to request that the system be set up to provide this report.)
- Call the plan administrator and request an explanation of the plan's poor payment habits. Most managed care contracts guarantee a 30-day reimbursement schedule if the claims are submitted in order. If you do not receive your payments as agreed, it may be a sign that the plan is in financial trouble. If the payment problems persist, you may wish to terminate the contract.
- Make contractual adjustments at the time payments are received.
- Conduct a periodic review of Explanation of Benefits (EOB) forms. An EOB statement, similar to a check stub, accompanies every insurance payment. Compare the EOB with the filed claim to assure that the insurer is paying claims appropriately, without reductions or denials.
- Consistent follow up is the key to satisfactory reimbursement. If insurance claims are produced on a file-and-forget method, you may find yourself with a cash flow shortfall. Give employees a copy of the written policy. Make them accountable for following these routines.

Managing Your Accounts Receivable

At the end of each business day you create an account of all the services you have provided and billed for that business day. The cumulative total of that account is your accounts receivable (A/R). As each billed service is paid or adjusted for write-offs, your A/R changes. A/R therefore refers to the charges you have sent as claims to insurance companies and to the patient balances you have billed to patients. Most practices bill higher charges than insurance companies will allow, so A/R amounts are usually higher than what you will finally collect. For example, if your charge for a procedure is $800, but the insurance company only allows $400, your A/R for that procedure will be $800 once the claim is filed. If you receive a payment of $320 from the insurer, you would write off $400, post the payment of $320 and your remaining A/R for that claim would be $80, which you would then bill to the patient. Until you receive payment from the patient, your A/R for that claim would be $80; when the patient pays the bill your A/R would go to zero for that procedure.

Some practices match their charges to their insurers' allowables, so that their A/R very closely reflects what they should collect, but this requires consistently tracking allowables and then setting up and maintaining multiple fee schedules.

Tracking your "days in A/R" is a good way to measure how well your collection policies and practices are working. Days outstanding in A/R is a measure of how long it is taking to collect your money. It is calculated by dividing your total charges for a year by 365 to figure your average charges per day. You then divide your average charges per day into your total accounts receivable (how much you are owed) to calculate how many days of charges you have in accounts receivable. For example:

> Total annual charges: $730,000
> Days in the year: 365
> Charges per day: $2000
> A/R: $90,000
> Days in A/R: 45
> (also called *Days Sales Outstanding*)

The lower the days in A/R the quicker you are collecting your money and the less pressure there will be on your cash flow. Typically the days in A/R range from 25 to 45; anything over 60 days warrants immediate attention. In general, if days in A/R are less than 45 your billing staff should spend about 10% of their time following up on past due claims. If your A/R days are more than 45, 20% or more of the staff's time should be spent following up on claims. In some cases it may be best to add some temporary help to the billing department to catch up on past due claims.

When the number of days in A/R begins to climb, your cash flow is immediately affected, and lack of attention in this area can create a situation in which you do not have enough money in your bank account to meet your expenses, so this figure should be tracked monthly.

Most insurance companies have a time limit for providing a clean claim, from as little as 90 days to as long as 18 months. If you do not submit a clean claim (incorrect claims do not count) within the time frame allotted the insurance plan will refuse to pay you even if you can prove that you provided the service. For this reason it is critical to follow up promptly on every claim you submit.

Setting Collection Targets for Each Payor Class

Most practice management computer systems can provide a report of the amounts due from each different insurance plan, with an aging spread showing how much is current

(0–30 days since date of service), 31–60 days out, 61–90 days out, and 91–120 days past due. This report is helpful in identifying which payors are taking too long to pay claims or are denying too many claims—in some cases, your practice may not be following insurers' billing rules correctly. Focusing on the payors that have the most money in the past due columns will help you determine how to better handle their claims so that you get paid promptly.

Some payors have longer collection cycles than others. For example, if you have a number of senior patients with a particular Medigap policy, those claims will be delayed because Medicare has to pay first before the claim gets sent to the secondary insurer. As you track the reasons for denials for each insurance company, you will be able to set collection targets individually for those companies and to track your progress in meeting those objectives.

Tracking Payor Denials

When you understand why payors are denying payment, you may be able to modify your procedures. Here's an example. A three-doctor practice showed more than $1.2 million in A/R, almost $900,000 of which was past due. The billing manager had no idea what the major reasons for payment denial were, and therefore was not in a position to modify procedures, coding, or other systems. She assumed part of the problem was due to patients who changed insurance companies without telling the practice. When asked if the practice had a procedure for checking current insurance coverage at the start of an office visit, she did not know.

Tracking and analyzing the reasons for insurance company denials is the single most important task you can do to make your collections easier. Once you determine the reasons for denials, you can fix those areas within the practice so that bad claims never get sent to insurance companies. Those practices that never send bad claims have far fewer complaints about collecting from insurance companies than those that consistently send faulty claims.

Table 5-2 shows an actual payor denial report. These figures were compiled from data received from several insurance companies and illustrates why some claims had not been paid. Note the following problems that can be seen by careful examination of this report:

- The denial reasons marked with an asterisk may have been caused by the practice.
- The insurance company did not receive 30% of these past due claims. This may be a problem with a specific insurer, but when every insurer is missing claims, that usually indicates a problem within the practice.
- Of the overall claims, 22% should have been billed to the patient. There may be someone in the billing office of the practice who does not know how to send the amount due to the patient balance bucket of the practice management software once the insurance has paid its portion.
- Of the overall claims, 6% were incorrect, but over a fifth of the claims for Insurer C were incorrect, meaning that the practice probably is not following some guideline for billing claims to Insurer C.

Table 5-2 Common Reasons for Denied Insurance Claims

Reason for Denial	Ins A	Ins B	Ins C	Ins D	Ins E	Medicaid	Medicare	Average
Missing claim*	15%	29%	14%	33%	32%	50%	42%	30%
Patient responsibility*	22%	43%	24%	11%	18%	0%	31%	22%
Incorrect claim*	12%	0%	21%	0%	0%	0%	11%	6%
Insurer will reprocess claim	10%	29%	10%	11%	12%	0%	0%	9%
Nonprovider*	12%	0%	10%	0%	0%	0%	6%	3%
Policy canceled prior to services*	2%	0%	7%	0%	6%	0%	0%	2%
Incorrect policy number*	10%	0%	2%	0%	0%	0%	0%	2%
Coordination of benefits issue	0%	0%	2%	0%	3%	0%	6%	1%
Secondary needs primary insurance EOB*	5%	0%	2%	0%	3%	0%	0%	1%
Noncovered service*	0%	0%	0%	0%	6%	0%	3%	1%
Op report/chart notes needed	7%	0%	0%	0%	0%	0%	0%	1%
Preauthorization needed*	2%	0%	0%	22%	0%	0%	0%	3%
Practice needs more info from patient*	0%	0%	0%	0%	3%	0%	0%	7%
Medicare payment greater than MCD allowable	0%	0%	0%	0%	0%	50%	0%	6%
Duplicate claim	2%	0%	0%	0%	0%	0%	0%	0%

* Indicates the denial may have involved practice error. See the text for more details.

- For insurer D, 22% of the claims were denied because of a lack of pre-authorization. Clearly, the practice needs to research this problem and figure out why preauthorizations are not being received for insurer D's patients.
- When called, the insurance companies reported 9% of the time that there did not seem to be any reason why the claim had not been paid. In those cases, the person contacted would put the claim in for processing and payment. That happened with insurer B on almost 30% of their claims. If the contact had not been made with the insurance companies, none of those claims would have been paid, so it is critical that your billing staff follow up on every unpaid claim.

Collections Issues

The payments you receive may come from insurance companies, credit card companies, or patients themselves. Controlling the A/R process will help assure that your practice is financially successful.

As many a business can attest, collecting monies due is not a process that runs on its own. Establish measurable goals and make employees accountable for responsibilities in the process. It is hoped that most of your payments are made without difficulties, but as the following text describes, there are steps to take when payments are not received in a timely manner.

Collecting Payments through Insurance Companies

When everything works the way it should, you send in claims and they get paid; you collect the patient's portion on the day of service and all is well. Unfortunately, as illustrated in the preceding section, everything does not always work the way it should. If you are sending clean, correct claims to the insurance companies and you understand their policies and what they will and will not pay, and you still have trouble collecting from a particular insurer or group of insurers, it may be time to escalate matters. Most of the people your staff deals with in following up on past due claims have very limited authority to make changes within the insurance company. If you can establish a pattern of improper denials, downcoding, or faulty payment patterns on the part of an insurer, you may have to open a dialog with someone at the health plan who has authority to resolve the issue.

You may want to start with the supervisor of the employees who answer the telephone when you call the insurer for problems that seem simple, but in many cases you will need to delve into the executive ranks. The medical director can sometimes be helpful because he or she is a doctor who may understand your frustrations. However, at some insurers the medical director has little or no true authority. If all else fails, and maybe before that point, you may want to contact the CEO of the health plan, either by phone or by registered letter. Sometimes an inquiry to lower levels of the company from the very top will get things moving and changes made. As a last resort, you may want to contact the insurance commissioner from your state with your complaints against the health plan. Some state medical associations have committees whose purpose is to help practices work through issues with insurance companies, so it may be worth investigating that option. Many state ophthalmologic organizations have a third-party payor committee that can be very helpful. In general, aim to work through insurance company problems in a collaborative and cooperative way; save confrontation for those cases where it is the only method that will work.

Collecting from Patients

Patients are personally responsible to you, the physician, for the payment of medical services that were rendered, even if they have insurance. You are not obligated to file the patient's insurance claims unless you have a contract with the insurance company. These contracted agreements include Medicare, Medicaid, and managed care plans. Agreeing to file a patient's insurance claim and wait for the reimbursement is a service you provide to your patients. This service is important, and it is one that most practices provide. However, make sure your patients understand that payment is ultimately their responsibility.

As with insurance filing and billing, a structured process for patient billing and follow up is the most important factor in achieving reimbursement. Establish a written financial policy that you can present to your patients before they receive treatment. This financial policy should explain payment expectations and your policy on filing insurance claims (see the box, "What to Include in the Written Financial Policy").

Statements sent to patients should itemize the procedures and include the entire amount due, even if an insurance company will pay most of it. Many practice manage-

What to Include in the Written Financial Policy

- Payment for services is expected at the time of service unless arrangements are made prior to treatment.
- The office will file insurance claims for services rendered, but the patients are not relieved of responsibility for payment because they have insurance.
- Patients must pay co-pays or deductibles due before surgical procedures are performed and at the time services are rendered.
- Statements are mailed every 30 days. Any balance left unpaid after 90 days will be turned over to a collection agency.
- Financial arrangements can be made for payment of bills that are more than a certain dollar amount, which each practice must set.

ment software programs produce statements that show both the amount presumed covered by insurance and the portion for which the patient is responsible.

Patients should receive statements regularly for any outstanding amount. Your billing cycle can be set up in several ways. The traditional method is to send all statements at the end of each month. Other methods include sending statements twice monthly, one half on the 15th and one half on the 30th. The third method is to send some statements out each week according to letters of the alphabet, or based on insurance payments received. These last two billing methods spread the cash flow and the associated payment posting work more evenly throughout the month.

The following are a few suggestions for billings and collections:

- Send each patient a billing statement within 30 days after the date of service. If insurance has not paid yet, indicate insurance has been billed and payment is pending.
- Call each patient who has an unpaid bill 45 days after the date of treatment. Ask if a problem has prevented payment of the bill. Make notes of any comments made by the patient.
- If the patient says that he or she cannot pay the full amount of the bill, offer to set up a payment schedule. There are companies that can set you up so that you can make automatic bank account or credit card withdrawals each month from the patient's account and this is the best way to handle monthly payments, since receiving the money is far more probable. Some practices make this the only option for patients who want to make monthly payments of amounts due.
- Offer the patient a payment envelope.
- If the patient wants to make a partial payment, set up (and record) a payment agreement.
- Remember to say "Thank you!"
- At 60 days, send a second statement as needed.
- At 75 days, if the bill remains unpaid, call and remind the patient of a previous balance, and record the patient's comments.
- At 90 days, send a third statement.
- At 100 days, send letter stating that payment is due within 10 days or the account will be turned over for collection.
- At 110 days, review the account. If payment has not been received, turn the matter over to the collection agency.

Officially terminating the patient/physician relationship is important when a patient does not meet financial obligations. The physician cannot refuse to treat an established patient who owes the practice money unless the relationship has been formally terminated. See Chapter 7 for further discussion and a sample patient care termination letter.

Using a Collection Agency

Approximately 2% of patients do not pay their medical bills. After you have exhausted all your in-house collection techniques, it may be best to turn some accounts over to a collection agency.

Choose a collection agency carefully, being mindful that the agency's collection methods reflect on your practice. Talk with other physicians or office managers to see which agency they are using. Ask if they are satisfied with the services they receive and what percentage of accounts turned over for collection are paid. Collection agencies typically show a collection success rate of less than 25%.

Besides the items just discussed, the following points should be considered:

- Get copies of all the letters the agency will send to your patients.
- Do not turn over accounts of less than $20.
- Make a note on the patient's ledger card that you have turned over the account.
- Never pay a collection agency a commission up front.
- Make sure patient accounts can be recalled any time.
- Have a written agreement. Read the fine print.
- Do not allow the agency to litigate an account without your permission.
- Report changes in the collection status of an account to the agency.
- Keep a log of all accounts in collection. Enter the name, date turned over, amount due, amount the patient paid, and the net back.
- Use two agencies simultaneously so their efficiency can be evaluated.
- Establish a time limit on how long an agency is entitled to a percentage of amounts collected after an account is withdrawn.

Accepting Credit Cards

Most offices routinely accept credit cards for payment of medical bills. This method brings funds into the practice immediately and transfers the risk of nonpayment to the credit card companies.

Almost every bank offers vendor/merchant accounts that allow you to deposit your credit card payments into the bank for processing. Some credit card companies transfer the funds to your bank electronically so that you have access to the money immediately.

Each bank sets its own service charge for processing credit card transactions; the charge is generally based on a percentage of your overall credit card deposits and ranges from 1.5% to 8%. The service charge is often negotiable. If you have no deposit history with the bank, your negotiating clout may not be very strong. If the bank accepts electronic transfers of your funds from the credit card companies, the service charge should be lower.

Your credit card merchant account does not have to be in the same bank as your checking account. However, you will find that it is more convenient, and you will generally receive favorable service charge rates from your own bank. To set up your practice to accept credit cards, see the box, "Establishing a Credit Card Account."

Establishing a Credit Card Account

- Visit the bank where you have your office account and inquire about setting up a merchant account for the acceptance of credit card deposits. Ask the rate of their service charges. (Do not accept their first offer; attempt to negotiate the lowest rate possible.)

- Once an account has been established, you will be assigned a merchant number. The bank typically provides all necessary materials for accepting credit cards such as charge slips, credit slips, deposit slips, and electronic card reader. They also provide the machine that allows you to obtain approval from the credit card companies and have the funds electronically transferred into its account. This process may vary; every bank's credit card department has established protocols for merchant accounts.

- Ask the bank representative if a bank employee can come to your office to set up the electronic transmittal unit and explain to your staff how the credit card process works.

CHAPTER 6

Regulations and Licensing Requirements

Medical practice involves many rules and licensing requirements; in fact, health care is one of the most highly regulated industries in the nation. You are responsible for keeping informed on the issues and noting changes as they occur through announcements and bulletins as they are released by regulatory agencies. Further, rules are constantly changing, which requires continuous education for the practitioner and practice staff. However, with the proper resources, you can figure out how to maneuver your way through the minefield with few wounds.

These laws and regulations originate from many sources and would require a huge volume to explain in full. This chapter, therefore, serves as a resource directory for regulations required for starting a practice and ongoing compliance. Bear in mind that in some cases the regulation may not be entirely applicable. For example, Joint Commission on Accreditation of Healthcare Organizations (JCAHO) regulations apply only if your practice is owned by a JCAHO-approved hospital. Also keep in mind that the addresses and web sites cited herein are subject to change.

> ✓ **KEY POINT**
>
> **Regulations can be overwhelming. The Academy and AAOE offer several resources to enhance your understanding of this important area of knowledge. See Appendix I for product information.**

Certification by the American Board of Ophthalmology

Board certification is required for many insurance plans, and it is an important step along your career path. Without board certification you will find some professional options closed to you, so take the time to prepare for the requirements of the board certification examinations.

The American Board of Ophthalmology (ABO) is an independent, nonprofit organization responsible for certifying ophthalmologists and protecting the public. The certifying evaluation is designed to assess the knowledge, skills, and experience requisite for the delivery of high standards of patient care in ophthalmology. The basic educational requirements for board certification, as listed by the American Board of Ophthalmology's web site (www.abop.org), are the following:

- All applicants must have graduated from an allopathic or osteopathic medical school.
- All applicants, both graduates of allopathic and osteopathic medical schools, entering ophthalmology training programs must complete a postgraduate clinical year (PG-1) in a program in the United States accredited by the Accreditation Council for Graduate Medical Education (ACGME) or a program in Canada approved by the appropriate accrediting body in Canada.
- The PG-1 year must be comprised of training in which the resident is primarily responsible for patient care in fields such as internal medicine, neurology, pediatrics, surgery, family practice, or emergency medicine. At a minimum, 6 months of this year must consist of a broad experience in direct patient care.
- In addition to a PG-1 year, all applicants must satisfactorily complete an entire formal graduated residency training program in ophthalmology of at least 36 months duration (PG-4 or higher) in either the United States accredited by the ACGME, or in Canada accredited by the Royal College of Physicians and Surgeons of Canada.

In 2003, about 66% of the candidates passed the written qualifying exam and about 80% passed the oral examination. More information on the board certification process, including maintaining certification, can be found on the ABO web site.

Additional Requirements at the State and Federal Level

In starting out your practice, take time to determine that all of the necessary state and other licenses, identification numbers, and privileges are in order.

Acquiring Documents, Numbers, and Privileges

State Medical License

Call your State Board of Medical Examiners to obtain the necessary forms and a list of any backup documents that may be needed to apply for your state license. For a complete Internet listing of contact information for the Board of Medical Examiners in your state, visit the Federation of State Medical Boards web site at www.fsmb.org. If you move from one state to another, you may not wish to relinquish your prior state licenses; it is easier to keep a license active for the future than it is to reapply.

State Tax Identification Number

A state tax number may also be needed for your practice, and some states require different numbers for payroll withholding, unemployment insurance, etc. Check with your accountant to be certain that all required identifying numbers for establishing a medical practice in your state have been received.

Employer Identification Number

As an employer, you will need a federal employer identification number (EIN). All correspondence with the Internal Revenue Service (IRS) and all tax payments must reference this EIN. To apply for an EIN, fill out Form SS-4, which may be obtained at any IRS or Social Security Administration office. You can also apply for an EIN online (visit www.irs.gov and search on the keyword EIN for application instructions) or by phone (see the federal listing for the IRS in the phone book). Complete the Form SS-4 before calling the IRS Service Center for your state. When the EIN is obtained by telephone, the completed form must be mailed or faxed within 24 hours.

When you apply for an EIN, the IRS sends you a payment coupon book (Form 8109) to use when depositing withholding taxes. The following is the EIN contact information:

Internal Revenue Service (Treasury Dept.)
1111 Constitution Ave., NW
Washington, DC 20224
(800) 823-1040
www.irs.gov

Medical Staff Privileges

Before hospital medical staff privileges are awarded, you must be licensed to practice medicine in your state. Many facilities require a federal Drug Enforcement Administration (DEA) license (see the next section) and state registration before privileges will be extended. Visit each hospital in the area where you need to obtain staff privileges. Complete the necessary credentialing forms and collect any other documents that may be needed for attaining admitting privileges. If you are joining a group practice and need to be on call, temporary privileges may be awarded until a license is received.

Be sure to plan adequate time to receive hospital staff privileges; in some cases it can take several months to get on hospital staffs and it may be difficult to be accepted on insurance panels until you are on the staff of at least one hospital.

Federal Narcotics License/Drug Enforcement Administration Number

Under the Controlled Substances Act of 1970, if you have never had a DEA number, you need to contact the Department of Justice for a license to dispense narcotics. New applicants will use DEA Form 224, Application for Registration. This form is for the retail pharmacy, hospital/clinic, practitioner, teaching institution, or mid-level practitioner categories only. The current fee is $210 for 3 years. For more information, write to or visit the following:

United States Department of Justice
Drug Enforcement Administration
Central Station
P.O. Box 28083
Washington, DC 20038-8083
(202) 307-7725
(800) 882-9539
www.deadiversion.usdoj.gov

All registrants must report any changes of professional or business address to the DEA. Notification of address changes must be made in writing to the DEA office that has jurisdiction for your registered location. For a list of DEA offices, call the DEA or visit the DEA web site. Send your requests for the following actions to the address that is listed for your state: request a modification to your DEA registration (address change), request order form books, or check the status of a pending application.

State Narcotics License

Some states require that physicians have a state-issued narcotics license in addition to the federal license. Check with your state.

Credentialing Services

For a fee, companies can assist you in becoming credentialed with hospitals, health plans, and medical licenses. To find credentialing services, ask other doctors or practices for recommendations or do a search on the Internet using the words "medical credentialing services." Computer software is also available for organizing and simplifying the credentialing process.

Universal Provider Identification Number

The Centers for Medicare and Medicaid Services (CMS), formerly Health Care Financing Administration (HCFA), assigns every physician a universal provider identification number (UPIN). The number you are assigned will be your provider number for as long as you are a practicing physician, regardless of where you practice. CMS assigns this number when you apply for a Medicare provider number. No extra forms are required. Write to CMS or visit the CMS web site for information about CMS regional offices and the information available for a new physician:

Centers for Medicare and Medicaid Services
P.O. Box 26676
Baltimore, MD 21207
(410) 786-3000
www.cms.gov

Medicare Provider Number

If you are starting your own practice and plan to provide medical services to Medicare recipients, you need to apply for a provider number. The Medicare program has two parts: Part A covers hospital services, and Part B covers physician services. If you already have a Medicare provider number and you are moving to another state, you will be assigned a new provider number for that state. You will need your state medical license to obtain your Medicare provider number. To apply for the Medicare provider number, contact CMS as noted in the preceding paragraph. For questions you may have about who is the Part B carrier (ie, payor and administrator) in your area, call CMS or visit their web site.

Medicaid Provider Number

If you plan to treat recipients of Medicaid services, you need a Medicaid Provider number. It can be obtained from CMS when applying for a Medicare number. If you are joining a group practice or becoming an employee of a hospital, the Medicare and Medicaid numbers will be linked with a group number for that group or employer. Your employer will help you obtain this provider number. To apply for the Medicaid provider number, contact CMS as noted in the preceding section.

Retired Railroad Employees' Coverage

Travelers Insurance Company covers all retired railroad employees regardless of where they live. Once Travelers assigns a provider number, it remains the same anywhere you practice. For a listing of all the Railroad Retirement Board locations in the United States, visit the Railroad Retirement Board web site (www.rrb.gov).

Business License

Before opening your office the first time, you need a business license from your city or county, depending on where the practice is located. If the practice is within the city limits, go to the city hall to purchase your license. If the practice is outside the city limits, most likely you can obtain the license by applying at the county courthouse. In rare instances, both a city and a county license may be needed. The cost of the license varies by city and state but the general range is $100–$300 annually.

Laboratory License

The Clinical Laboratories Improvement Act (CLIA) of 1992 requires all physicians' office laboratories to be licensed according to the complexity of the tests they perform. If you are a solo practitioner and plan to do any laboratory testing on site, you will need a CLIA number. The CLIA license can be obtained through CMS in your state or visit the web site (www.cms.hhs.gov).

If joining a group, ask what CLIA license the group holds. If you are starting your own office, determine what tests you will be performing in the office, and apply for the appropriate level of license. Costs are involved in having an in-office laboratory. Each level has a registration fee and an annual inspection fee. Other costs are in proportion to the level of the laboratory and the annual test volume.

Ongoing Compliance and Documentation

The physician must be cognizant of ongoing issues and agency policies that regulate the practice of medicine. Particular attention must be paid to decisions and actions by the Center for Medicare and Medicaid Services (CMS); rulings on the Health Insurance Portability and Accountability Act of 1996 (HIPAA); accreditation standards of the Joint Commission on Accreditation of Healthcare Organizations (JCAHO); and activities of the Office of the Inspector General (OIG) and the Department of Justice (DOJ). As an employer, other important agencies to the medical practice are the Occupational Safety and Health Administration (OSHA), the Department of Labor (DOL), and the Equal Employment Opportunity Commission (EEOC). Each of these initiatives is described on the following pages.

Each regulatory agency has certain requirements for the documentation that must be kept to show compliance with its regulations. For example, Medicare requires accurate and complete documentation of the work you perform on Medicare patients. If you fail to do that and you undergo an audit, you may be required to refund money, pay fines, and possibly lose the ability to see Medicare patients. Likewise, the DOL has requirements for documenting employee hours and pay. Failure to keep good records can cause enormous grief and expense if you run afoul of that agency.

Center for Medicare and Medicaid Services

The Center for Medicare and Medicaid Services (CMS) provides health insurance through Medicare, Medicaid, and the State Child Health Insurance Program (SCHIP). CMS also performs several quality-focused activities, including regulation of laboratory testing (ie, through CLIA); develops coverage policies; maintains oversight of the survey and certification of nursing homes and continuing care providers; and makes available to beneficiaries, providers, researchers, and state surveyors information about these activities and nursing home quality. For more information, visit the CMS web site (www.cms.hhs.gov).

Health Insurance Portability and Accountability Act

The Health Insurance Portability and Accountability Act of 1996 (HIPAA) has different meanings to different people. Its mission is to improve portability and continuity of health insurance coverage in the group and individual markets; to combat waste, fraud, and abuse in health insurance and health care delivery; to promote the use of medical savings accounts; to improve access to long-term care services and coverage; and to simplify the administration of health insurance. More recently, HIPAA has come to represent privacy initiatives that physicians in medical practice must meet on behalf of their patients.

In some way, the entire health care industry is affected by HIPAA in how a patient's health information is transmitted or maintained. Extensive information on HIPAA's impact on the medical practice is available on the Department of Health and Human Services web site (www.hhs.gov, keyword search HIPAA). To learn more about resources available from the Academy to help you with HIPAA issues, refer to Appendix I.

Joint Commission on Accreditation of Healthcare Organizations

The Joint Commission on Accreditation of Healthcare Organizations (JCAHO) evaluates and accredits nearly 18,000 health care organizations and programs in the United States. JCAHO is an independent, nonprofit organization and is the nation's predominant standard-setting and accrediting body in health care. Its mission is to continuously improve the safety and quality of care that is provided to the public through the provision of health care accreditation and related services that support performance improvement in health care organizations. For more information on JCAHO and its effect on the medical practice, visit the web site (www.jcaho.org).

Joint Commission on Allied Health Personnel in Ophthalmology

The Joint Commission on Allied Health Personnel in Ophthalmology (JCAHPO) is an international nonprofit corporation that certifies and provides continuing education opportunities to ophthalmic allied health professionals. JCAHPO's organization is a commission with 16 ophthalmologic and ophthalmic allied health societies/associations in the United States and Canada. Each organizational member selects two individuals who agree to represent their society or association to JCAHPO.

JCAHPO certifies ophthalmic allied health professionals at the following levels:

- Certified Ophthalmic Assistant (COA)
- Certified Ophthalmic Technician (COT)
- Certified Ophthalmic Medical Technologist (COMT)
- Subspecialty: Ophthalmic Surgical Assisting

The COA exam is at the entry level, the COT is at the intermediate level, and the COMT at the advanced level. Certification at one of the three core levels is a prerequisite for certification in Ophthalmic Surgical Assisting. Certification in COA, COT, COMT or Ophthalmic Surgical Assisting requires completion of a computer exam, and for the COT or COMT certification, completion of a hands-on test.

Since 1969, JCAHPO has certified over 14,000 ophthalmic allied health professionals. Employers and peers recognize the COA, COT, and COMT credentials as validation of an individual's knowledge and experience in, and commitment to the ophthalmic allied health profession and quality patient care. More information about JCAHPO is on the web site (www.jcahpo.org).

Office of Inspector General

The Office of Inspector General (OIG) protects the integrity of the Department of Health and Human Services (HHS) programs, as well as the health and welfare of the beneficiaries of those programs. The OIG's responsibility is to report to the Secretary of the Department and to Congress all program and management problems and to offer recommendations to correct them. The OIG's duties are carried out through a nationwide network of audits, investigations, inspections, and other mission-related functions performed by the OIG components. The most common inspection by the OIG is the Medicare audit to identify inconsistencies in billing, coverage, and payment of bills for particular services. Each year, the OIG publishes a work plan that outlines the areas that will receive investigative priority.

Often, the results of the OIG work plan for a particular year are not evident for several years. Areas where entities appear to be taking advantage of the Medicare or Medicaid programs are often the targets of the OIG work plan. For more information on activities of the OIG and its effect on the medical practice, visit the OIG web site (www.oig.hhs.gov). Also see "Fraud and Abuse" in Chapter 7.

Department of Justice

The Department of Justice (DOJ) enforces the law and defends the interests of the United States according to the law by providing federal leadership in preventing and controlling crime, seeking just punishment for those who are guilty of unlawful behavior, and ensuring fair and impartial administration of justice for all Americans. The DOJ works with HHS to prevent Medicare fraud and abuse and to bring charges against those who would violate the Medicare and Medicaid programs. Be aware of the implications of "physician courtesy discounts" and similar write-offs. For more information, visit the DOJ web site (www.usdoj.gov).

Occupational Safety and Health Administration

The Occupational Safety and Health Administration (OSHA) aims to save lives, prevent injuries, and protect the health of America's workers. OSHA and its state partners have approximately 2100 inspectors, plus complaint discrimination investigators, engineers, physicians, educators, standards writers, and other technical and support personnel spread over more than 200 offices throughout the country. This staff establishes protective standards, enforces those standards, and reaches out to employers and employees through technical assistance and consultation programs. Medical practices are subject to OSHA guidelines for blood-borne pathogens and adherence to OSHA's hazard communication standard. For more information, visit the OSHA web site (www.osha.gov).

Department of Labor

The Department of Labor (DOL) fosters and promotes the welfare of the job seekers, wage earners, and retirees of the United States. Its mission is to improve working conditions, advance opportunities for profitable employment, protect retirement and health care benefits, help employers find workers, strengthen free collective bargaining, and track changes in employment, prices, and other national economic measurements. In carrying out this mission, the DOL administers a variety of federal labor laws including those that guarantee workers' rights to safe and healthful working conditions; a minimum hourly wage and overtime pay; freedom from employment discrimination; unemployment insurance; and other income support. Visit the DOL web site (www.dol.gov) for more information, including advice on the laws that require employers to display official DOL posters where employees can readily observe them. Also see "Employment Law Posting Requirements" in Chapter 9.

Equal Employment Opportunity Commission

The Equal Employment Opportunity Commission (EEOC) protects the civil rights of those in the workforce through enforcement of various employment laws. Employers may not discriminate against employees based on race, sex, religion, national origin, physical disability, and age. Visit the EEOC web site for more information on the EEOC's application to small businesses such as medical practices (www.eeoc.gov).

CHAPTER 7

Risk Management

This chapter explores risk management, which is at the core of successful practice management. The practice must prioritize its risk plan and create operational consistency. Without a good risk management program, you may pay some grave consequences, such as being removed from the Medicare program, being hit with fraud and abuse charges, or facing noncompliance with other government regulations.

Risk management is more than a program to prevent lawsuits: it is how a medical practice provides quality care for patients and improves the quality of life for physicians and their staff. Successful risk management requires close attention to building strong physician-patient relationships and capable physician-administrator teams.

Overview

Following are the critical steps involved in risk management:

1. Maintain legal compliance with your corporate structure. Business entities (eg, sole proprietorships, partnerships, corporations, S corporations) have specific requirements for governance and tax reporting. Once the business entity is established, make sure that you maintain compliance with the legal and tax guidelines applicable to your organization. Seek professional advice and assistance from your attorney and accountant.

2. Develop record-keeping procedures. Maintain records for your practice in relationship to your organizational structure. If yours is a corporation or partnership, you must live by your bylaws and articles of incorporation or by the decisions of the partners. Your attorney and accountant can advise you on record-keeping requirements.

3. Develop conflict resolution and grievance procedures. Managing risk encompasses personnel management, operational policies and procedures, OSHA compliance, and labor laws. The ability to resolve internal and external conflicts is important. Set up the necessary processes to anticipate, address, and resolve problems before they become issues that put your practice at risk of lawsuits, fines, or penalties.

4. Obtain liability insurance. Liability protection includes coverage for professional malpractice, directors and officers (for corporations), errors and omissions, and medical, disability, and property insurance for your employees, business, and

> **✓ KEY POINT**
>
> Risk management has evolved beyond reducing exposure to professional liability actions to include more complex issues. Now, risk management has grown to protecting the practice's financial and physical assets through insurance and proper management techniques and behaviors. A good risk management program reduces practice expenses and limits exposure.

property. Before purchasing such insurances, assess the level of risk. A reputable and trustworthy insurance agent or broker can help you do this. Chapter 8 goes into more detail about insurance matters.

5. Establish personnel and property security plans. Establish a policy for unauthorized or inappropriate use of the Internet and resources such as computers, telephones, and other technology that are available to practice staff. These policies and protections should be a part of your employee handbook (see Chapter 9) and administered consistently.
6. Develop and implement quality assurance and patient satisfaction programs. (Also see "Developing Patient Satisfaction" in Chapter 10.)
7. Establish confidentiality policies. Protect your practice by having employees sign confidentiality agreements from the employee handbook stating that violations of practice confidentiality and breaching patient confidentiality will be cause for termination. Medical records must also be protected as a part of the practice's policies and procedures. The policy must address federal, state, and local regulations surrounding privacy and confidentiality, medical records policy and distribution, and organizational information flow.
8. Negotiate and comply with contractual arrangements. The practice is responsible for negotiating contracts, performing due diligence on them, and understanding them. If you are unable to get enough information on the company or understand the contract language or its implications, seek outside assistance from a third party, such as a reputable consulting firm.
9. Maintain compliance with government mandates. Many laws result in somewhat nebulous policies and procedures, such as self-referrals and safe harbors. Thorough knowledge of federal, state, and local laws and regulations regarding human resources, OSHA, self-referral, fraud and abuse, Medicare fraud and abuse, ADA, antitrust, and research is mandatory—regardless of the vagueness of their interpretations.
10. Develop a network of advisors. Seek advice and assistance from trusted professionals (eg, accountants, lawyers, insurance companies, coding experts, local Medicare office, and consultants) for knowledge about the rules and changes that are continually occurring.

Protocols for Managing Risk

The following sections individually address many areas of practice operation and provide suggestions for developing risk management and loss prevention protocols.

Identifying and Remedying the Risks

Scheduling

A common source of patient dissatisfaction and subsequent increase in the risk of a professional liability claim is the length of time the patient must wait for an appointment with the physician. The busy practice staff may not realize that when patients endure long waits, they perceive a lack of concern. See "Scheduling Patients" in Chapter 4 for details to consider in managing the flow of patients through your office.

Documentation of appointment information is almost as critical as the progress note itself in relation to managing risk. Always track all appointment questions and concerns using the following guidelines:

- Record missed or canceled appointments in the patient's chart.
- Do not erase, white out, or otherwise obliterate any appointment in the appointment book or computer schedule.
- Document any attempts to reach the patient to reschedule a missed appointment. If the patient's condition warrants, send a certified letter.

Billing and Collections

Many malpractice claims are partly a response to collection efforts that are offensive. A written collection policy assures that all practice staff members know what the policy is and how to handle each billing and collection. In addition, also consider addressing the following issues in the policy as a measure of risk management:

- Patient education—including letting the patient know before the first appointment about fees and payment requirements
- A review procedure for circumstances that require special action
- The patient's past payment history
- The quality of care
- The patient's satisfaction (If the patient has a complaint about paying a bill, discuss it to reach an agreeable payment arrangement, if possible.)
- The cost of legal action vs how much money the patient owes (Obtain information from the appropriate small claims court in the area.)
- Having the physician review every chart before initiating aggressive collection procedures
- Understanding of patients' rights concerning privacy and the physician-patient relationship (Do not send any medical information to a collection agency.)
- Awareness of the Fair Debt Collection Act (Periodically evaluate the collection agency's practices. Also see "Payment for Services" in Chapter 5.)

The Work Environment

Just by stepping into the office, the patient develops a first impression of the kind of medical care that the practice is likely to provide. If the surroundings are pleasant, clean, and convenient, patients will more likely view you as competent and providing quality care. Consider the following suggestions as a part of your risk management plan:

- To prevent patient injury, evaluate the facility to ensure easy access. Check all patient care areas, including the parking lot, to identify potential safety hazards.

- Provide comfortable office furnishings to allow the patient to feel at ease. Check furnishings periodically to assure that they are in good condition. Take steps to ensure cleanliness and good housekeeping. Messy or dirty offices create a negative impression and significantly affect the patient's perception of quality of care.
- Have furnishings that meet the needs of various patients. Soft or low seating is problematic for women who are pregnant, senior citizens, and persons with disabilities. Remove obstacles that could cause tripping or falls. Breakable and small objects can be hazardous to children.
- Keep the room at a comfortable temperature and provide plenty of lighting.

Medical Equipment

Patients are often injured because of faulty or improper use of equipment. The practice administrator should institute a policy of regular maintenance and use of all equipment, in addition to the following training practices:

- Train all employees on the proper use of equipment.
- Document the training, time, and place in each employee's personnel file.
- Calibrate all equipment as recommended by the manufacturer.
- Maintain a log of all equipment maintenance and service.
- Report to the malpractice insurance carrier any patient injury associated with a piece of equipment. Remove the equipment and all its collateral equipment from service.
- Avoid tampering with the equipment or sending it to the manufacturer for repair until the insurance company has been notified and the manufacturer offers instructions.
- Do not document any assumptions about an equipment malfunction or improper usage in the medical record.

Emergencies

Your risk management plan should also include a written protocol for handling a medical emergency, such as the following:

- Post emergency numbers (eg, ambulances, hospitals, poison control) next to all telephones.
- Require all staff to stay current on cardiopulmonary resuscitation (CPR).
- If the office has emergency equipment and medications, train all staff members on their use. Not having this equipment on hand is better than having it and having untrained employees use it improperly. There is often less liability in doing nothing than in doing something incorrectly.
- Conduct periodic emergency drills to role-play various emergency scenarios.

Confidentiality

Communication between patient and physician is confidential and critical to the patient-physician relationship. The patient's right to confidentiality extends to all members of the practice staff. Many suits are filed based on breach of confidential information. Only the patient has the right to decide what information may be revealed to others.

A risk management plan will institute the following constraints for the practice staff:

- Do not communicate personal data, medical notes, and billing information to anyone without the patient's written consent, unless it is for purposes of treatment, payment, or operations as defined in the HIPAA regulations. This type of information is confidential.
- Do not discuss a patient's illness with any staff member who does not need to know.
- Do not discuss a patient's illness with family members or friends except as authorized by the patient.
- Watch your voice volume and pay attention to who is nearby. Loose talk that is overheard by others can be the basis for a defamation or invasion of privacy suit. Train staff to do likewise.
- Conduct a confidentiality audit of your office. Test to see how easy it is to overhear conversations. If necessary, install some soundproofing or white noise measures.
- Avoid discussing a patient's medical care on a cellular telephone with either the patient or anyone else. Sometimes police scanners and radios intercept cellular telephone conversations.

Patient Care Complaints

A patient usually shows dissatisfaction and intentions to sue long before the legal papers are served. A staff member may be the first to be aware of a patient complaint. All complaints must be brought to the physician's attention, no matter how minor the incident may seem. No complaint should be ignored. The risk management plan should include the following guidelines:

- Institute a formal complaint policy in the office. Use an incident report form and a complaint log to track the occurrence and disposition of all patient complaints. Do not enter this information in the patient's medical record.
- Notify the physician of the complaint on the day it is received.
- Respond to the complaint quickly and follow up with the patient.

Termination of the Patient-Physician Relationship

The inferred contract between a patient and physician begins not when the appointment is made, but when examination or treatment begins. Once a patient-physician relationship has been established, the physician is not free to terminate the relationship without formal, written notification. The patient-physician relationship continues until it is ended by one of the following circumstances: the patient has no need of further care; the patient terminates the relationship; or the physician formally terminates the relationship. Failure to formally terminate may constitute patient abandonment and bring about fines or legal action if the patient is harmed by the abandonment.

There may be circumstances in which it is deemed necessary to terminate the patient-physician relationship. For example, perhaps the patient is noncompliant, and it is believed that continued treatment would increase the chances of a complication or poor outcome. Maybe the patient is rude or abusive, or maybe the physician and the patient just do not get along. Or, perhaps the patient routinely fails to pay his or her bills. Any of these reasons and many others may be a basis to terminate a patient from the practice. A physician, however, cannot refuse to give a patient an appointment because the patient has not paid the bill without first terminating the patient-physician relationship. Terminating the patient-physician relationship can be accomplished by sending the patient a certified mail, return-receipt letter.

Once the patient is released, be sure to follow some specific guidelines to minimize the chance of being sued for abandonment. Observe the following principles as a matter of your risk management strategy. First, put the notice in writing. The reason may or may not be stated, but can be one of the following. If for noncompliance, say so clearly in the letter. If for personality conflict, an unpaid bill, or for a reason not to be made public, avoid stating the reason in writing. Send the letter by certified mail, with return-receipt requested. Keep the receipt in the patient's file, along with a copy of the letter. Figure 7-1 shows a sample patient discharge letter; Figure 7-2 shows a sample letter to a patient who had been noncompliant.

The amount of time a physician is required to give a patient to seek alternative health care varies in each state. Contact your local medical society or seek counsel from an attorney to find the answer. This termination process protects you from having to see the patient who fails to follow your suggested treatment plan.

Patient Bill of Rights

The patient-physician relationship is the foundation of medical law. Upon it rests the legal rights and obligations of both patients and physicians. The physician and staff members must be aware of certain legal rights that belong to the patient. They include but are not limited to the following:

- The right to choose the physician from whom to receive treatment, although in some cases the patient's health plan may not pay for services by nonpaneled physicians
- The right to say whether medical treatment will begin and to set limits on the care provided
- The right to know before the treatment begins what it will consist of, what effect it will have on the body, what are the inherent dangers, and what it will cost

Recent years have seen some efforts to codify more extensive patients' rights, so make sure you stay abreast of any new developments in this area and that you train your staff in any significant changes or additions.

Consent to Treatment

Legal consequences for treating a patient without properly informed consent include charges of assault and battery and negligence. For emphasis, take note of the following:

- Treating a patient without permission is grounds for an assault and battery charge.
- Treating a patient with the patient's consent, but failing to explain the inherent risks of a procedure, could result in a charge of negligence.

Implied consent is reflected in the patient's actions, such as having a prescription filled or accepting an injection. *Expressed consent* is an oral or written acceptance of the treatment.

[CERTIFIED MAIL-RETURN RECEIPT REQUESTED]

[Doctor's Name]
[Street Address]
[City, State ZIP]

[Patient's Name]
[Street Address]
[City, State ZIP]

[date]

Dear [Patient]:

After careful consideration, I feel it would be in your best medical interest to seek the services of another ophthalmologist. I have decided to discontinue as your ophthalmologist effective 30 days from the date you receive this letter for the following reason(s):

[Indicating the specific reason(s) for termination is optional although if it involves your medical treatment, such as failure to take prescription medication, you may wish to do so.]

I strongly urge you to make arrangements for the services of another ophthalmologist as soon as possible to maintain the continuity of your care. If you need a referral, you might contact your health plan, the local ophthalmological society [give number] or the [state or county] medical association [give number]. My office will transfer a copy of your records to your new physician upon receipt of a signed authorization to do so.

If you should have a medical eye emergency before you have been able to secure the services of another physician, I will be able to provide such emergency care for 30 days from the date you receive this letter.

In closing, I wish to remind you of the importance of seeking regular eye care and maintaining the continuity of services by another qualified ophthalmologist. [If the patient has a condition that requires specific care, state the care AND the consequences of no care in clear, patient-friendly language. If the patient has a condition that needs regular follow-up, state the frequency and urgency of the follow-up, AND state the consequences of not getting the follow-up at the recommended time in clear, patient-friendly language.]

I appreciate your understanding and assistance in this matter and assure you we will do all we can to facilitate a smooth transition in your care.

Sincerely,

[Ophthalmologist's Signature and Name]

Figure 7-1 Sample letter of termination of care. This sample letter is provided as a guideline only and should be modified according to the situation. Be sure to place a copy of the letter and the signed return receipt in the patient's chart, but realize that a letter of termination does not automatically offer a defense against a charge of abandonment.

Obtain the written form of expressed consent when the proposed treatment involves surgery, experimental drugs or procedures, or high-risk diagnostic or treatment procedures.

Informed Consent to Treatment

The fiduciary relationship between the physician and the patient is based upon trust and confidence. The nature of this relationship obligates the physician to act for the benefit of the patient. Contained in this obligation is the physician's duty to voluntarily inform the patient of all relevant information concerning the treatment being offered, including potential hazards and risks. This duty and legal principle that a mentally competent adult

---

[CERTIFIED MAIL-RETURN RECEIPT REQUESTED]

[Doctor's Name]
[Street Address]
[City, State ZIP]

[Patient's Name]
[Street Address]
[City, State ZIP]

[Date]

Dear *[Patient]*:

You have canceled your follow-up appointment on *[date]* without rescheduling. We have tried multiple times to reschedule your missed appointment. To date, you have not responded to our efforts. It is our understanding that you may have terminated your care with our office.

Continued care is essential to the health of your eyes. You have an eye condition that will worsen without proper care. *[If the patient has a condition that requires specific care, state the care AND the consequences of no care in clear, patient-friendly language. If the patient has a condition that needs regular follow-up, state the frequency and urgency of the follow-up, AND state the consequences of not getting the follow-up at the recommended time in clear, patient-friendly language.]* Permanent damage may occur, resulting in visual loss or blindness. Kindly realize this letter is not meant to alarm you. We only wish to inform you of the seriousness of your condition, as it was also explained during office visits, and encourage you to seek proper care.

If we have not heard from you within three weeks, we will assume that you have transferred your care to another physician and have terminated your relationship with this office. We will transfer a copy of your medical records to your new physician upon receipt of a signed authorization to do so. An authorization form is enclosed for your convenience.

With best regards,

[Ophthalmologist's Signature & Name]

Figure 7-2 Sample letter to a noncompliant patient.

has control over his or her own body requires a physician to obtain the patient's informed consent before beginning medical treatment.

Informed consent develops from the patient's understanding of the following factors:

- General nature of the treatment and consequences involved
- Normal risks and hazards of inherent treatment
- Side effects or complications known to occur
- Alternative treatments

Patient Follow Up

For obvious patient care reasons, it is very important to follow up with patients if issues remain after a visit. For example, if a patient is expecting to hear test results, he or she can get very anxious if no communication is forthcoming from your office. Even if test results are normal, patients still deserve to know so that they do not worry. Likewise, the resolution of billing problems needs to be communicated to patients for their peace of mind.

When patients have chronic problems that need regular care or monitoring, it becomes even more important to make sure your follow-up processes are functioning well.

> ✓ **KEY POINT**
>
> Informed consent: Refer to Rule 2 of the Academy's Code of Ethics, discussed in Chapter 15. The rule states, "The performance of medical or surgical procedures shall be preceded by appropriate informed consent."

> ✓ **KEY POINT**
>
> To reinforce the informed consent form, always document information disclosed during the informed consent process. Also, offer patients a copy of the signed informed consent for their own records.

For example, a glaucoma patient who needs regular exams requires more reminders and monitoring than a healthy person with myopia. Many ophthalmology practices have developed systems for recalling patients who need additional care. Although all patients should have regular eye health exams, it is critical that those with chronic problems understand their need for ongoing care and that they be reminded of that need regularly. Because of medicolegal considerations, some practices dismiss chronic patients who do not follow recommendations for treatment (see "Termination of the Patient-Physician Relationship" above).

Patient Recall Processes

Patient recall processes are important for building and maintaining your practice, but more importantly for making sure patients get the care they need. In most practices, patients who need a return visit within several months are given an appointment for the follow-up exam when they check out of the office. If the exam is further in the future, or if the patient does not want to commit to an appointment at check-out, the recall system should be activated.

Most recall systems involve sending a written notice to patients around the time of their needed appointment that asks the patient to call and make a follow-up appointment. Some offices telephone patients to offer appointments, and that method is usually more effective, although more costly. Most of the computer systems in use in ophthalmology practices print a list of patients needing recalls each month—either in report form for telephone recalls or in labels for addressing written recalls.

Of course, some patients who receive a recall notice do not respond. The best recall processes also track who makes an appointment and who does not, and keeps those who do not come into the office on the recall list for further action.

However your recall process works, it is important to document your recall efforts for every patient. Some malpractice plaintiff's attorneys have argued in court that their client's health would not have been compromised if the doctor had made more effort to get their client into the office for further examinations or treatment. If a doctor knows that a patient has a condition that needs to be followed with regular exams, he or she has some responsibility to make sure that patient understands the consequences of neglect. Although a doctor may feel that it is not the practice's responsibility to nag patients to take care of their health, if efforts are made to educate patients and to remind them of their need for care, the responsibility to follow up is at least in part transferred to the patient.

Be careful to follow HIPAA regulations in your recall efforts. Your HIPAA disclosure document should include a notice to patients of how you will handle your recall process, including sending notices of recall through first class mail or over the telephone. Be sure that any postcard recalls you send do not reference specific care or reveal the patient's diagnosis or treatment. Also make sure that staff members making telephone recalls only speak to the patient directly or to those the patient has approved for dealing with his or her health information. If you leave recall notices on a patient's voice-mail, make sure your HIPAA disclosure document includes that as a part of your recall policies.

Maintaining Medical Records

A well-documented, legible, structured medical record is absolutely critical for good patient care and is the physician's first line of defense in a malpractice legal action. The medical record is a form of communication among health care professionals about the patient's condition. This documentation identifies the patient, supports the diagnosis, justifies the treatment, and documents the results of treatment.

The medical record is confidential. The information is private; it should remain secure and not made public. While the physical parts of the record belong to the physician, the information belongs to the patient.

See Appendix I for information about forms that can help you in documenting examinations with patients. Software with modifiable forms is also available.

Paper Records and Electronic Medical Records

Most offices still use paper records, although the use of an electronic medical records (EMR) program is becoming more popular each year (Figure 7-3). Whether you use paper or the computer to keep track of patient information, the principles of privacy, accuracy, and complete documentation in patient charts hold true. The information in this chapter is written with paper charts in mind, and although electronic medical records actually make some aspects of patient charting easier, there are some things to keep in mind specifically for EMR systems:

- *Security is paramount.* Ensure password protection so that only those with appropriate authority can access patient records.
- *Backing up your EMR database every day is absolutely imperative.* The daily backup tape should be removed from the premises each night to protect it from damage in case of a fire. Periodically test that the backup tape system is working. One practice that used an EMR program to completely replace their paper charts had their computer hard drive crash. They found that their backup tapes had not been working for over 6 months! They had no patient chart information for that entire period, and the process of how to recover from that tragedy was very difficult. EMR systems can be extremely efficient, but you must ensure that all systems are functioning properly.

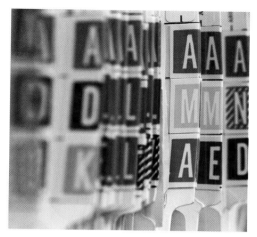

Figure 7-3 Whether electronic or paper, medical records must be organized, maintained, and protected as a part of the practice's policies and procedures.

- *Some EMR programs claim to help you code appropriately for eye examination and evaluation and management codes.* This can be a big help in proper coding, providing the software is accurate in its code suggestions. Keep in mind that in an audit you will still be responsible for any improper coding, even if you are just following the software's suggestions.

Authorization to Release Records

Sole authority to release information from the medical record belongs to the patient. The office should be prepared with a printed release form that the patient signs to release the medical record to a third party. The release form need not be complicated or full of legal language.

As a word of caution, HIV/AIDS information is not included in a standard release form. The release form must specifically state that the release includes this information. Any mention of HIV/AIDS testing or treatment is extremely sensitive and should be maintained in a separate part of the medical record. Some attorneys suggest it should be maintained in an envelope marked, *CONFIDENTIAL! DO NOT RELEASE.*

Elements of a Good Medical Record

Records are the heart of systematic patient care. Excellent record keeping is one of the most effective tools in patient care and in preventing claims. Many physicians have been unsuccessful in malpractice suits because of incomplete or illegible medical records. Malpractice insurance carriers and risk management experts recommend the following tips as loss prevention initiatives:

- Fasten all materials into the chart.
- Dictate progress notes and have them transcribed, if possible.
- Clearly identify allergies on the chart.
- Enter the patient's name on every page in the chart.
- Initial every entry in the medical record.

Note: do not keep financial data in the chart. See Table 7-1 for areas to think about in creating and maintaining a thorough paper medical record.

Figure 7-4 shows a sample medical records checklist form that can be used when checking a patient's chart. To minimize risk, check 10 to 20 charts every other month to ensure that these guidelines are being met.

Documentation to Support Level of Service

Most health insurance plans have guidelines for documenting patient encounters. Sometimes they conduct post-payment audits in the physician's office to assure that the documentation on the patient's medical chart supports the service that was charged, and to assure that the physician took the proper steps to reach a satisfactory diagnosis. Medicare also conducts post-payment audits and usually request that the physician mail in photocopies of specific patient records. Both health plans and Medicare will require the physician to repay any amount paid for a service that is not supported by proper documentation. These repayments can sometimes amount to thousands of dollars.

To avoid this type of risk, begin during the start-up phase to set up the patient records according to the guidelines in this chapter, and make thorough documentation as convenient and efficient as possible. Existing charts (inherited from other practitioners) can be converted over time and information organized for efficiency. Preprinted forms are recommended for progress notes, medication records, telephone calls, and other reports.

Charting the Patient's Progress

Using a standard format to record the patient's visit assures that every encounter includes all the components that are necessary for complete documentation.

In the example of the basic patient chart, utilizing the well-known "SOAP" format, the physician records the patient encounter as follows:

> S = Subjective findings
> O = Objective findings
> A = Assessment of problem/complaint
> P = Plan of treatment

This format, although not widely used today, is easily followed by any health care provider and should be complete if the record is ever subpoenaed in a legal case.

One efficient way to organize a chart is to include patient demographic information on the left side of the folder medical information—organized by office visits, tests, and surgeries—on the right. This approach allows for quicker and more complete review of historical information, which leads to better care.

Fraud and Abuse

Any medical practice treating Medicare patients must be aware of the strict fraud and abuse rules governing Medicare billing. The Office of Inspector General (OIG) is responsible for identifying and eliminating fraud and abuse. The OIG carries out this

Table 7-1 Elements of a Good Medical Record

Element	Characteristics
Uniformity of records	Structure charts by inserting dividers for lab, ancillary tests, and progress notes, and use a problem list. In this format, subsequent health care professionals can scan information easily.
Securing pages	Fasten pages together in chronological order to prevent pages from being lost. Most offices use two-prong fasteners with holes punched in the top of the pages.
Organization	File patient charts for easy and accurate retrieval. Practices typically file a chart by last name and then first name, or by the patient's account number. Whatever system is used, it should be logical and clear to all staff members and physicians (eg, active vs inactive patients, color coding for chronic problems or frequent diagnoses, stickers or different color folders for patients referred by other doctors).
Timeliness	Make all entries in the record, whether written or dictated, at the time of the patient contact. Include the date and the time of the exam or contact. The greater the time lapse between the exam and the entry, the less credible the medical record becomes.
Legibility	Ensure legibility. Health care professionals with illegible handwriting should dictate notes so they can be transcribed or use electronic medical records (EMR). This helps to avoid misinterpretations that result in improper treatment.
Dictated notes	Proofread and sign dictated notes. The statement "dictated but not read" does not relieve the physician from responsibility for what was transcribed. At best, the statement alerts another health care professional that the note has not been proofed and may not be correct. This phrase is difficult to defend in a professional liability claim.
Accuracy	Record all information in objective, concise terms. Never include extraneous information, subjective assessments, or derogatory comments. Include direct quotations from the patient.
Corrections	Never improperly or unlawfully alter a medical record. Do not obliterate an entry with a marker or whiteout. If an error has been made, draw a single line through the inaccurate entry and enter the necessary correction. Add the date and time, and initial the correction in the margin. Making an addendum to a medical record is also acceptable. It should be made after the last entry noting the current date and time, and both entries should be cross-referenced. A record that appears to have been altered implies that a cover-up has occurred.
Jousting	Never criticize or make derogatory comments about another health care professional or organization to the patient or in the medical record. A negative comment can undermine a patient's confidence in the previous health care worker and contribute to or cause a decision to pursue a legal claim regardless of causation and/or who was responsible.
Patient telephone calls	Document all patient telephone calls in the medical record. When speaking to a patient while you are away from the office, and the medical record is not available, record notes on a call pad regarding any prescriptions or medical advice given over the telephone. The sheet must be entered into the chart when you return to the office.
Conversations	Address and document all patient/family worries or concerns in the patient record. Record the source of the information, if other than the patient.

(continued)

Table 7-1 Elements of a Good Medical Record (continued)

Element	Characteristics
Important instructions	Always document important warnings and instructions given to the patient at the time of discharge. Documenting discharge instructions may help prove a patient's noncompliance if a question or a trial arises. In particular, if a patient's best corrected vision makes him or her an unsafe driver, make sure to alert the patient, warn him or her not to drive, and document that warning in the medical record. Make sure you know and follow your state's regulations regarding notifying state government of patients who cannot qualify for their drivers license.
Informed consent	To reinforce the signed informed consent form, always document information disclosed during the informed consent process.
Potential complications	Document all possible complications that might occur. Failure to recognize a complication in time to prevent injury is a common basis for a lawsuit. Proving negligence is difficult if the record shows prior awareness that a complication might occur.

mission through a nationwide network of audits, investigations, and inspections of physicians' offices.

The most common inspection by the OIG is the Medicare audit to identify inconsistencies in billing, coverage, and payment of bills for particular services. The Centers for Medicare and Medicaid Services (CMS) defines Medicare fraud as "knowingly and willfully making or causing a false statement or representation of a material fact made in application for a Medicare benefit or payment." Fraud occurs when a physician knowingly bills Medicare for a service that was not rendered or when the physician overstates or exaggerates a particular service.

Some examples of Medicare fraud are:

- An indication that there may be deliberate application of duplicate reimbursement
- Any false representation with respect to the nature of charges for services rendered
- A claim for uncovered services billed as services that are covered
- A claim involving collusion between the physician and recipient resulting in higher costs or charges

Medicare abuse refers to activities that may directly or indirectly cause financial losses to the Medicare program or the beneficiary. Abuse generally occurs when the physician operates in a manner that is inconsistent with accepted business and medical practices.

The most common types of Medicare abuse are:

- The overuse of medical services (eg, repeated lab testing when results are normal)
- Up-coding and overuse of office visits
- Waiving co-payments for a patient's deductible portion (Physicians are required to collect the 20% Medicare co-payment from the Medicare patient. Routinely waiving the co-payment, unless in a very unusual case such as extreme financial hardship, is considered a fraudulent activity.)

Medical Records Checklist

Check:	Yes	No	N/A
Patient name on all pages	[ ]	[ ]	[ ]
All pages secured with fasteners	[ ]	[ ]	[ ]
Forms organized with tabs for easy access	[ ]	[ ]	[ ]
Organized chronologically	[ ]	[ ]	[ ]
Legible entries	[ ]	[ ]	[ ]
Missed appoints documented	[ ]	[ ]	[ ]
Telephone messages documented	[ ]	[ ]	[ ]
Allergies uniformly documented	[ ]	[ ]	[ ]
Entries dated, timed, and initialed	[ ]	[ ]	[ ]
Dictation proofread and initialed	[ ]	[ ]	[ ]
Only standard abbreviations used	[ ]	[ ]	[ ]
Diagnostic reports initialed prior to filing	[ ]	[ ]	[ ]
Reason for visit documented	[ ]	[ ]	[ ]
Clinical findings (positive/negative) documented	[ ]	[ ]	[ ]
Treatment plan documented	[ ]	[ ]	[ ]
Entries are objective	[ ]	[ ]	[ ]
Patient instructions documented	[ ]	[ ]	[ ]
Patient education materials given/documented	[ ]	[ ]	[ ]
Medication List	[ ]	[ ]	[ ]
1. Current	[ ]	[ ]	[ ]
2. Prescriptions	[ ]	[ ]	[ ]
3. Refills	[ ]	[ ]	[ ]
4. Allergies	[ ]	[ ]	[ ]
Informed consent on chart	[ ]	[ ]	[ ]
Consultation reports on chart	[ ]	[ ]	[ ]
Problem list kept current	[ ]	[ ]	[ ]

Figure 7-4 Sample medical record checklist.

Medicare Audits and Appeals

Medicare audits physician practices for appropriate billing and documentation, and although it has been estimated that your chance of being audited in any given year is only about 3%, if you are audited it can be a harrowing experience, especially if you have deficiencies in your documentation processes. You can expose your practice to greater odds of a Medicare audit in the following situations.

- You have been audited before and problems were found.
- Your utilization of evaluation and management codes or other codes significantly differs from most ophthalmologists.
- Your utilization of diagnostic tests is higher than average given your number of patients seen.
- You use a higher than normal number of certain CPT codes that are under current scrutiny by Medicare.
- Your billing of claims reflects a high number of errors.
- An employee, patient, or other provider registers a complaint against your office.

A Medicare audit typically begins with a request for chart notes and documentation from a specific list of patients. The Medicare auditor then compares the codes billed with the documentation in the charts. If the physician has billed for work that is not documented in the patient's chart, Medicare will want those payments refunded. In addition, if a pattern can be detected, the doctor may be asked to refund money for services for all patients for whom the practice might have been overpaid. For example, if it is found that the doctor billed for level 4 codes but the documentation only justifies a level 3 code, Medicare may ask for a refund of the difference in payment between the two codes for all patients who fall in that category, even without an audit of every patient's chart. These refunds can amount to thousands of dollars, and if negligence or fraud can be proven, the punishment can involve additional fines or even imprisonment.

In addition, even though the physician is always responsible for what gets billed under the name of the physician or the practice, employees who knowingly participate in fraudulent Medicare claims can also be prosecuted. For this reason, it is much more likely that an employee will "blow the whistle" on the physician who is knowingly submitting incorrect claims. The employee who knows about the problem and ignores it risks prosecution.

Most doctors, when faced with a Medicare audit, are well advised to immediately contact a coding and reimbursement consultant who has been through the process before with other ophthalmology practices. If you face an audit, an experienced consultant can help you send appropriate information and explanations to the auditor and can guide you through the process of negotiating with Medicare if problems are uncovered in your documentation.

If you believe the results of an initial Medicare audit are incorrect, you have the right to appeal. At this point you will definitely want to involve a coding consultant. If the charges are serious you will want the advice of an attorney who is experienced in Medicare fraud and abuse statutes and has an understanding of coding issues.

Risk management is vital to the success of your practice. Be mindful of your liabilities in every aspect of your practice. In addition to having the proper insurance coverage for your liabilities, be sure to have the proper procedures and protocols in place to make a difference in your exposure to risk.

CHAPTER 8

Insurance Coverage

Among the most crucial decisions to make for the practice is the purchase of various types of insurance coverage. The purpose of this chapter is to address the many questions about insurance that arise in a practice startup and direct you to the appropriate resources to answer your needs.

Types of Insurance

Due to the many liabilities inherent with the practice of medicine, protecting yourself through insurance will be a vital part of running your practice. State law requires every physician to carry some types of insurance; hospitals or managed care plans require other types of insurance, and companies that finance your office or equipment leases require still others. Additionally, you need to assess the level of risk you are willing to take and what protections are financially feasible. For example, will you insure small losses that you might incur, or do you accept the risk and absorb replacement cost—and at what level? The box "Obtain All Necessary Coverage" specifies a few of the many types of coverage you might consider.

Knowing what to protect is another concern. For example, a patient who trips on loose carpet and falls at your office door may sue you, even if you lease office space in a medical building. If the fall occurs within your suite, you, not the landlord, may be at fault.

> **Obtain All Necessary Coverage**
>
> Every medical employer carries some form of insurance in addition to professional liability coverage (eg, malpractice). This might include property insurance, commercial general liability insurance (CGL), life insurance, overhead disability insurance, workers' compensation insurance, group health insurance, and fidelity bond insurance that protects the practice if there is embezzlement.

Professional Liability Insurance (Malpractice Insurance)

Professional liability insurance, or medical malpractice insurance, is available through various sources, including traditional insurance companies, physician-owned companies, self-insured companies, group purchasing programs, and risk retention groups. What is available to you depends largely upon how much coverage you plan to purchase and the vendors in your area. Not all carriers operate in every state, and some carriers have left the malpractice business in recent years. The Ophthalmic Mutual Insurance Company (OMIC), one of the largest risk retention groups in the United States, is the only professional insurance liability carrier endorsed by the American Academy of Ophthalmology for its members. OMIC provides coverage up to $5 million per claim, or $10 million annual aggregate, for the full scope of ophthalmic practice to members in 49 states and in the District of Columbia. For more information about OMIC, you may contact them directly at (800) 562-6642.

Professional liability insurance will be the most important insurance you can buy. According to The Doctor's Company, a national malpractice carrier owned and operated by physicians, there are 17 claims filed each year for every 100 full-time practicing physicians. Ophthalmologists are not sued as often as some other specialists, but eye doctors are certainly not immune from professional liability lawsuits, so a comprehensive malpractice insurance policy is one of the first purchases you will make for your practice.

Choosing a Professional Liability Carrier

Aspects to consider when choosing a carrier for medical malpractice insurance include:

- *Company's financial condition.* Because litigation takes 3–5 years, seek coverage from a company with financial stability that is likely to be around to defend you.
- *Risk management/loss prevention assistance and advice.* Concurrent with conducting risk assessments of your practice, your liability carrier should be a resource for training, education, and guidance for your staff in implementing loss prevention measures that strengthen the practice.
- *A comprehensive policy.* Make sure you know what your policy covers and what it does not cover. Review a copy of the policy, paying particular attention to the exclusions.
- *Experienced claim professionals and a strong legal network.* Just as you would research any professional you hired, research and scrutinize prospective malpractice carriers by checking references and evaluating credentials.

Purchasing Coverage for Malpractice Claims

Consider the following points when purchasing medical malpractice coverage:

- *Purchase adequate limits.* Many physicians purchase coverage based on the minimum requirements of the hospital(s) in which they practice, usually $1 million per occurrence and $3 million aggregate. However, a single occurrence can exhaust the coverage under an existing policy. The aggregate should be two to three times the occurrence limit. Usually higher limits do not cause a proportionate increase in premiums. However, higher limits encourage higher claims. Limits should be determined in consultation with your carrier.
- *Understand the difference between claims-made and occurrence policies.* Claims-made policies cover claims made while the policy is in effect, even if the incident happened before the policy was written, and if the policy lapses the coverage is no longer in effect. Occurrence policies cover anything that occurs during the coverage period. If you have a claims-made policy and choose to get a different policy, or

if you retire, you will need to purchase "tail coverage" to protect you from claims made after the original policy has lapsed. Sometimes the new insurer will include tail coverage in your new policy.

- *If you are structured as a professional corporation, name your professional corporation on your policy.* Most legal actions would name both you and your corporation.
- *Consider insuring the corporation separately.* By insuring the corporation separately, available coverage can be increased for a fraction of the cost of increasing your individual limits.
- *Make sure that other professionals are properly covered.* Your employees are usually covered under your policy except for optometrists, who will need their own policies. Of course, every ophthalmologist in your practice will need his or her own policy.
- *Check with your malpractice insurer for any available discounts.* Ask if they give a discount for using an electronic medical records system.

Note: If you are joining a medical group, most likely the group's policy will cover you, or the group will use a uniform carrier with uniform policy terms. The premiums may be a part of your compensation package. If you already have "claims made" malpractice coverage that you will cancel when you join the group, you will need to purchase tail coverage (malpractice insurance that covers you in the event of future claims on past acts) to cover any potential litigation stemming from actions prior to the new group coverage taking effect. Be sure you check with the new group/employer to find out who is responsible for payment of premiums for tail coverage. Leave nothing to chance!

Commercial General Liability Insurance

Commercial general liability coverage provides comprehensive protection from lawsuits brought against you by third parties. A third-party person is any individual other than the policyholder, the insurance company, or persons specifically exempted from coverage under the policy. The policy typically includes personal injury, product liability, advertising liability, and contractual liability. Look for policy limits of $1–$5 million. The cost for the higher limits often represents only a minimal increase over the cost of insurance at lower limits.

Also consider nonowned and hired automobile liability coverage for damages to a third party by an employee's vehicle used for the business of the practice, such as going to the bank or post office. This coverage would include damages to a third party incurred by an employee using rented automobiles while working on behalf of the practice.

Property Insurance

A considerable amount of money has been spent to purchase the furniture and equipment necessary to start your practice. Evaluate the cost to replace the tangible assets owned by the practice to determine the proper amount of insurance to purchase. Purchase an adequate amount of property insurance to replace fixed assets in the event they are destroyed by fire or another disaster. In addition, include office supplies, medical supplies, medical books and journals, artwork, files, and file contents.

You may purchase many options through your property insurance. Depending on locale, you may want to consider earthquake or flood coverage, which are usually excluded from property policies. Always request special or all risk coverage. Consider higher deductibles to reduce costs. For reliability, try to use companies rated "A" or better by A.M. Best.

Technology Insurance

Your property insurance will likely cover the computer hardware; however, you may wish to purchase additional coverage that includes loss due to power surges or loss of data. Consult a software vendor to see how much software insurance is needed for the practice's licensed software.

Business Interruption Insurance

Business interruption coverage, which is important and inexpensive, is somewhat like disability insurance for your office. If your office becomes inaccessible due to a covered property loss (eg, fire or hurricane), this coverage reimburses you for lost revenue, continuous expenses, and lost profit. Be sure that the coverage includes funds for a temporary office, expediting expenses, advertising the new location to your patients, and the expenditures to move back into your office once the damages are repaired.

Employee Dishonesty Insurance

Although you work hard to hire the best employees, you may want to protect yourself from the threat of criminal activity This coverage protects your practice from losses due to employee theft or embezzlement of funds.

Equipment Breakdown Insurance

This insurance covers the cost to repair or replace equipment that may be a means of generating significant revenue to your practice. Coverage also includes lost revenue for the period that the equipment is unusable.

Umbrella Policy

In addition to the standard office package, you may want to consider an umbrella policy, which provides comprehensive catastrophic coverage for claims beyond the normal limits of the regular policies. These policies generally start at a $1 million of coverage and go up from there.

Workers' Compensation Insurance

Workers' compensation insurance is mandatory in most states if you have three or more employees. Each state regulates benefits and costs so most policies have identical coverage. Make sure the policy you purchase is covered by your state's insurance insolvency fund. Premiums are based on payroll estimates for a 12-month policy term, subject to a final audit to adjust for changes. All wages should be included in the payroll estimates, including bonuses. When purchasing workers' compensation insurance ask about the insurer's provider network, safety program discounts, and caps for offers (which can offer big savings).

Some states do not require owners or principles of a business to cover themselves under workers' compensation plans. Because premiums are based on wages paid by the practice, a substantial sum can usually be saved by not covering yourself. This is only advisable, however, if you already have a good disability policy and health insurance plan in place.

Life Insurance

It is very important that you and any other physicians in your practice have adequate life insurance to protect your families in case of death. In addition, some practices purchase life insurance for each owner, with the practice named as the beneficiary so that if the physician dies the practice has some funds to replace lost income while another provider is recruited. Some practices also buy life insurance policies for their employees as a fringe benefit. There are limits as to how much life insurance the practice can provide to employees, so consult your tax advisor if you decide to provide this benefit.

Disability Insurance

Statistically, you are more likely to be disabled than to die during your working years, so it is just as important to have a good disability policy as to have enough life insurance. A disability policy pays you a monthly amount if you are unable to continue working. Short-term disability policies generally pay benefits up to a year, while long-term disability policies may pay you until retirement age. Some policies do not pay benefits if you are unable to continue practicing as an ophthalmologist, but you are still able to practice medicine in some form.

If your practice entity pays your disability premiums as a tax-deductible business expense, then your disability payments are subject to income tax. If you pay your premiums with after-tax dollars, any disability benefits you receive are not taxable.

Some practices provide disability insurance for their employees as a fringe benefit. Rates are usually not too expensive and the coverage can be a means of providing some security to staff members. Short-term and long-term disability policies are available with a variety of waiting periods; the shorter the waiting period, usually the higher the premium. These policies, and their respective waiting periods, should be considered in relationship to the sick leave policy in place at the practice.

Insurance as a Vehicle for Retirement Saving

Life insurance has long been touted as a vehicle for investment and retirement. In general, the returns on life insurance are not as high as on some other types of investments, but there may be a place for some cash-value life insurance policies in your financial strategy. Any unusual investment plans should be reviewed by an objective advisor such as your tax accountant. Over and over again, unscrupulous tax shelter promoters sell products to unsuspecting clients, including doctors, and when the IRS learns of the scheme the promoters disappear and the clients are left to pay the back taxes, fines, interest, and penalties.

Smart Shopping

Following are other guidelines for purchasing insurance products:

- Higher deductibles usually mean lower premiums.
- Avoid over-buying. Expensive add-ons are unnecessary if you have good coverage on your basic policy.
- Select appropriate policy limits and buy larger amounts of protection when it is economical. Increasing your limits under a liability policy is usually cheaper than adding coverage under a second policy.
- Self-pay smaller claims, adhering to legal parameters. Consult with your insurance advisor or plan on this option.
- Give prompt attention to any third-party claim.
- Pay premiums annually instead of monthly. Typically, an annual payment is less expensive than monthly installments.

Whatever type of insurance coverage you purchase, it is no substitute for risk management. Work with your insurance agent to help you develop a sound loss prevention program for all forms of practice liability. Conducting a regular loss prevention in-service education program keeps your employees aware of the importance of loss prevention and on-the-job safety.

Review your insurance program regularly. Read your policies and confer with your insurance agent or consultant (and with legal counsel, as appropriate) regarding your insurance program. Policies differ, needs differ, costs vary—a sound insurance program to achieve adequate protection of corporate and personal assets requires careful and continuous review.

The Insurance Plan Assessment in Appendix I can help you and your insurance agent to assess your insurance plan and protection.

CHAPTER 9

Personnel Management

As an employer, the ophthalmologist starting in medical practice must be knowledgeable about labor and employment laws that govern all businesses, in addition to knowing about customary compensation and benefits. Further, employers have responsibilities and standards that are a part of management. This chapter provides an overview of personnel issues you should begin becoming conversant with. The American Academy of Ophthalmic Executives offers a broad array of personnel management products and resources for physicians; see Appendix I for a list of these.

Overview of Rules and Regulations

Even as an employee, a physician is viewed as an authority figure in a medical practice. The ophthalmic assistants, receptionists, billing staff, and supervisors expect the physicians to understand and follow the rules. If you plan to become an employee of a group practice, hospital, or other entity, you should have a working knowledge of the laws and statutes regulating the medical practice, and a thorough understanding of the internal personnel guidelines that pertain to managing the employees.

Avoiding Discrimination

It may seem obvious, but it is important—and a legal obligation—for employers to avoid discriminating against employees and potential employees on the basis of age, sexual orientation, and presence of a disability. In some cases, special arrangements need to be made to accommodate certain employees. Following is a discussion of some of the most common discrimination issues.

Age Discrimination in Employment Act

Both Title VII and the federal Age Discrimination in Employment Act (ADEA) prohibit employers from disciplining or discharging because of age an employee who is more than 40 years old. The ADEA contains explicit guidelines for benefit, pension, and retirement plans. The ADEA does not regulate job-related discipline.

Other Types of Discrimination

Though not a part of federal law pertaining to civil rights, a growing body of law prevents or occasionally justifies employment discrimination based on sexual orientation. Employers should check with their state governments to see if there is legislation against discrimination for sexual orientation.

Americans with Disabilities Act

The Americans with Disabilities Act (ADA), which is broader than outlined by Title VII, protects persons with disabilities from discrimination in employment, public services, public accommodations, and telecommunications. The statute has two components that affect ophthalmology practices. The first one pertains to discrimination in hiring or employment and requires an employer to make reasonable accommodations for an employee with a disability if he or she can perform the essential functions of the job. The second component pertains to accommodations that must be provided for persons with disabilities to access your facility or services. These accommodations, for example, would include having a wheelchair ramp or a restroom that is large enough to accommodate a wheelchair.

Understanding Employment Issues

Employment Classifications

Part of the practice's responsibility when hiring the practice staff encompasses obtaining a working knowledge of the Fair Labor Standards Act (FLSA). This complex law determines whether an employer is subject to federal minimum wage and overtime requirements. Most medical employees are covered. For compliance, first ascertain the status of your practice. Then, conclude the exempt or nonexempt status of each employee—the descriptions below may help you understand how to classify employees.

It is important not to confuse the terms "salary" and "hourly" with the terms *exempt* and *nonexempt*. Some doctors think that if they just pay everyone on their staff a salary, then they do not have to pay any overtime. Nothing could be further from the truth. You can pay a receptionist a salary, but if he or she works more than 40 hours a week you would have to pay overtime based on that person's weekly salary divided by 40 hours times 1.5. Exempt employees are normally paid a salary, and nonexempt employees are usually paid on an hourly basis, but just paying staff members a salary does not make them exempt from overtime. It is very important that you follow the employment rules in this regard. It is painful to have to pay substantial back wages (sometimes reaching back years) to an employee who leaves your practice and then reports you to the labor board.

Exempt Status The following employment categories have been adapted for application to the medical practice for defining employees who are exempt from overtime pay requirements. These categories include executive employee, administrative employee, and professional employee.

Executive employees must meet all of the following definitions to be exempt (practice administrators are typically considered exempt):

- Minimum salary: $155 per week (subject to change)
- Primary duty: manages enterprise, department, or department subdivision

- Other job characteristics: directs the work of two or more full-time employees; exercises discretionary powers; is authorized to hire and fire or to recommend those actions; and must spend no more than 20% of working hours in nonexempt duties

Administrative employees must meet the following definitions to be exempt (administrative assistants, personnel directors, office managers, and laboratory supervisors are typically considered exempt):

- Minimum salary $155 per week (subject to change)
- Primary duties: performs office or nonmanual work; work relates directly to management policies or general business operations; and works directly in academic instruction or training
- Other job characteristics: uses discretion and independent judgment regularly; assists owner, executive, and other administrative employees; and must spend no more than 20% of time in nonexempt duties

Professional employees must meet all the following requirements to be exempt (physicians, registered nurses, registered or certified technologists, physician assistants, speech pathologists, and physical therapists are typically considered exempt):

- Minimum salary $170 per week (subject to change)
- Primary duties: work requires advanced knowledge acquired through specialized study of an advanced type in a field of science
- Other job characteristics: must consistently exercise discretion and judgment; job tasks must be intellectual in nature; and must spend no more than 20% of workweek on activities unrelated to professional duties

Nonexempt Status Common medical practice positions that typically are considered nonexempt are billing clerks, ophthalmic assistants and technicians, receptionists, opticians, licensed practical nurses, nurses' aides, laboratory technicians or assistants, clerical workers, orderlies, food service employees, and janitorial employees.

Wage Records Requirements

The FLSA requires that employers keep records on wages and hours worked. Wage records should include the following for each employee:

- Full name as used in Social Security Administration records
- Social security number, employee number or symbol, as used in payroll records
- Home address, including ZIP code
- Date of birth, if the employee is under the age of 19
- Sex
- Position title
- Time of day and day of week employee's work begins
- Regular hourly rate of pay
- Amount and type of pay for any pay that is not included in regular rate
- Hours worked by employee on each work day and total hours worked for week

- Employee's total daily or weekly earnings (not including any premiums paid for overtime)
- Employee's total payment of overtime for the workweek
- Total wages for employee for each pay period
- Date of each payment made to the employee and pay period covered by the payment
- Total amount of additions to or deductions from wages for each pay period
- For each deduction, the employer must show the date, amount, and nature of the deduction

Unless the employee is exempt from overtime pay, the employer must pay one-and-one-half times the employee's regular rate of pay for all time worked over 40 hours in one work-week (overtime in some states begins after 8 hours in a single day). Even if an employer pays every two weeks, there can be no averaging of hours in the pay period. For example, if the employee works 30 hours the first week of the pay period and 50 hours the next week, he or she is entitled to 10 hours of overtime pay for the second week. Overtime is based on hours worked over 40, not including vacation and sick leave taken during the same pay period.

The At-Will Employment Relationship

The most common type of employment agreement in the health care industry is the oral, at-will agreement. The concept is that an employee can quit at any time, or the employer can terminate the employee at any time, with or without reason.

At-will does not apply to a job in which a contract is in effect stating a specific period of employment. The right of the employer to apply the at-will doctrine does not override the restrictions placed on the employer, such as the discriminations defined in Title VII of the Civil Rights Act of 1964.

By using the term *at-will* vs *just cause*, an employee serves at the discretion of the medical practice and therefore may be dismissed with or without "cause." Using the term just cause sets a prerequisite that justifiable cause must be shown in order to discharge an employee. The practice's employee handbook should use specific language indicating that employees of your practice are employees at-will. Please note that state law can be more restrictive in this regard than federal law, so be sure to understand your state statutes.

Employment Law Posting Requirements

Federal and state laws often require employers to post a notice about a particular law. Usually provided as posters or permits, these notices should be in a conspicuous place easily accessible to all employees (eg, typically, the break room). Table 9-1 lists the posters that employers are required to display under current federal law.

Posters may be obtained from the government agency charged with enforcing a particular law. Most agencies have developed a single poster that satisfies the requirements of several different laws administered by that agency. Also, private companies publish posters that employers are required to post. Contact the following agencies to obtain these posters:

Table 9-1 Employer Posting Requirements*

Area	Title	Availability
Age Discrimination, Disability Discrimination, Equal Employment	Equal Employment Opportunity is the Law	Department of Labor, Employment Standards Administration (www.dol.gov/esa)
Child Labor, Minimum Wage, and Overtime	Federal Minimum Wage (wage-hour poster 1088)	Department of Labor (www.dol.gov/esa)
Family and Medical Leave	Your Rights under the Family and Medical Leave Act of 1993	Department of Labor (www.dol.gov/esa)
Polygraph Testing	Notice: Employee Polygraph Protection Act (wage-hour poster 1462)	Department of Labor (www.dol.gov/esa)
Safe and Healthy Workplace	You Have a Right to a Safe and Healthful Workplace (Occupational Safety and Health Act poster 3165).	Occupational Safety and Health Administration (www.osha.gov)
	Summary of Work-related Illnesses and Injuries (OSHA Form 300A, required annually)	Occupational Safety and Health Administration (www.osha.gov)

* Posting requirements and web site addresses are subject to change.

Equal Employment Opportunity Commission Office of Communication
1801 L Street, NW
Washington, DC 20507
(800) 435-7232 or (800) 669-3362

U.S. Department of Labor Posters
200 Constitution Avenue, NW, Room S-3502
Washington, DC 20210
(866) 4-USA-DOL

Workers' Compensation

Physicians may think of workers' compensation insurance with regard to the medical care it provides to other employers' workers. However, as noted in Chapter 8, the physician-employer must cover his or her own employees with this type of coverage. Information that outlines your responsibilities can be obtained by contacting the Workers' Compensation Board in your state. An insurance agent is also a good resource for information about workers' compensation requirements.

OSHA Workplace Requirements

The Occupational Safety and Health Administration (OSHA) was enacted in 1970 to assure safe, healthful working conditions for employees. Employers are required to furnish employees with a place of employment that is safe from recognized hazards. In the medical office, blood-borne pathogens are the hazard of greatest concern.

It is the responsibility of every medical employer to obtain complete information for compliance with OSHA regulations. The *OSHA Handbook for Small Businesses,* which includes self-inspection checklists, is available from local OSHA offices or online (www.osha.gov).

Termination of Employment—Laws and Guidelines

If your state's laws specify that employment is "at-will" unless otherwise contracted, and you do not have a verbal or written contract with an employee, you do not have to give an employee a reason to terminate their employment. However, be careful that you do not give reasons that could be considered discriminatory, or you may find yourself being sued for wrongful termination.

Some practices have found that seemingly innocent comments such as "You do a great job. You can work here as long as you want" can create a verbal contract of employment that can be enforceable at law. Do not hesitate to compliment employees on work well done, but be careful not to commit to anything that would supersede your "at-will" employment relationship.

Of course, it is illegal to terminate employment for reasons of race, color, religion, sex, national origin, or physical or mental disability, so be sure to protect your practice by not considering any of those factors in the decision to terminate an employee.

Staffing Your Practice: A Primer

Hiring employees will be one of the toughest, and can be one of the most rewarding things, you do as an employer. Practices that consistently do well financially also tend to have the best employees, and those two factors are inextricably linked. Good employees can make going to work a pleasure; difficult employees can try the patience of even the most forgiving employer. The key to having good employees is in finding the best candidates and then providing good management to keep their motivation and dedication to the practice at a high level. (See Appendix I for a list of concise resource guides available to help you with this all-important goal.)

Finding and Hiring Good People

It is evident by the contents of this book that modern ophthalmology practices must deal with complex, difficult, and potentially perilous business issues. These issues are likely to be handled inappropriately unless someone is actively managing the practice. Some physicians manage their own practices, but such an approach is very difficult, since most ophthalmologists have neither the time nor the inclination to deal with the numerous problems that surface in practices on a day-to-day basis.

Also, most ophthalmologists can be more productive by examining patients than by spending a lot of time managing their staff and overseeing all of the details of the practice. A practice that is just starting may not need a "manager" immediately although a capable person can help you avoid early errors and get your practice organized from the start. The cost of a good manager or administrator is small compared to the cost of having chaos in your office due to a lack of management.

In addition, employees need guidance, support, and occasionally redirection and discipline. If a management vacuum exists because the doctor is the only one in charge, and he or she does not have time to attend to all of the details of the practice, that vacuum will fill with employee arguments, power plays, and manipulation. Practices with good managers are far more financially secure and less stressful for physicians than those with poor management. Give a great deal of thought to the duties of the office manager and prepare a job description before beginning the advertising or hiring process.

Roles and Responsibilities

There are various levels of interaction between managers and physicians, but the physician-owners always maintain ultimate decision making authority. There are three basic levels of practice management personnel in ophthalmology practices: supervisor, office manager, and administrator.

A supervisor usually is responsible for organizing the work of a small practice (two to four employees or a department within a larger practice (eg, billing or optical). Supervisors arrange work schedules, do employee reviews, and provide some training but usually do not have responsibilities for hiring, firing, or accounting. Supervisors often spend most of their time working beside those they supervise and only a lesser percentage of their time actually managing staff.

Office managers usually manage an entire office, either the practice's main location or one of its satellites. Office managers often spend part of their time doing the billing or filling in as a tech, and then try to handle all of the other tasks a manager must do in the rest of the time. Office managers have more authority than supervisors, but usually clear major decisions (hiring, firing, expenditures) with the owner(s) of the practice.

Administrators—sometimes called executive directors, chief executive officers, or chief operating officers—have responsibility for the success of the entire practice, both in day-to-day operations and in long-term planning. Administrators typically have broad authority, including deciding staffing levels, hiring and firing staff, and reporting financial results. Administrators typically manage larger practices with several doctors and one or two levels of management.

The foregoing categories are not hard and fast; some office managers have the authority of an administrator; others operate at a lower level of authority. Whoever runs the practice, you as the owner are still ultimately responsible for what goes on in the practice, so you need to keep apprised of all of the major issues. It is axiomatic that if things fall apart in a practice, the employed management can find work elsewhere while the owners stay and pick up the pieces.

Personnel Files and Access to Them

Every employee, including the physicians, should have a well-maintained personnel file containing the following documents. The typical file should contain all government-mandated forms and employee benefit enrollment forms, as applicable:

- Resume
- Employment application
- Reference checklist
- W-4 form (tax withholding)
- State income tax form, if applicable
- I-9 form (employment eligibility verification)
- Payroll set-up information
- Health insurance enrollment form
- Long-term disability enrollment form

- 401(k) enrollment form
- Flex benefits form
- Personnel policies acknowledgment form (disclaimer)
- Attendance records
- Employment letter
- Salary change information
- Performance reviews
- Warning or disciplinary letters
- New employee checklist
- Training checklist
- Confidentiality pledge
- Contact list in case of an emergency

Personnel files should be kept in a locked cabinet, accessible only to the designated employee responsible for maintenance. Employees have the right to access their files during regular business hours, in the presence of a designated employee.

Personnel files should be retained for 3 years following termination. Applications of persons not hired should be maintained for 1 year.

Developing Job Descriptions

All employees need to understand what is expected of them. A well-written job description is the best way of communicating a description of the duties for which an employee is responsible.

A job description usually includes the following elements: the name of the job, a one or two sentence summary that defines the overall function of the job, a brief listing of educational and experience qualifications, and a list of the major job tasks describing what is to be accomplished.

You can get job descriptions from other practices or from professional associations (including the American Academy of Ophthalmic Executives web site at www.aao.org/aaoe) or from consultants, although these forms will always have to be customized to your practice. One good way of developing job descriptions for your practice is to provide each employee with a blank job description form and have them fill it out with what they see to be their job description, and to use that as a beginning point for developing a full job description. It is always interesting to see how different a staff member's idea of what his or her job is can be from what you think that job should be.

Sample Job Descriptions

Figures 9-1 and 9-2 are samples of job descriptions for positions that can be found in a medical practice. These job descriptions can be used for preparing specific descriptions for jobs in a practice. They can also be used for performance appraisals and employee counseling. As responsibilities change, revise the descriptions accordingly.

Staff Compensation

In general, administrators are paid more than office managers, who are paid more than supervisors. All three categories tend to have higher pay when they manage more people. In most cases, an administrator of a 50-employee practice will make more than the administrator of a 20-employee practice.

Position: Office Manager

Reports to: Physician(s)

Job Summary:

Responsible for all medical office activities, including accounting and financial procedures. Supervises all office personnel.

Specific Requirements:

- Furnish physician and accountant with account aging each month
- Conduct regular staff meetings
- Responsible for accounts payable system
- Supervise, train all front office personnel
- Assist in creating, updating business administration policies
- Update office personnel policy manual as needed
- Maintain controls on accounts receivable system
- Prepare financial reports at end of month for physician, accountant
- Approve all Medicaid, Medicare, and other write-offs in consultation with physician
- Approve credits, refunds to patient accounts
- Arrange personnel schedules and vacations
- Responsible for all hiring and terminating of office personnel
- Conduct performance, salary reviews for office personnel

Job Qualifications:

Previous medical office experience required. Supervisory experience preferred. Knowledge of medicolegal principles and medical ethics is necessary.

Figure 9-1 Sample job description for an office manager.

Position: Certified Ophthalmic Assistant

Reports to: Office Manager

Job Summary:

Assist physician with patient examination and treatment. Also responsible for patient histories, ancillary tests, routine lab procedures, and collection and preparation of specimens for transport to lab.

Specific Requirements:

- Maintain general appearance, cleanliness of exam rooms
- Sterilize instruments, maintain diagnostic equipment
- Prepare, replenish supplies; maintain inventory
- Prepare patients for examination
- Take patient histories, visual acuities, intraocular pressures and other test as deemed appropriate by physician
- Give certain medications (eg, eye drops) under physician supervision
- Record laboratory, ancillary test and other clinical data on patient charts
- Receive and organize the handling of medication samples
- Dispose of contaminated and disposable items
- Return patient phone calls, call pharmacies for prescriptions
- Perform other tasks as requested by office manager or physician

Job Qualifications:

Graduate of ophthalmic assistant training course; COA certificate. Previous clinical experience and knowledge of anatomy, physiology, and terminology also required. Medical office experience helpful.

Figure 9-2 Sample job description for a certified ophthalmic assistant.

It is difficult to give specific ranges for compensation for these positions because of large variations from region to region, and even within the same city. It is best to do some research to determine appropriate compensation for your managers, but you will find that supervisors typically make 10%–20% more hourly than those they supervise, managers' salaries range from $35,000 to $70,000 per year, and administrators make from $60,000 to $160,000. Good managers prove their worth and the value of their services to observant practice owners. Personnel salaries and benefits will be your largest single expense. You will want to hire the person with the best skills at the most affordable pay. Developing a salary range for each job title is the recommended way to set salaries. Staff salaries should be predicated on the following:

- How much the practice can afford to pay now and what you can probably pay next year
- The average salary for the same job within the community where your practice is located for staff with the same level of experience and education

Before comparing salaries with other offices, make sure the job description is compared as well.

Posting Position Requirements

You will find the best success finding good candidates for a position when you use a number of different channels to notify potential candidates of your opening. For example, visit the Academy's web site (www.aao.org) and review the Professional Choices information, which includes information on practices seeking physicians. This is a very good place for you to advertise because it has become a popular place for ophthalmologists to check for openings. The Academy also offers a job fair at its Annual Meeting, bringing together more than 100 practices seeking physicians with several hundred job-seeking young ophthalmologists. The following are other sources for developing a pool of candidates for a position at the practice:

- Office managers' professional associations
- Community colleges
- Private vocational schools
- Local chapters of health care organizations, such as the American Association for Medical Assistants or the Medical Group Management Association
- Medical societies' placement service
- Pharmaceutical representatives
- Hospital personnel department
- Employment agencies
- Online help wanted ads
- Newspaper help wanted ads

Be sure to list any mandatory requirements in your advertising. If you want an experienced technician, make that requirement very clear or you will be sifting through many resumes from unqualified applicants.

Placing an Effective Classified Advertisement

The Civil Rights Act of 1964 (Title VII) also applies to the advertising, application, and hiring process. Ads must be carefully written to avoid any appearance of discrimination based on sex, age, race, religion, national origin, or disability. Use the basic components of the job description to write the ad, focusing on what the job requires and the work habit characteristics that are needed. Read the ad before placing it and ask yourself how you would feel about working for your practice. Ads that list only stern requirements sound unappealing and will not get as many good applicants as ads that make the position sound appealing.

For screening purposes, when placing a newspaper advertisement, have candidates send their written resumes to a box number or to your fax machine rather than listing your office address. If you are advertising for the position of a person who will be terminated, be careful to be discreet in how you publicize the job opening.

Interviewing to Hire High Performers

Review the written resumes received, choose at least five qualified candidates, and rate each resume by priority. It may save time to screen the top five applicants by telephone first, or you may decide to have all five candidates come in for a face-to-face interview, so that the choices can be narrowed down to two or three candidates. Those two or three should be brought back for more in-depth second interviews.

Be organized in the face-to-face interviews, having a prepared list of questions to ask each candidate. This will allow you to compare the candidates on the same basis. Give each candidate a copy of the job description and have him or her complete an EEOC-approved application form. Using an EEOC form will assure that you are not violating any of the Title IV statutes. These forms are available through the American Medical Association's publications department, office supply stores, and most mail order catalogs offering forms for the medical office.

It is a good habit to use a simple form to grade candidates in the areas you deem most important for their position. For example, if you are hiring a billing clerk, you might grade the applicants in the following areas:

- Experience in medical billing
- Experience in ophthalmology billing
- Experience with your computer system
- Experience with insurance and patient collections
- Work habits
- Initiative
- Ability to work cooperatively with other staff members

Each of those seven areas would have a maximum grade of five points and the two or three candidates with the highest total scores would be invited back for a second interview. The one who did best in that interview would be offered the job. It is especially helpful if you have two or three people interview the applicants and then compare their scores for each person.

Every employer develops a unique interviewing style. You may want to begin your interviews by telling the candidate a little about yourself or your specialty. Share with the candidate why that particular geographic area was chosen, where you went to school, and what your philosophy is about the practice of medicine. Next, the following topics could be addressed (also see the box to the right, "Interview Questions"):

- Ask if the candidate has reviewed the job description and whether there are questions about the essential functions of the job.
- Ask about the applicant's experience with each task listed on the job description. Ask how he or she performs these tasks in the current position or in former jobs. Write the answers on a separate piece of paper. Do not write on the job description, application form, or resumes to avoid any comments that may be perceived as discriminatory.
- Ask open-ended questions that require the applicant to provide information. Avoid questions that can be answered simply with yes or no.
- Spend more time listening in the interview than talking.
- Remain neutral in your responses. Do not show approval or disapproval.
- Watch for nonverbal clues that indicate unusually high tension or anxiety.
- Zero in on topics of interest to you and investigate further.
- Quickly review your objectives.
- Document key points.
- Let the candidate know what happens next.

Asking questions in certain areas can get you in trouble with the Department of Labor or with the Equal Employment Opportunity Commission. The following are some sample legal and illegal areas of discussion:

OK to Discuss	Not OK to Discuss*
Name	Maiden name
Address and duration	Birthplace
If over 18	Age (except "if over 18")
US citizenship status	High school or college graduation date
Proficiency in English	Religion
Education	Race
Experience	Height or weight
Criminal convictions	Marital status
Contact person	Gender (Mr., Ms., Mrs.)
Professional organizations	Disability if not directly job related and lawful
Employed relatives	Citizenship, national origin
	Relatives
	Arrests

* Although some practices like to take or get a photograph of candidates so they can remember who they saw, this is not advisable.

References

Reference checking is vitally important to medical employers, especially since they are increasingly being held responsible for negligent hiring decisions. The following are steps that can be taken to ensure a smooth hiring process:

Interview Questions

Use the same list of questions with each candidate, making notes on a separate piece of paper, not on the resume or application. Some questions you may want to include:

- What did you like best about your last (current) position? What did you like least about it?
- Which of your past positions did you find most satisfying? Why?
- How would your last (current) supervisor describe you? In what area would he or she say you need the most improvement?
- What is one of your most significant on-the-job accomplishments?
- What academic areas of study interest you the most? What, if any, helped prepare you for your field?
- What did you like best about your last supervisor? What did you like least?
- What change would you (or did you) make in the last office you worked in?
- Describe your experiences in collecting money for medical bills.
- Which of your skills do you think you could develop here?

- Request that each applicant provide you with two or three references from former jobs, preferably from former employers or supervisors rather than just co-workers.
- Call the references instead of accepting letters of reference at face value.
- Ask to speak to the applicant's immediate supervisor.
- Ask if the applicant is eligible for rehiring.
- Listen for what they do not say.

For additional guidance on interviewing, obtain *The Ophthalmic Executive's Resource Guide: Interviewing to Hire Smart* (see Appendix I).

Orientation and Training

How the new employee is integrated into the practice makes a difference in the long-term relationship with that staff member. The following key points will help you start out right with the new employee:

- Make sure the employee understands the offer of employment. Before starting work the employee should know the hours, pay, benefits, duties, supervisor, and start date. It is usually a good idea to make the offer in writing so there is less chance of a misunderstanding, but be careful not to make a written offer commit you to any irreversible long-term employment.
- Make sure the employee receives all of the necessary documents on their first day of work. These documents include the personnel manual, retirement plan and insurance plan brochures, and so on.
- Make sure the employee fills out all of the necessary forms on the first day of employment. These forms include the IRS forms, immigration forms, health and disability insurance forms, and so on.

- Make sure the employee gets a complete orientation to the practice including explanations of key policies, a tour of the facilities, introduction to other staff members, and a meeting with that person's supervisor.
- Make sure the employee gets appropriate training in their job responsibilities. Too often, a new staff member's training consists of sitting for several days with the person who is leaving the practice. That person usually has little incentive to make sure the training is done well. Training should follow a specific, organized curriculum so that all pertinent areas are covered and bad habits are not passed on from departing to arriving employees.

For additional guidance in getting a new employee off to the right start, obtain a copy of *The Ophthalmic Executive's Resource Guide: Helping New Employees Succeed* (refer to Appendix I).

Probationary Employment Period

When hiring, inform the new employee that he or she will be subject to a 90-day trial period to be used for orientation and training. During this period, monitor the employee's attitude, work habits, and capabilities, and assure that he or she is receiving the proper instructions. The employee or employer may end the employment relationship at-will at any time during this initial period, with or without cause, and without advance notice. Employees will assume regular status upon satisfactory completion of the orientation period.

Developing and Enforcing Personnel Policies

Although during the start-up phase of a medical practice, all policies are not likely to be in a handbook or manual yet, developing written policies should be addressed in the earlier stages. If these policies are in place on the first day, present the employee with a copy of the policies, taking time to explain the basic work rules and regulations.

As your practice grows, you should add new policies to the personnel manual and give copies of those new policies to all employees. It is also critical that employment policies be enforced fairly and evenly for all employees. For example, if one staff member is allowed to "borrow" vacation time before it is earned, then you must extend that courtesy to all employees or you may find your practice being accused of discrimination. Routinely waiving employment policies can have the effect of making all of the policies in your employee manual unenforceable. *The Ophthalmic Executive's Resource Guide: Developing Your Employee Handbook: Protective Shield of Legal Minefield* can assist you in this important process (refer to Appendix I). This publication comes complete with a CD-ROM containing a template and content for a solid employee handbook. While this handbook addresses federal employment laws, you should be prepared to incorporate any pertinent laws for the state in which you practice.

The Employee Handbook

As discussed in "Setting Policies and Procedures" in Chapter 4, the employee handbook is a key part of an employer's communication program. Handbooks give employees a sense of security. With all the rules and policies in one place, each person knows what is expected. When benefits are listed and explained, each person knows what is provided. Handbooks can also help motivate employees.

Handbook Format Choose a size for the handbook that is easy to use. The typical sizes are 5 × 7 or 8 ½ × 11 inches, either loose-leaf or bound. Loose-leaf notebooks allow for replacement of pages when policies change. Some employers use both formats—a small bound handbook for employees, and a loose-leaf policy and procedures manual for managers. Both books should include an employee acknowledgment form that the employee signs indicating that he or she received the handbook.

Make the booklet attractive; put it together in such a way that employees will want to read it. Consider these suggestions for making the contents easy to read:

- Limit the use of words with three or more syllables.
- Keep each sentence 20 words or less.
- Limit discussion of subjects to one page.
- Use drawing, charts, and cartoons where applicable.
- Leave at least one-quarter of each page blank.
- Be concise.
- Limit the number of pages.

Choose a writing style and be consistent throughout. Use gender-neutral terminology. A handbook should cover what employees need to know to get along on the job—the policies and procedures that employees will encounter almost every day. Avoid subjects that change frequently, such as a lengthy and detailed description of benefits plans.

Handbook Content Employee handbooks vary considerably due to individual needs and circumstances; therefore, the amount of information provided varies. A medical practice may also consider publishing Occupational Safety and Health Administration (OSHA), Clinical Laboratories Improvement Act (CLIA), and other government-regulated guidelines in its handbook. For the overall purpose of a handbook, however, mentioning these rules in passing is appropriate, while covering them more extensively in other documentation (eg, policy manual). Regardless, be sure the practice's acknowledgment form covers all policies. See Appendix I for a sample table of contents that can be helpful in formulating a handbook. It is always advisable to have an attorney review your employee handbook to make sure you do not state anything that could make commitments beyond what you intend. For example, in the past it was sometimes recommended that formal disciplinary steps be detailed in the employee handbook. Now, most attorneys lean toward discouraging that since it can lead to problems if it is necessary to terminate an employee without going through all of the disciplinary steps. General disciplinary guidelines and reasons for termination should be included, but exact disciplinary procedures may come back to haunt the practice unless you make sure you follow those procedures exactly.

Managing Personnel

There are many philosophies of personnel management, and thousands of books have been written on how to manage your employees. To start you out with basic principles, the following steps describe a simple yet effective process for supervising employees and helping them achieve their optimum productivity.

Supervisor's Responsibilities

1. *Provide the tools.* Employees must have the tools they need to be able to effectively do their jobs. The tools required may include adequate space, computer equipment, written forms, telephone, etc. If employees do not have the proper tools, they cannot be held accountable for accomplishing their work.

2. *Provide training.* Employees must be properly trained in their responsibilities, and it is management's responsibility to provide opportunities for receiving training and then it is the employee's responsibility to take advantage of those opportunities. You need to make sure that you provide training to each employee in each of the positions that they are expected to work.

3. *Set goals.* Practice ownership and management should set overall goals for how it wants to position itself and for what it wants to accomplish. Then, each department or work group should set complementary goals which, when accomplished, will help the practice reach its goals. Employees then should focus on the practice and departmental goals in setting goals for their own performance improvement. Management should review and approve all employee goals, and may at times ask individual employees to work on specific goals to improve performance.

4. *Become a resource.* Once employees have the tools and training they need, and they have set goals for improvement, management needs to become a resource to help the staff when they have done everything they can and reach an impasse or an obstacle which they cannot overcome by themselves. For staff to look to management as a resource, managers must be available, approachable and ready to listen with an open mind and to coach the employee in their responsibilities. However, managers must also be careful to let the employee retain responsibility for accomplishing their goals; the manager is only a resource—she or he should not take the responsibility away from the employee.

5. *Hold employees accountable for progress towards their goals.* Since goals are often set without full knowledge of all the factors that will be faced in accomplishing the goal, it is appropriate to measure success by progress made rather than by whether or not the goal has been accomplished in the projected time frame. Employees can be held accountable through regular reviews and individual interviews. These are also good opportunities to give employees feedback, correction and commendation where appropriate.

Employees' Responsibilities

1. *Use the tools.* Employees are responsible for using the tools they are given.
2. *Apply the training.* Employees are responsible for applying the training they receive from the practice.
3. *Work to accomplish goals.* Employees are responsible for setting goals for improvement of their work and for working toward the accomplishment of those goals.
4. *Ask for help when needed.* Employees must ask for help if they cannot do their job or reach their goals. They are responsible for using their supervisor as a resource as needed.

5. *Be accountable for progress on their goals.* Employees are responsible for making an accounting of their efforts in reaching the goals they have set.

Monitoring and Rewarding Performance

Someone once said "The trouble with not having a goal is that you can spend your life running up and down the field and never scoring." To be effective, goals must be written down and communicated between employee and supervisor. They must also follow the SMART pattern:

- **S**pecific: clearly stated, one at a time
- **M**easurable: stated so that it is measurable in time and quantity
- **A**chievable: able to be accomplished with a person's given abilities
- **R**elevant: able to bring about positive change and a sense of accomplishment
- **T**rackable: so that progress can be checked

It is best if your employees set their own goals, subject to management's approval. Employee goals should complement the objectives of the practice. Management needs to interview each employee at least quarterly to see how they are progressing on their goals, and the performance review meeting is a good time to review the past year's goals and set new goals for the coming year.

Reasons Employees Fail

If you use the system of management presented earlier in this section and teach your employees their corresponding responsibilities, you could avoid many of the personnel problems that plague some practices. However, you may still find employees who are not progressing in accomplishing their goals and improving their work. The reason will almost always be one of these three:

- *The employee is untrained.* Employees simply may not know what they are supposed to do, or how to do it. The solution here is to provide additional training.
- *The employee is unable.* Some employees will simply not be able to do the job the way it needs to be done. A shy employee, for example, may simply be unable to perform the work of a refractive surgery coordinator, due to his or her personality. The solution in this case is to move the employee to a job where he or she can be successful, and in some cases that may mean releasing the person from your employment.
- *The employee is unwilling.* Some employees have the training and are capable of performing the work required, but they decide they are not going to do what you need them to do. The solution in this case is to counsel with the employee, make their unwillingness explicit, and get a commitment for change. If no commitment is forthcoming, or if the person commits but doesn't follow through, termination is the only alternative.

Establishing goals with employees in your practice has enormous benefits, but ongoing focus and follow up takes some discipline on the part of ownership and management.

Performance Evaluation and Management Systems

Each employee should have a performance appraisal every year, either at a designated time for annual reviews or on the anniversary of the employee's hire date. Following are pointers on conducting a successful performance review:

- *Use a preprinted form.* Give the employee a copy a week or two in advance and ask for a self-evaluation on performance.
- *Conduct performance reviews separately.* Do not conduct a salary review during performance reviews. By combining the two, employees will concentrate on dollars rather than performance.
- *Allow adequate time.* Give the review process enough time to address the necessary topics; avoid rushing through!
- *Choose a quiet location.* Conduct the appraisal in a confidential atmosphere.
- *Give positive feedback.* Whenever possible, point out to the employee areas where he or she has grown and helped the practice.
- *Highlight needed improvements.* Set specific goals and timelines for improvement.
- *Get a signature.* Ask the employee to sign off on the form acknowledging that the review was conducted.
- *End the review on a good note.* Close the discussion with a compliment.

Salary Reviews

As a matter of necessity, salary increases must be based on practice profits. When funds are available, salary increases should be based on merit. Based on an employee's performance, merit raises can be motivators in that they recognize special effort or provide an incentive to improve. Know who is contributing, what they add to the practice, and how much. Do not be afraid to make a distinction; this is the point of merit raises.

At the time salary reviews are conducted and raises are given, it is good practice to review salary ranges for similar positions in your city, state or region. Many medical associations, state societies, and private and government groups survey businesses for salary ranges, so there is usually some information available that you can use to compare with your pay scales. It is important not to underpay employees or you will suffer from high turnover and low morale. Remember that pay is not only a financial necessity for employees, but it is also a message that you send to them. If you gave a $1 per hour raise last year and only 50¢ per hour this year, be prepared to discuss the reasons. Make sure all employees understand how salary increases are calculated and how they are given. Explain the process in the employee handbook.

Pay for Performance Systems

A good bonus system allows the staff to financially participate in the success of the practice and can motivate them to change habits to assist in that success. Unfortunately, many bonus programs have unintended side effects:

- In one practice, the optician was paid 4% of the optical "profits" each month if the profits were under $5000, 6% if the profits were $5000 to $10,000, and 8% if the profits were over $10,000. The trouble was, that's an easy system to game— the optician simply bought all supplies every other month, and nothing on the alternate months. On months when she didn't buy any supplies, profits were usually over the $10,000 mark, and when she bought supplies there would be no profits. You can see that it would mean more money to her to get an 8% bonus on $10,000 in profits every other month than 4% on $5000 every month.

- Sometimes practices pay bonuses to their billing staff based on the amount of outstanding accounts receivable. This can be a quick way to reduce your A/R since the staff can just write off any old debts, but it does not do anything to help cash flow.

- One practice developed an elaborate bonus system that would have required miracles for the staff to receive any money. What was an attempt to motivate the employees backfired and resulted in a decline in morale and trust between staff and management.

Some simple performance bonuses can work fairly well. A practice with lots of cancellations and no-shows decided that for every day when the appointment schedule was full of patients that were actually seen in the office, each staff member would get $5. Suddenly, the schedules were full, and staff members would call patients on a waiting list to come in for an exam if they had any holes in the schedule.

The best performance systems put the incentive on what the practice really wants to improve. One model works something like this:

1. All practice expenses plus doctors' regular salaries are subtracted from total collections.
2. The remaining money, called the "profit," is split 50/50, or with some other ratio, between the doctor and the staff.
3. The doctors split their share based on production.
4. The staff share is split based on pay level, years of service and the results of their confidential written grade done by other staff members.
5. In this system everyone has the incentive to control costs and to increase revenues and to be individually productive so that their bonus is maximized, and those are exactly the attributes that the practice wants.

A nice, healthy bonus demotivates when it fails to meet expectations. Be wary of annual bonuses that you subjectively decide, because they are fraught with peril. An administrator of one practice got a $5000 bonus from his doctors and that would have been a very nice gesture, except that one physician had told him it would be about $10,000 so he ended up being disappointed. Remember, compensation isn't just money, it is also a message you are sending to your employees—be sure to send the message you intend.

Employee Dispute Resolution, Counseling, Discipline, and Termination

Managing a staff requires counseling, discipline, and some eventual terminations. Make every effort to work with your employees so that they may give their best to their duties. Note and file in the personnel file any disciplinary discussions held with the employee, documenting what was said and the subsequent response. These records will substantiate the reasons for termination, if this action becomes necessary. Having proper documentation reduces your exposure to loss from claims brought by a disgruntled staff member.

Before beginning the termination process, keep the following points in mind:

- Often, potential grounds for dismissal are present at the time an employee is hired. Be sure to check all past references thoroughly and have an understanding of how the applicant got along with previous coworkers, supervisors, and patients.
- Employees must understand the terms of any probationary period. It is important that they know the grounds for dismissal; that no advance notice will be given; and that severance pay and unemployment benefits may not be extended. (Check your state statutes.)
- All policies governing grounds for dismissal, disciplinary procedures, grievance procedures, etc, should be clearly outlined in the employee handbook. Be sure that all standards are equally and impartially applied to all employees.
- Any decision to terminate should be the final step in a clearly documented and well-defined process. Make sure all alternatives have been exhausted first.

You may have a host of reasons for instituting a disciplinary process for an employee. The employee must be made aware of unsatisfactory performance or behavior and be given a chance to improve. After giving ample opportunity to no avail, you need to terminate the employee without delay. In some cases it is best to get legal counsel to make sure your documentation process has been adequate to protect you in the event of a wrongful termination suit.

Handling disputes between employees can be difficult at times, but one of the best methods involves the following steps:

1. Train your employees in appropriate ways of dealing with each other. For example, staff members need to know it is inappropriate to "triangulate," meaning the situation where staff member A complains to staff member B about something that staff member C did instead of going directly to staff member C.
2. If an employee comes to you with a problem that involves another employee, ask him or her to discuss the situation directly with that employee.
3. If needed, have both employees meet with you privately and let the two of them discuss the problem in front of you. It is best if you do not solve the problem for them, but let them agree together on an accommodation.
4. Make sure employees take problems to their supervisor first and only approach the managing doctor if that does not result in a solution.
5. In cases of accusations of harassment or other legal issues, be sure to take the complaint very seriously and follow the guidelines in your employee handbook.

Most employee problems can be solved by increasing communication between staff and management. In some cases, however, an employee just refuses to change and a termination is necessary.

Staff Development

As your practice grows, be sure to budget for staff development. The field of medicine changes so rapidly that employees who do not have the benefit of regular training in their job tasks fall behind. Appropriate investment in staff development yields:

- Billing staff who will find you more money

- Technical staff who will be better able to help you see patients
- Receptionists who will be better with your patients
- Opticians who will be better able to help patients get the best vision from their glasses
- Managers who will keep you abreast of the latest necessary changes in all aspects of the business of ophthalmology
- Employees who take more interest in the success of the practice

It is very discouraging to staff to see their doctors go off to meetings every year to receive additional training and to never have the opportunity to develop their own skills.

CHAPTER 10

Strategies for Building Your Practice

The rapidly changing health care environment constantly challenges physicians to adopt strategies to attract new patients and maintain the loyalties of existing patients. If the term *marketing* is a concern and it contains negative connotations, think of these strategies as building or expanding the practice. Whatever the description, these actions are a vital part of your success. This chapter introduces effective ways to market and build your practice.

Ethics Regarding Marketing

As you consider your overall marketing strategy, keep in mind the Academy's Rule 13 of the Code of Ethics on Communications to the Public. The rule states:

> "Communications to the public must be accurate. They must not convey false, untrue, deceptive, or misleading information through statements, testimonials, photographs, graphics or other means. They must not omit material information, without which the communications would be deceptive. Communications must not appeal to an individual's anxiety in an excessive or unfair way; and they must not create unjustified expectations of results. If communications refer to benefits or other attributes of ophthalmic procedures that involve significant risks, realistic assessments of their safety and efficacy must also be included, as well as the assessments of the benefits or other attributes of those alternatives. Communications must not misrepresent an ophthalmologist's credentials, training, experience or ability, and must not contain material claims of superiority that cannot be substantiated. If a communication results from payment by an ophthalmologist, this must be disclosed unless the nature, format or medium makes it apparent."

See Part II of this book for a closer look at ethical issues.

Building Your Practice Through Marketing

Building a medical practice takes a concerted effort and careful planning. Typically, in the early stages of practice startup, marketing funds are limited. Be sure to spend all marketing dollars thoughtfully in the area and specialty. If help is needed, get assistance from a reliable and experienced health care consultant who can keep the practice focused on initiatives that are most likely to be beneficial.

Overall Marketing Strategy

Strategies employed to attract new patients are generally very tangible, such as phone directory or newspaper advertisements, or even a web site. These are called *external marketing strategies*. Internal strategies are directed toward retaining the patient base and increasing loyalty through activities conducted within your existing patient base. The physician and staff accomplish these through friendliness and efficiency, expressed by communication and concern. This chapter provides some suggestions on both internal and external marketing strategies.

Developing the Marketing Budget

As the first year's operational budget is established, include a specific amount for marketing expenses. Establishing a marketing budget is an extremely important step in the development of the practice's promotional efforts. There are many ways to advance your practice, and every method has its costs. Do not consider these expenditures as optional; they are as vital to your success as having the proper equipment. If you do not expend the necessary time and money, you may suffer the consequences in loss of patients to the competition.

Obtain quotes on the development and printing of a practice brochure, appointment and business cards, letterhead, other stationery, and educational materials. The Practice Forms Master product available through the Academy allows you to create customized forms for your practice, including the ability to incorporate your own logo and other artwork. A variety of patient information brochures are also available. Refer to Appendix I for further details on these and other products for practice management. Factor the costs for obtaining the necessary forms, stationery, and patient information brochures into the first year's budget, and include the costs of any other marketing expense you might have such as a newspaper announcement and a phone directory listing.

Developing the Marketing Plan

Just as you have planned for the furniture and equipment needs in starting your practice, you will want to establish a marketing plan. The plan need not be complicated or formal, but it is imperative that it is committed to paper. Share this plan with your staff. They will become an integral part of your marketing efforts.

Four Months Before Opening

- Check sources that present information to new residents (eg, Chambers of Commerce). Supply handouts for their distribution.
- Set up a system to track how patients are referred to the practice. One method is to use a referral log, a simple grid that lists the various sources of referral. Referrals come from various sources (eg, the newspaper, a phone directory, a presentation made to a civic group, or another physician or patient). Always ask patients the name of the patient, physician, or other individual who referred them to you. Send a note to that person saying, "Thank you for the referral." Be sure your thank-you notes are HIPAA compliant.

- Attend meetings and join civic groups that will enhance your presence in the community. If you have children in the local school system, join the parent-teachers association. Offer to speak to these organizations on ophthalmic topics. Tell the medical staff secretary at your hospital(s) that you are available for public speaking engagements.
- Check with local hospitals to see if these institutions have planned health fairs or health screenings in the future. Offer to participate.

Three Months Before Opening

- Develop a practice brochure. An attractive, well-prepared brochure provides your patients with all the information they need about the practice. Include a short paragraph about yourself, your specialty, and your education. Add a photograph for a good touch. If the budget does not permit a professionally prepared brochure, use computer software and a laser printer to print information about your practice. (See "Brochure Contents" later in this chapter for an outline of a practice brochure.)

Two Months Before Opening

- Design and place an order for announcement cards to send to local physicians and other health care professionals. These announcements should show your name, specialty, address, and telephone number; mail at least 2 weeks before opening.
- Order stationery and appointment cards with the letterhead and logo if one has been developed. Order only small amounts to begin with. Changes may need to be made later.

One Month Before Opening

- Order patient education materials. The American Academy of Ophthalmology has a variety of patient education brochures and CD-ROM educational products available, and customizable for your practice. Be sure your name and address are on every piece of educational information that is handed out or placed in the waiting room. This information may find its way to another potential patient.
- Visit the hospital(s) where you will be on staff. Introduce yourself to the department heads and nursing staff.
- If you are providing treatment for work injuries, industrial glasses, company eye exams or other occupationally related services, visit the employers in the area; introduce yourself and the services you provide. Take copies of your practice brochure and your business cards. Meet with the person responsible for workers' compensation injuries or treatment, and the benefits coordinator.

Two Weeks Before Opening

- Draft a newspaper advertisement and submit it to the local newspaper(s). The advertisement should give your name, address, and telephone number. It should define and briefly describe your specialty and services that will be offered. Also, indicate the hours of operation.
- Meet with your staff to share the marketing plan and ask for ideas. Patients who call for an appointment will want to know a little about you. Give each employee

a copy of your curriculum vitae and outline your specialty training. Tell them about yourself so they can discuss your credentials with potential patients. Explaining to your staff the types of services provided by your specialty is also helpful. Keep in mind that your staff is marketing the practice's services to patients as well.

- Conduct office staff training on telephone communications to patients and referring physicians. If you receive a referral from a physician you have not previously met, it is a good idea to speak to that physician yourself. Put these protocols in writing and make them a part of the policies and procedures manual. Tell your staff how much time is needed for specific types of appointments. Allow extra time for any first visit; you will be building relationships during this time.

Guidelines for Building the Practice

With any marketing effort, developing guidelines is important. Clarify your thoughts and plans on paper and follow these suggestions:

- Define your objectives for the short term (less than one year) and the long term (more than one year). Express them in a way that they can be quantified and tracked so that successes and failures can be measured.
- Caution! Practically all professionals automatically say, "I'd like to double my practice." It is not as simple as that. Determine how much time and energy can be spent to achieve that goal.
- Remember cash flow. Many strategies call for 50%–75% of the marketing budget to be spent in the first 25% of the program. This usually means that the first large sum of cash needs to be in the bank at the start of the program, so it cannot come out of unexpected cash flow.
- Identify the target groups. Define the groups that the practice is trying to reach. Describe the target populations by the chief characteristics that are most important, usually income, education, sex, age, and location. If business is targeted, describe it by industry, industry position, yearly sales, number of employees, and location.
- Create a different, one-page marketing plan for each of your target groups. For example, set up a plan to reach your target populations, such as senior citizens or other practitioners, from whom to generate referrals. Then rank those groups, targeting the easiest first.
- Define what the target groups want. What are the characteristics most important to the target group in selecting a physician in that specific field? Is it experience, specific services, hours, location, or pricing?
- Define what distinguishes the physician's education, expertise, years of experience, and credentials. What does the practice offer in terms of location, hours, pricing, and special equipment?
- Analyze the main competitors within your service area. Do not ignore the indirect competitors outside the profession to whom prospects could turn as a substitute, such as chain optical shops. Chart each competitor's strengths and weaknesses. How does the practice rate against those main competitors? Where can the practice

best compete? List primary points, then secondary points. Can the targets be serviced well, or is the practice going too far outside its area of expertise? Assume the physician has good, solid experience, but that a competitor has more. If that competitor does not promote experience and the practice does, the practice will have the reputation for experience with the public. The same is true for any other advantage.

- Determine the budget. How much can the practice afford now? Reconcile the budget with the goals.
- Choose a strategy. Should it be internal promotion? Phone directory listings? Newspapers? Seminars? Is this strategy the most effective one? Weigh the pros and cons of various vehicles against each other.
- Choose the timing. List events, both external and internal, that will affect the campaign over the period that has been specified. Choose the time of year, which months, and what week to act. If the practice has seasonal peaks, promote heavily upon entering those busier periods, not during the practice lows. Dollars and efforts must work a lot harder in low periods when prospects are not already looking for services.
- Plan the execution. Assign responsibilities. Set deadlines for all steps on a master time line.

Developing Patient Satisfaction

In a pure fee-for-service market, a patient's dissatisfaction with a physician generally amounts to the departure of that one patient and possibly his or her family members. In a market dominated by managed care organizations, patient dissatisfaction can result in the defection of an entire patient population.

Managed care organizations gather a tremendous amount of data from their enrollees and use this information as a component in grading the plan's physicians. If a physician fails to make the grade, he or she may be dropped from the plan.

Be proactive in attempts to increase patient satisfaction. After the practice has been established about 6 months, conduct a patient satisfaction survey. Survey at least 100 patients or, if possible, every patient for a period of 2 weeks. Invaluable opinions about the practice, the staff, and the physician's own success up to this point can be gained. Take the patients' suggestions seriously. Carry out any changes that will increase patient satisfaction.

Some of the basic considerations of patient satisfaction might include ease of parking, time spent waiting in the office, and the doctor's ease of communication. As simple as these areas might seem, they are major factors in creating a satisfied patient—which often can translate into a patient for life, who refers friends and family to your practice. The

---

✓ KEY POINT

Understanding what makes a patient "satisfied" will allow you to establish an office culture that proactively considers the satisfaction of your patients.

Practice Forms Master product available from the Academy (see Appendix I) includes an electronic template for a patient satisfaction survey. Another sample follows in Figure 10-1.

Be sure to leave plenty of room for patient comments, which are often the most enlightening part of a patient survey. The key to a good satisfaction survey is to keep it short, no longer than one page. You can use this tool to identify areas that need attention, create a plan to deal with the problem, and follow up with subsequent surveys to document your success in dealing with identified issues.

Services and Amenities for Patients

Marketing can be as simple as making every patient feel comfortable and appreciated. Differentiate the practice from others by providing a personal touch to patient relationships. Follow these guidelines as a part of the practice's approach to patient service:

Patient Satisfaction Survey

Thank you for answering the following questions:	Yes	No
Do you have trouble getting an appointment when you would like?	[ ]	[ ]
Are our office hours convenient for you?	[ ]	[ ]
Is the location of our office convenient?	[ ]	[ ]
Are our parking facilities adequate?	[ ]	[ ]
Do you find our waiting room comfortable?	[ ]	[ ]
Is your wait too long in the reception area before you see the doctor?	[ ]	[ ]
Do you find our receptionists friendly and courteous?	[ ]	[ ]
Are your telephone calls handled in a prompt, courteous manner?	[ ]	[ ]
Are you receiving adequate help with your insurance?	[ ]	[ ]
Have our payment and billing policies been explained to your satisfaction?	[ ]	[ ]
Do you find our doctors' assistants friendly and courteous?	[ ]	[ ]
Do you have to wait too long in the examination room before you see the doctor?	[ ]	[ ]
Does the doctor spend enough time with you?	[ ]	[ ]
Does the doctor answer your questions adequately?	[ ]	[ ]

How were you referred to this practice?

Your additional comments:

Figure 10-1 Sample patient satisfaction survey.

Content to Cover in the Brochure

- The name, address, and telephone number of the practice
- A brief history of the practice
- The practice's philosophy and approach to patient care
- Professional profile of each physician in the practice, including photograph and details on training, board certification, areas of special interest, and perhaps personal information
- Explanation in simple terms of all of the services an ophthalmology practice provides
- Office hours, especially if appointment times are beyond the typical practice hours (eg, evening or Saturday hours)
- How to schedule and cancel appointments, including a different telephone number for scheduling appointments, if you have one or a customary fee in the event of a no-show or a late cancellation
- Hospital affiliations
- Policy related to patients' financial responsibility
- Forms of accepted payment and whether payment is expected when services are rendered
- A listing of the insurance plans in which the practice participates and whether or not the practice accepts Medicare assignment
- Billing information such as statement periods, policy about collection, and telephone number to call regarding billing questions
- A listing of all services the practice offers
- Policy regarding prescription refills, so that patients know how to handle routine prescription refills
- Notice that an answering service will respond to calls after normal office hours
- A map of the office location that includes nearby landmarks such as a hospital, a lake, or a park

For your site it is best to begin by figuring out what you want your site to do and how you want it to look. See the box, "Resources for Building a Web Presence" for additional guidance. Visiting other ophthalmology and medical practice web sites is a good way to understand the Internet's potential. Once you have a list of the most important characteristics you want in your own site, you will need to find someone to design and set up the web site for you.

If you find a site that really appeals to you, you may want to contact that practice to find out who did their programming. Although it is a little more convenient to have someone working for you who can sit down in your office and discuss your plans, in some cases it may be best to work with a programmer who is at a distance from your office if he or she is the one who understands what you want and can best provide it. Get several bids from companies on your web site design—the cost can vary dramatically. Look for a company or people with good track records and enough business that they are likely to stay in business, because web sites require ongoing maintenance.

Resources for Building a Web Presence

The Ophthalmic Executive's Resource Guide: Making the Most of Your Practice Web Site, produced by the American Academy of Ophthalmic Executives (AAOE), teaches you how to implement web site design improvements, make your practice HIPAA compliant, improve search engine rankings, and market an online presence to patients (see Appendix I).

Another resource to consider is The Medem Network. Together with leading health care partners, Medem has established a physician–patient communications network designed to facilitate online access to information and care for more than 90,000 physicians, their practices and their patients. Members of the Academy are currently eligible to have a web site developed for their practice without cost through a relationship with Medem. For more information, visit the Academy's web site (www.aao.org).

E-Mail Etiquette

Some practices use e-mail to communicate with patients. A simple e-mail newsletter is less expensive than a printed version sent through the regular mail. Be sure you send marketing e-mails only to patients from whom you have secured permission.

E-mail may eventually be a good way to remind some patients of their appointments, but many people do not check their e-mail every day. Automated appointment reminder systems that use your computer appointment logs to call patients are a more efficient way to accomplish this task.

The Web Advantage If you put resources into a web site, make sure that your stationery, brochures, appointment cards, business cards, and other written materials all display your web site address. In addition, work with your site designer or your web hosting company to get your listing to appear at or near the top of Internet search engine results, which will lead interested patients to your site.

CHAPTER 11

Technology for Optimal Business Performance

With all the options available today, it is easy to get confused about how best to equip a medical practice with information technology. This chapter presents an overview of the fundamental options available and considerations to think about as you make your technology decisions.

The health care industry is often considered burdened with inefficiency and laced with labor-intensive processes to accomplish even a simple function. As practices continue to face these challenges, and with added pressure to their bottom lines, processes will need to improve and become more time-efficient for a practice to survive. Now, and even more in the future, ophthalmology practices will need to use technology and use it well to keep up with the demands of the medical business climate.

Overview of Infrastructure and Applications

When building the technology infrastructure, consider two factors: cost and features.

Weighing Costs

While money drives many decisions, higher costs must be weighed against increased revenue and benefits. Select technology based on its ability to save you money and time. For example, should the practice spend thousands of dollars every year ordering encounter forms or superbills, or purchase a practice management system that will allow the practice to design and print its own forms at minimal cost? Can the process be taken a step further and all charges captured electronically on a personal digital assistant (PDA) and synchronized back into the billing module? By taking this extra step or investing in a tool to eliminate the paper superbill and the charge entry process, operating cost is reduced.

The initial cost of a computer system may be modest in comparison to the ongoing expenses of maintaining and upgrading the technology (see the box "Hidden Technology Costs Beyond the Initial Sale").

> **Hidden Technology Costs Beyond the Initial Sale**
>
> - Your systems and software require ongoing maintenance and support.
> - Fees may apply to electronic transactions such as electronic claims, insurance eligibility, remittance, and statements. Avoid arrangements that require a per-transaction fee unless the cost is justifiable.
> - Most medical software vendors develop a new version every 12–18 months, necessitating continuous upgrades. Some vendors make customers pay for each new release; others include all continuous upgrades at no additional cost.
> - Customization typically costs $100–$200 per hour, depending on the requirements.
> - Most vendors charge $2000–$5000 to convert data from another system; they may be willing to negotiate this fee to get your new business.

Picking Features That Fit

While most functions are possible, in theory, one must be realistic. For example, some practice management systems incorporate rules into their processes. Such systems are known as *rules-based systems.* Rules are useful because they alert the end user before a mistake can be made. However, the rules must first be put into place and kept up to date before the benefits can be realized. Some systems allow the practice to link directly with the payors for obtaining eligibility and payor-specific rules. Do not assume the rules come with the system you are considering.

Voice recognition is another function that sounds good in theory. While this technology continues to improve, it generally requires months to train the application to become familiar with the user's voice. Even then, achieving 100% accuracy with this system is unlikely. When involved in a demonstration of voice recognition software, be mindful that presenters spend considerable time training their systems. Ask for permission to speak into the system yourself, and you will instantly see a difference.

Integrated vs Interfaced Systems

Integrated systems generally run on a single database with all of the functionality and workflow converging through a single application. Integrated systems, which usually have lower licensing costs and do not require costly interfaces, are usually less expensive than interfaced systems. However, if the integrated system cannot perform all the desired functions, it will require an interface to another application that would provide those functions.

Interfacing or combining applications allows buyers to build their ideal system. This approach means, for example, buying an insurance billing system from one company and an electronic medical records program from a different company. The disadvantage of interfacing is in having to deal with multiple vendors. This requires them to communicate with one another and, at times, share their technical expertise. It can lead to disagreements about which company is responsible for a problem, with each one thinking the other is at fault.

Working with an ASP

The ASP approach includes the following steps:

1. Select an ASP that offers the desired software applications and services.
2. Agree on terms. (The fee is fixed and there is nothing to buy; thus, the process is straightforward.)
3. Establish connectivity. (This can take 30 days or more and varies by location.)
4. Determine the number of workstations and users needing to access the system.
5. Determine if any data conversion or migration is required.
6. Connect a dedicated data communications line or virtual private network (VPN) to the ASP's data center. (The ASP will handle this for you.)
7. Have the application turned on and training started 1–5 days after connectivity. (Expect training to last 2–5 days.)
8. Go live with the new ASP.

Lessons in Installation and Training

A financial management program can be installed in minutes; most of the retail products work much like a paper checkbook, so they are relatively easy to learn. The most popular ones have video, CD-ROM, and classes for training. On the other hand, a practice management or EMR system requires a lot of work to prepare for its use in your practice.

If you are installing new hardware and software, the installation process can take from several days to several weeks, so make sure you plan for extra time to install and test the equipment.

Practice management programs must be customized with your data such as provider numbers, tax ID numbers, insurance company addresses, and physician names. This process is extensive and may take a week or more. It is absolutely imperative that you review a printout of all of the practice data once it has been entered into the system (usually by the software vendor) and check it for accuracy. If provider numbers are not properly entered, all of your claims will be denied.

EMR programs must be customized to your method of seeing patients. Although the software vendor can and should assist you in this, be prepared to spend a lot of time working on customizing your templates so that they are as efficient for you as possible.

Training can seem expensive, but do not shortchange yourself or your staff. Before you sign the purchase contract, make sure the vendor gives you details about how much training is included in the purchase and how much extra training will cost. One of the most frequent problems with implementation of software systems is inadequate training of the staff.

If you install a new insurance billing program, all of your staff members need to know they must learn the system or find another job. EMR systems are different in that they are often designed to be used by the doctors, and if a doctor resists learning the EMR system he or she may not face the same consequence. In one practice that installed an EMR system several years ago, the oldest doctor spent a couple of hours on the system, got frustrated, and then refused to use it. The middle partner would use the program only if the patient was already registered in the EMR system from a previous visit; otherwise she would document in the paper chart. The youngest partner used the EMR program for all of his patients. The practice spent large sums trying to accommodate all three physicians, but many of the benefits of EMRs were not realized in that practice. The lesson to learn from this practice's experience: If you decide to install an EMR system, be prepared for the lengthy learning curve and make sure all of the doctors are committed to making the system work.

Data Conversion

If you are changing from one system to another, you need to convert the data in the old system and put it into the new system. For practice management software, the process to convert patient demographics (eg, name, address, phone, insurance ID number, and insurance plan) is relatively straightforward. Because every system handles financial information differently, it is often inadvisable to try to convert old account balances to the new system. If that is the case, you have two choices: Keep the old system running until the claims are paid by insurance and then convert the remaining patient balances to the new system by manually entering them; or manually enter all of the information on claims into the new system.

If your former software vendor will not convert the data to a format usable by your new system, you may have to start fresh, entering every patient seen as a new patient in the system. Some practices choose to do this in order to clean up inaccurate old information, but be prepared to have your staff work lots of extra hours if you must choose this option. Most data conversions cost between $2000 and $5000, but typically these costs are more economical than having your staff re-enter all of the old information into the new system.

practice is doing in meeting its goals. Some practices conduct these retreats on their own while others invite a consultant familiar with ophthalmology practices to moderate and to give an objective viewpoint.

- *Billing process review.* See Table 5-1 in Chapter 5 for a tool to help you perform a review of your billing processes and to make sure you are getting the maximum reimbursement for your work.
- *Patient flow analysis.* Taking a close look at the flow of patients in your office, from reception area, through the exam process, to check-out can be very revealing as you optimize the time spent examining patients and providing other services. Even having a staff member use a stopwatch to time how long you and your technicians take to perform different types of exams can be a start in understanding the vagaries and difficulties of keeping patient appointments on time.

Internal Benchmarking

Measuring the key financial and patient flow statistics within your practice and comparing them to previous benchmarks for your own office is a way of seeing the progress that your practice is making. Comparing your practice against its own internal benchmarks is often more helpful than using national averages because every practice is different and faces different challenges in its managed care environment, its competitive landscape and its own capabilities. Some typical benchmarks are included in Chapter 4.

External Benchmarking

External benchmarking can be helpful, provided you use those national or regional figures in appropriate ways. Striving to meet a particular national benchmark can be damaging to a practice if it is done without understanding how it should apply to your practice. For example, if the national average occupancy expense ratio (total rent or mortgage expenses divided into the collected revenues) is 6% and your occupancy ratio is 9%, it may be due to your location more so than anything else. Obviously, leased space is more expensive in Manhattan than in Missoula, so a higher occupancy ratio in New York would not be surprising, even though the reimbursements might be a little higher there.

Working with Practice Management Consultants

Many physicians and physician groups go through the entire practice cycle without ever seeking the assistance of an experienced practice management consultant. Unfortunately, these physicians probably spend many hours of their own valuable time and effort on projects that a consultant could handle in a fraction of the time. In particular, a physician new to practice or in a practice transition will benefit greatly by using an experienced consultant. Besides offering operational advice and organizing the practice setup, the seasoned consultant can develop policies and procedure manuals, fee schedules, employee handbooks, and job descriptions for the practice. For established or existing practices, engaging a consulting firm to complete an operational assessment can uncover areas where practice efficiencies can improve and where revenue can be enhanced for improvements in billing and collections procedures.

When selecting the practice consultant, ask candidates for the names of other physicians the consultant has helped. Talking with these references provides a feel for the

---

✓ KEY POINT

You do not have to go it alone. There are many practice management consultants available to ophthalmologists. Check the American Academy of Ophthalmology web site for a list of consultants who have qualified for inclusion in the Consultant Directory.

---

consultant's knowledge, the nature of the assignments, and the success of the project in which the physician received assistance. Most consultants have areas of special interest or qualifications, so be sure to find a consultant whose skills match your needs. If you contract with a large consulting company, be sure you know in advance who will handle your project and what his or her qualifications are.

It is often a good idea to use a written agreement (between the physician and the consulting firm) listing, as specifically as possible, what you expect to be achieved. Corresponding to this list, the consulting firm should state exactly what work will be provided, including a timeline for completion. Most consultants will send you an invoice for their work once a month; in some cases they may ask for a deposit before beginning work, but you should not have to pay in advance for a major project.

Next Steps

Ophthalmology practice in today's world is challenging, exciting, difficult at times, and complex. Part I of this book has given you an overview of some of the main issues you will deal with as you embark on your career as an ophthalmologist and it has shared with you some ideas about the options you have in your practice.

You will quickly learn that the pressure to offer the highest quality medical care will never end, and the demands will stretch your heart and your mind. It won't be long before the satisfaction of serving your patients continuously motivates you to incorporate the best systems into your practice as you aspire to having the best staff, the most satisfied patients, and a reputation for quality and compassion that sets you apart from others.

PART II

Ethics in Ophthalmology

Introduction

Why is ethics important to ophthalmology and why should we study ethics? The simplest answer is, "To become a more competent physician." While technical skills and knowledge are the *sine qua non* of the medical doctor, the competent physician also requires an understanding of the fundamental purposes of medical practice, that is, an awareness of the ethical behavior that the profession, the patient, and the society believe is proper. The fact is that ethical concerns are not limited to occasional events we might describe as crises. Ethical principles and behavior are an integral part of the practice of medicine, and they permeate even the simplest decisions we make in relation to our patients. For this reason, the ability to recognize and act on ethical issues is an essential qualification of the competent physician, the competent ophthalmologist, and the whole person.

Although there is no objective standard by which to assess ethical awareness and behavior, there should be no question that these attributes are an essential part of the competent physician. Many would argue that ethical behavior cannot be learned from an instruction course; but ethical behavior *is* indeed learned. Much as we learn how to behave among family, friends, and schoolmates, we discover as physicians what is acceptable and what is not, what is correct and what is not, what is caring and what is not. Correspondingly, we can learn the standards of ethical behavior that are considered appropriate by our society, our profession, and our natural instincts. We can learn to be more aware of the ethical considerations in what we choose to do and how we choose to behave. This, at least, can be taught by didactic means, as well as by the example of our peers and role models.

With that in mind, this part of the book reviews the historical background of medical ethics, offers case studies in the practical applications of ethical behavior for today's physician, and reprints a selection of fundamental ethics documents of the past two millennia. If the concepts presented here have a central goal, it is to help physicians become better healers of their patients, better participant-members of their communities, and better people themselves.

Appendix II lists additional resources related to the topic of medical ethics. It includes publications and other offerings from the Academy and from other sources.

Background and Practical Applications

The paramount guideline for ethical behavior for physicians is not *Primum non nocere* ("First, do no harm"); nor is it "Put the best interests of the patient above all else." The truly paramount guideline is "Do what is in the best interest of the patient." The difference in emphasis between the latter two statements is critical. The former is sacrificial, while the latter includes developing and caring for one's professional self as well as participating in the advancement of the profession. In the historical development of medicine and its component ethical structure, one can see the creation of professionalism as an important goal of practitioners. Important milestones include the Hippocratic Oath, the formation of guilds, the development of various codes of ethics, the establishment of education guidelines, and professional certification. All of these advance the ideals of refining the profession of medicine and medical ethics. The historical figures and the development of medicine as outlined in the following chapter are an important element of your medical education. You cannot be a true medical professional without the knowledge of the development of your profession and its ethical imperatives.

CHAPTER 13

History of Medical Ethics

Since the time of Hippocrates (ca. 460–375 B.C.E., Figure 13-1), codes of medical ethics have been formulated to represent physicians' loftiest moral philosophy. Physicians' ethics have been derived from their religion, their education in the humanities, and their medical tradition. In addition, ethical standards have been imposed on physicians by their governing professional bodies and by the state. The value of various codes of medical ethics to the physician is that they provide a systematic and well-reasoned framework to assist in the making of moral decisions about the complex clinical problems confronted in patient care. In addition, as early as the time of Hippocrates, codes of medical ethics have served to protect groups of physicians from unfair competition. In other words, medical ethics has always involved elements of fairness and "good business."

Until well into the twentieth century, medical ethics focused on the scope of knowledge of the physician and on personal conduct, behavior, and manners. Starting in the

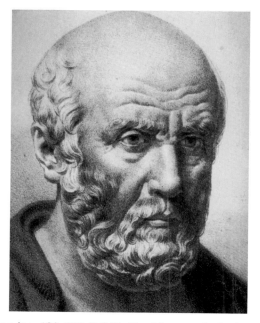

Figure 13-1 Hippocrates (ca. 460–375 B.C.E). The Hippocratic Oath stresses kindness, courage, a refusal to cheat the patient, a willingness to set a fair fee, and a lifestyle that lacks ostentation and extravagance. *(Etching courtesy of Museum of Vision & Ophthalmic Heritage.)*

late 1960s and the early 1970s, a new wave of complex and subtle ethical problems and issues began to appear, as a result of advances in medical and scientific technology, economic factors, and social change. Examples include the use of evolving or unproven surgical and technical procedures; shared responsibilities among diverse health care and eye care providers; advertising and marketing; evaluation and treatment in the managed care setting; and the use of anticipated quality of life improvement in clinical decisions. One thing is certain: The principles of medical ethics are as pertinent today as in the past, and they serve as a valuable touchstone for physicians encountering the questions and crises of the twenty-first century.

The Hippocratic Oath

The Oath of Hippocrates establishes a code of ethics separate from the laws of the state. We have little first-hand knowledge of Hippocrates as a historical figure. Many writings have been attributed to him, but it is difficult to determine which are really the works of the "Father of Medicine" himself. As with the books of the Bible, different Hippocratic writings seem to have been composed by different scribes at different times, setting down a concrete record of what had previously been an oral tradition of belief and practice. These writings have shaped the development of Western medicine and continue to affect its practice to the present day.

In *The Evolution of Modern Medicine* (New Haven, Conn: Yale University Press; 1921), Sir William Osler describes the two features of the Hippocratic writings that have influenced the evolution of medicine. The first of these Osler termed "the note of humanity." This can be seen in the Hippocratic phrase "In purity and holiness I will guard my life and my art." The second feature is the directness with which Hippocrates addressed medical and ethical issues. Osler noted: "Everywhere one finds a strong, clear common sense, which refuses to be entangled either in theology or in philosophical speculation." Hippocrates was largely responsible for developing a new way of looking at nature, and he changed forever the way disease was viewed. Western medicine as we know it began to develop with Hippocrates.

The Hippocratic Oath was probably written between 450 and 370 B.C.E. It consists of both a pledge to uphold a high ethical standard in medical practice and an indenture to share the earnings received by the candidate with his teacher, to help the teacher financially when necessary, and to teach student signatories of the Oath in the manner that one would teach one's own child. (See Chapter 16 for two versions of the Oath.)

The Oath stresses kindness, courage, a refusal to cheat the patient, a willingness to set a fair fee, and a lifestyle that lacks ostentation and extravagance. The physician is to help the sick and to respect the art of medicine and, in addition, to refrain from poisoning, gossip, and sexual misconduct. There is a clear implication that the healer who practices ethically will have a return on his moral investment. It is clearly indicated that adherence to medical ethics differentiates the good healer from the bad.

The Oath was written at a time when the medical marketplace may have been highly competitive and unregulated and when competing physicians could produce their own ethical rules. The code helped establish the fact that morality and technical competence were closely associated and that adherence to the code required medical competence. It should be noted that the medical ethics of ancient Greece were not confined to a single document formulated by consensus, but existed as competing codes of ethics developed by various medical sects.

Medieval and Renaissance Developments

By the beginning of the medieval period (ca. 1100 A.D.), the Western Roman Empire had fallen, Greek science was moribund, and Greek philosophy (neo-Platonism) had proven a total failure. Loose tribal groups were becoming organized into nations. The Christian church had emerged as a major force with its spiritual appeal, compelling symbolism, and formidable organization. The spread of the Judeo-Christian virtue of compassion toward weakness and suffering led to initiatives in medicine, particularly in nursing the sick and establishing hospitals for their care. Popes and emperors generated legislation for chartering and building medieval universities.

By the end of the fifteenth century, there were well-organized hospitals and medical schools with laws governing the practice of medicine. Severe penalties were prescribed for those who practiced without the necessary license. The medical physicians, known as Masters or Doctors in Medicine, were regarded as academicians and occupied university chairs. Popes and princes sought their services in the healing arts as well as in nutrition, herbs, and lifestyle. Medical physicians viewed the skills of the surgeon as an inferior art, unworthy of scholars. On occasion they might give written surgical advice, but they abstained from any practice of surgery. In fact, surgery was considered so demeaning that fourteenth-century medical students in Paris had to swear that they would not perform any surgical operations.

Surgeons evolved as an order of professionals lower than physicians. These professionals seldom had formal or higher education, but they had the ability to operate for urinary calculi, hernias, and cataracts and to extract diseased teeth. At the top of the hierarchy of surgeons were those who were gifted in the art of surgery, although ignorant of the works of Hippocrates, Celsius (ca. 25 B.C.E.–50 A.D.), and Galen (ca. 130–ca. 200 A.D., Figure 13-2). They maintained rooms where they treated patients and trained their apprentices in the surgical arts. Of lower status than these surgeons were the barbers, who were important figures in medicine from medieval times into the eighteenth century. The barbers gained importance in about 1100 when the monks who required their hair-cutting services also used them for bloodletting. Eventually, they were charged with the treatment of boils, lumps, and open wounds, and they performed cupping, pulled teeth, and gave enemas.

At the bottom of the hierarchy were the itinerants, who disappeared before the results of their treatment became apparent. The management of cataract and other eye diseases tended to be relegated to the more irregularly trained practitioners. By the sixteenth and seventeenth centuries, the skills of trained physicians and surgeons were so deficient that even the irregular practitioners were countenanced and legitimized. The army of ophthalmic and other quacks who practiced at this time operated within the law. Under Henry VIII in England, through Act 34-35, it became lawful "for any person being the

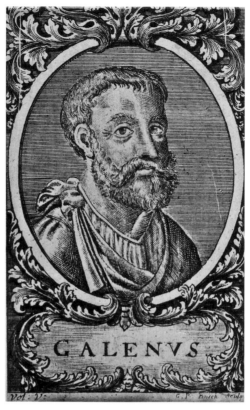

Figure 13-2 Galen (ca. 130–ca. 200). Anatomist, surgeon to gladiators, and author of several ophthalmic texts that described the eye as the most divine organ. *(Engraving by GP Busch. Courtesy of U.S. National Library of Medicine.)*

King's subject, being no common surgeon, but having the knowledge and experience of the nature of herbs, roots, and water, etc. to practice and minister to any outward sore and for the stone, strangury, and ague, not withstanding any statute to the contrary." This act became known as the Quack's Charter and remained in force into the twentieth century.

The Renaissance (1453–1600) was a remarkable transition period from medieval to modern civilization. It is associated with a number of major events, including the discovery of America, the introduction of gunpowder into Europe, Magellan's circumnavigation of the globe, the establishment of heliocentrism by Copernicus, the Reformation, and the invention of the printing press by Gutenberg in 1454. In the sixteenth century, medical oaths began to be sworn by medical students, and it is thought that the Hippocratic Oath gained primacy because of its ethical compatibility with Christianity.

In ophthalmology, the Renaissance was signified by a series of textbooks dealing with the eye. Most of these reflected a return to medicine's classic past: Grasus, *De Oculis* (11th century); Aetius of Amida, *Librorum Medicinalium tomus primus* (1534); Leonhart Fuchs, *Ein newes Hochnutzlichs Buchlin* (1538) and *Alle Kranckheyten der Augen* (1539);

Stromayer, *Die Handschrift des Schnittund Augenartztes* (1559); Bartisch, *Ophthalmodouleia* (1583); Guillemeau, *Traité des Maladies de L'Oeil* (1585); and Bayley, *A Briefe Treatise* (1586).

George Bartisch

Bartisch's book (Figure 13-3) deserves particular attention because it alone captured the Renaissance spirit of individual achievement. Often called the "Father of Modern Ophthalmology," George Bartisch (1535–1606) was an itinerant barber surgeon and oculist who became court ophthalmologist to the Elector of Saxony. In 1583, he wrote a treatise based on his 36 years' experience treating eye diseases. This was the first "modern" work on ophthalmology.

Medical Ethics and the Guilds

The guilds were initially formed in Europe in the Middle Ages as associations of working men in the various crafts, such as weavers, bakers, goldsmiths, and so on. Their purpose was to establish standards of quality for the products they made and sold and to preserve their monopolies. The guilds were usually authorized by local community or city governments, but some obtained their charters from the sovereign of their country. In London, Paris, and the larger European cities, there were as many as 50 or more guilds by the fourteenth century.

By the eighteenth century, medical practice and ethics had become inseparably connected with guild organization in Europe. As with other guilds, codes of regulations evolved for medical guilds governing performance and ethical standards. In England these codes were influenced by the Royal College of Physicians, founded in London early in the sixteenth century. An established contractual relationship developed between the king and the physicians (see the box, "Henry VIII Establishes the Royal College of Physicians"). The physicians received a charter granting a strict monopoly on defined goods and services, while the sovereign received a guarantee of a high standard of service. Much of the impetus for the development of modern medical ethics arose from the conflict between those who were protected by the guild and those who were not (the latter being surgeons, apothecaries, midwives, various "irregulars," and quacks).

John Gregory

It was during the eighteenth century that two English physicians, John Gregory and Thomas Percival, laid the basis for modern English medical ethics. John Gregory (1724–1773) was a Scottish physician. In 1770, he published a treatise entitled *Observations on the Duties and Offices of a Physician*. In 1772, this was expanded into a new work entitled *Lectures on the Duties and Qualifications of a Physician*. Gregory's goal was to "advance the art of medicine by freeing its practice of imposture and its science of conjecture" (Haakonssen L. *Medicine and Morals in the Enlightenment: John Gregory, Thomas Percival and Benjamin Rush*. The Wellcome Institute Series in the History of Medicine. Atlanta, Ga: Clio Medica; 1997). According to Lester Haakonssen, "[Gregory's] task, as he saw it,

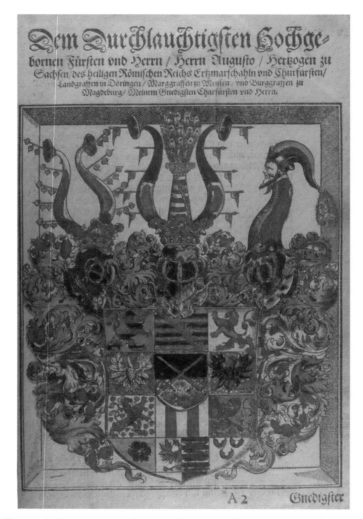

Figure 13-3 Cover of *Ophthalmodouleia, das ist augendienst,* by Georg Bartisch, published in 1583 in Dresden by M. Stockel, page A2. The book is the first extensively illustrated account of any surgical specialty. Bartisch, who served as court oculist to Duke August I of Saxony, was known for his skillful operations on cataracts using a clean needle to depress the lens through the sclera. *(Courtesy of the Clendening History of Medicine Library, University of Kansas Medical Center.)*

was to convince a new generation of physicians that it was indeed in their own as well as in their profession's best interest that they should 'labour to be wise.' "

Thomas Percival

Thomas Percival (1740–1804) is best remembered by medical historians today for his pioneering work as an epidemiologist in the field of communicable diseases. He also provided the most important work in medical ethics in Britain during the late eighteenth and early nineteenth centuries in his *Medical Jurisprudence* (Figure 13-4).

Henry VIII Establishes the Royal College of Physicians

The Royal College of Physicians was founded by Henry VIII by royal charter in 1518. The Roll of the Royal College of Physicians describes the founding of the College by Henry VIII in the following terms:

> Henry the Eighth, with a view to the improvement and more orderly exercise of the art of physic, and the repression of irregular, unlearned, and incompetent practitioners of that faculty, in the tenth year of his reign founded the Royal College of Physicians of London. To the establishment of this incorporation the King was moved by the example of similar institutions in Italy and elsewhere, by the solicitations of at least one of his own physicians, Thomas Linacre, and by the advice and recommendation of his chancellor, Cardinal Wolsey.

Samuel Bard

As American medicine developed, it drew heavily on the traditions of England and Scotland. This can be seen in the earliest American treatise on medical ethics, entitled *A Discourse Upon the Duties of a Physician*, which was delivered by Samuel Bard (1742–1821), professor of the Theory and Practice of Medicine at King's College, now Columbia University. His *Discourse* was presented at the King's College commencement in 1769 and published the same year.

Benjamin Rush

Samuel Bard's contemporary in Philadelphia, Benjamin Rush (1745–1813), had a more profound impact on the formative medical ethics of the United States. Rush was a signer of the Declaration of Independence and was surgeon general for a period during the American Revolution. Rush studied medicine in Edinburgh, London, and Paris and when he returned to Philadelphia, he carried with him the ideas of John Gregory and Thomas Percival and gave them the stamp of his country's culture. The pursuit of happiness, a right guaranteed in the Declaration of Independence, meant to Rush the moral, intellectual, and physical well-being of the individual in society.

American Medicine after the Mid–Nineteenth Century

By the mid–nineteenth century in America, physicians were independent general practitioners who acquired business through a lay referral network. The social and financial status of the majority of doctors was insecure and ambiguous. Physicians were a heterogeneous group. Those at the top of the profession had graduated from recognized medical schools and had often received at least part of their training in Europe. The vast majority in the middle had served apprenticeships and had often taken a course of lectures or had obtained a two-term medical degree, but had received little general education. The lowest ranks were practitioners who had attended small proprietary schools with ungraded curricula and who were largely self-taught.

32   MEDICAL JURISPRUDENCE.

XV. Some general rule should be adopted,
by the faculty, in every town, relative to the
pecuniary acknowledgments of their patients; and
it should be deemed a point of honour to ad-
here to this rule, with as much steadiness, as
varying circumstances will admit. For it is
obvious that a medium fee, as suited to the general rank of patients, must be an inadequate
gratuity from the rich, who often require attendance not absolutely necessary; and yet too large
to be expected from that class of citizens, who
would feel a reluctance in calling for assistance,
without making some decent and satisfactory
retribution.

But in the consideration of fees, let it ever be
remembered, that though mean ones from the
affluent are both unjust and degrading, yet the
characteristical beneficence of the profession is
inconsistent with sordid views and avaricious
rapacity. To a young physician it is of great
importance to have clear and definite ideas of
the ends of his profession; of the means for their
attainment; and of the comparative value and
dignity of each. Wealth, rank, and indepen-
dance, with all the benefits resulting from them,
are the primary ends which he holds in view;
and they are interesting, wise, and laudable.
But knowledge, benevolence, and active virtue,
                                           the

Figure 13-4 Reproduction from Percival, T. *Medical Jurisprudence; or, A Code of Ethics and Institutes Adapted to the Professions of Physic and Surgery* (1794), p. 32. Percival's work in medical ethics influenced the AMA's first adopted code of ethics in 1847. *(Reproduced with permission, Library of the College of Physicians of Philadelphia.)*

The American Medical Association

The American Medical Association (AMA) was organized in 1847, following a convention of delegates from medical societies and colleges that gathered in New York to plan a national medical association for the United States. In its early years, the AMA was engaged in a long struggle against two formidable challengers of "regular" physicians, the homeopaths and the eclectics. These alternative groups found wide acceptance among the public and politicians. The homeopaths maintained that diseases could be cured by drugs that produce the same disease symptoms when given to healthy persons, and that the effect of drugs could be heightened by administering them in minute doses. The other alternative medical group, the eclectics, agreed with most of the conventions of medical science, but campaigned against the excessive "drugging and bleeding" done by the regular profession.

The AMA's first code of ethics was published in 1847. After several revisions it was rewritten as "Principles of Medical Ethics" in 1912; it was last modified in 2001. (See "American Medical Association Principles of Medical Ethics" in Chapter 16.)

The American Ophthalmological Society

The American Ophthalmological Society (AOS) was founded in 1864 "to assemble physicians dedicated to determining the best methods of diagnosing and treating eye diseases." Of note, this was the first medical specialty society to be founded in the United States, and it brought together the founders of the eye infirmaries of New York, Boston, Philadelphia, and Chicago. The principal organizers, however, were ophthalmologists younger than the founders of these institutions; they had attended medical schools affiliated with universities and had college degrees. Also, most had studied in the major European medical centers under the most outstanding eye specialists of the period. The founders and early members of the AOS were thus the professional elite who did not necessarily identify their interests with those of the ordinary practitioners.

The Founding of the American Academy of Ophthalmology

In April 1896, Dr. Hal Lovelace Foster sent letters to 500 ophthalmologists and otolaryngologists inviting them to come to Kansas City to participate in forming a national organization. A group of approximately 50 ophthalmologists and otolaryngologists accepted the invitation and met in Kansas City and formed the Western Ophthalmological, Otological, Laryngological, and Rhinological Association. In 1898 this group renamed itself the Western Ophthalmological and Otolaryngological Association, and 5 years later the organization recognized its national character by changing its name to the American Academy of Ophthalmology and Otolaryngology. It remained a combined organization until October 1978, when the members at the Ophthalmology Division meeting in Kansas City voted to form a separate and independent American Academy of Ophthalmology starting on January 1, 1979.

Developments in Medical Education and Certification

In 1910, the Carnegie Foundation commissioned a study by Dr. Abraham Flexner to investigate educational conditions in the 155 medical schools in operation in the United States. In graphic terms and with considerable detail, his report brought to the public's attention the substandard educational conditions in many medical schools. Only Johns Hopkins, Western Reserve, and Harvard received clean bills of health. The Flexner Report had an immediate and lasting effect on medical education in the United States. Many of the severely criticized schools undertook extensive revision of their programs, facilities, and faculties; others closed; and still others merged with existing institutions. The AMA's Council on Medical Education extended its concern from undergraduate pre-med education to graduate medical education and continuing medical education. The states and the federal government took action as well. The medical curriculum became standardized, uniform licensing examinations for physicians were adopted, and physicians could go into practice only after successfully passing state board examinations or the National Board of Medical Examiners examination.

The American Board of Ophthalmology

At about the same time the Flexner Report was published, the three major eye organizations in the United States—the Academy, the American Ophthalmological Society, and the AMA—recognized the need for more comprehensive training and higher standards for eye specialists. The AMA, by this time, had recognized the need for support of the various specialty areas and had created an Eye Section. As early as 1914, Dr. Edward Jackson spoke out on the need for examination and certification of ophthalmologists. The severity of the problem can be seen by the fact that 51% of ophthalmologists entering the military service in World War I were found unqualified to practice their specialty. The effort to improve standards for ophthalmology culminated in the establishment of the American Board of Ophthalmic Examinations. The first examination was held in 1916 at the Medical School at the University of Tennessee in Memphis and consisted of a written test in the morning and an oral examination in the afternoon. In 1933, the name of the Board was changed to the American Board of Ophthalmology.

Ethics in Ophthalmology

Ophthalmologists and other physicians who practice medicine are beholden to two distinct ethical codes: One is a largely self-enforced personal code of values, developed during childhood from parental values and influenced by the physician's education, training, and professional experience. The second ethical code is that imposed upon physicians by their hospital, professional organizations, terms of licensure and certification, and government regulations and statutes. Physicians have a responsibility to the public to ensure that moral and ethical conduct is maintained by themselves and their colleagues. The Academy's Code of Ethics (reprinted in Chapter 14) embodies the basic tenets of ethical care, which have been enunciated through the centuries and which remain applicable in today's complex and changing medical world. In June of 1983, the Federal Trade Commission (FTC) approved the Academy's Code of Ethics. The Academy is the only health sciences organization to have sought and obtained approval for a code of ethics by the FTC.

Past, Present, and Future Concerns

Ethical problems that have existed in the past must still be dealt with in modern ophthalmic practice. These include the following:

- Achievement and maintenance of clinical competence
- Respect for patient autonomy
- Acting in the patient's best interests
- Sufficient communication and provision of information to patients
- Understanding of appropriate reimbursement issues

Complex new developments and changes have added a difficult gray zone to our understanding of medical ethics. These include the following:

- The devaluation of medicine from a *profession* or *guild* and its reemergence as a trade
- Increasing regulation by the government of physicians' practices; for example, new laws such as the Health Insurance Portability and Accountability Act (HIPAA) and the Emergency Medical Treatment and Active Labor Act (EMTALA)
- The activist role of the business community in the economics of health care
- Public awareness of health care options and information
- The emergence of poorly controlled advertising as a primary marketing tool for health care providers
- The economic impact of managed care and capitation on health care decisions and on access to health care
- The threat of malpractice lawsuits and its impact on physicians' decisions and options
- The ethical complexities of clinical trials and experimentation and the need for a definition of informed consent for participants
- The importance of alternative medicine as a complement to traditional medicine
- The importance of gender, race, and generational differences on the delivery of health care
- The importance of organizational ethics and an appreciation of ethical concerns in other countries

CHAPTER 14

Ethics and the American Academy of Ophthalmology

The Academy maintains an Ethics Committee whose charge is to help articulate and uphold ethical standards in ophthalmic practice. This chapter introduces you to the composition, history, and ongoing efforts of this important Academy committee. The Principles and the Rules of the Code of Ethics are reprinted at the end of the chapter, to serve as a ready reference both while you read the rest of Part II and as you encounter ethical challenges in your practice.

The Ethics Committee and the Code of Ethics

The Ethics Committee reports to the Academy's Secretary for Ophthalmic Practice, except in disciplinary matters, when it reports directly to the Board of Trustees. The Committee is directed by a chair, a vice-chair, and an ethics program manager, with a complement of up to nine committee members total (see the box "Composition of the Ethics Committee").

Members are chosen for their representation of the broadest possible cross section of Academy membership. Current responsibilities of the Committee include:

- Teaching of ethics in formal and informal programs, including visits to residency programs
- Contributing to Academy policy development in matters of patient care and professional conduct
- Investigation and adjudication of complaints about a member, or other allegations of a member's malfeasance

These activities in education, policy development, and enforcement are guided by the Academy's Code of Ethics, as described below.

History of the Ethics Committee

Significant changes in ophthalmology have occurred in the past several decades, most notably a shift from inpatient to outpatient surgery, the rapid proliferation of new devices and technologies, and the wider offering of elective refractive procedures to the public. Aware of these changes in the practice environment, Academy members in 1979 un-

Composition of the Ethics Committee

The Administrative Procedures section of the Code of Ethics describes the composition of the Ethics Committee as follows:

The Committee. The Board of Trustees appoints at least five (5), but not more than nine (9), ophthalmologists who are Voting Fellows or Members of the Academy to serve three (3) year, staggered terms as members of the Ethics Committee. The Board of Trustees makes its appointments to the Committee from among respected ophthalmologists who will, to the extent practicable, assure that the Committee's composition is balanced as to relative age, diversity, and experience and as to the emphasis of the appointees upon practice, education, research, or other endeavors within ophthalmology.

ambiguously expressed a strong desire to develop and codify standards for ethical practice. In response, the Board of Trustees established a new Committee, naming Jerome W. Bettman, Sr, MD, as chair. The new Ethics Committee was charged with developing a Code of Ethics specific to ophthalmic practice. While the new Code was to be inspirational and educational (by analogy to existing codes such as that of the AMA), there was also a consensus that it should contain enforceable rules, with specific sanctions that could be levied against those found in violation.

Development, Structure, and Implementation of the Code of Ethics

To accomplish the goal of creating the Code of Ethics, local and national committees were set up to generate concepts that warranted inclusion in the Code. Because it was strongly believed that the Code must represent a consensus of the views of the membership on ethics for it to become maximally accepted, the Ethics Committee also sought direct input from the membership at several critical points as the document took shape. Throughout this process, all efforts were guided by a recognition that the primary purpose of the Code would be to protect each individual patient, with each article designed to guide ophthalmologists in respecting and advancing the individual patient's best interests.

The Code was developed in three sections. The *Principles of Ethics* were intended to be general, aspirational standards of exemplary conduct. The *Rules of Ethics* were to be more specific, mandatory, and directive standards of minimally acceptable conduct. Lastly, the *Administrative Procedures* described the structure of the Committee itself, its operation, and the detailed procedures for enforcement of the Code (including guidelines for conducting investigations and hearings), as well as a system of appeals in the event of findings of Code violations.

The draft Code of Ethics was submitted to the FTC to ensure that it minimized the potential for conflicts with federal antitrust law, a concern inherent in a document that might be used to restrict or limit members' actions. Negotiations with the FTC continued for about a year, with approval granted in June of 1983. Securing this approval distinguished the Academy as the first organization of its kind to obtain an FTC Advisory Opinion for a professional code of ethics, an endorsement critical to the legitimacy of any future enforcement action. The Code was subsequently approved by the Academy Board of Directors and the membership in November of 1983 and became effective January 1, 1984. The current document applies to all Academy Fellows and Members and must be accepted as a condition for membership in the Academy.

The Current Code of Ethics—A "Living" Document

Since its initial approval, the Code has undergone revisions to accommodate and adapt to changes in health care as they have arisen. For example, with the advent of managed care, it became necessary to add to the existing prohibition against overproviding services that it is also unethical to withhold necessary services, a potential abuse that was not common before capitation and similar arrangements. Although changes have been infrequent, the Code remains a "living" document through the publishing of supplementary formal Advisory Opinions as guides for applying or interpreting the Rules in specific situations. The need for a new Advisory Opinion may be prompted by an important inquiry from a member, or by a recurring problem or pattern being identified in case submissions. The Advisory Opinions are reviewed periodically, with modification or retirement as necessary. Although the Code has almost exclusively concerned patient care issues, in 2004 a new Rule (Rule 16) became effective, which governs a nonclinical activity of some members: expert witness testimony (see the box "Expert Testimony Rule").

Additional Committee Activities

After reading the Code and the Administrative Procedures, it is easy to assume that investigation and adjudication of complaints is the primary function of the Ethics Committee. On the contrary, policing members, while important, is not the most effective method of meeting the long-term goal of encouraging ethical and professional practice. Instead, it is preferable to help the profession understand and voluntarily meet its ethical responsibilities, rather than to modify behavior through threat of sanctions. To this end, the Committee continuously introduces and revises educational materials and disseminates them in a variety of ways. Advisory Opinions on specific issues are available through the Academy office or web site. Courses are offered at the Annual Meeting addressing current issues, and the Breakfast with Experts program is popular as an interactive conversation on ethics topics. In addition to these offerings, the Academy's Online Ethics Courses and the Ethics Audio CD Courses can be used to satisfy specialty board recertification and continuing medical education (CME) requirements.

Expert Testimony Rule

Rule 16, the latest to be added to the Academy Code of Ethics, reads as follows:

Expert testimony should be provided in an objective manner using medical knowledge to form expert medical opinions. Nonmedical factors (such as solicitation of business from attorneys, competition with other physicians, and personal bias unrelated to professional expertise) should not bias testimony. It is unethical for a physician to accept compensation that is contingent upon the outcome of litigation. False, deceptive, or misleading expert testimony is unethical.

Because "an ounce of prevention is worth a pound of cure," the Committee also supports and endorses the mandate of the Accreditation Council for Graduate Medical Education (ACGME) for residency programs to include ethics in their formal curriculum. The Committee's text, *The Ethical Ophthalmologist: A Primer,* was widely used from 1993 to the initial date of publication of this *Basic and Clinical Science Course* companion volume. The Ethics Education Lecture Program brings ethics education to residency programs (see the box "The Ethics Education Lecture Program").

Members of the Ethics Committee remain alert to ethical issues that arise in their own diverse practice settings and share this information among themselves informally. Their observations help the Academy to recognize emerging contemporary ethical issues and to be better prepared to develop effective policies as these issues evolve.

What the Committee Cannot Do

Despite all its effort, the Ethics Committee regularly receives submissions related to potentially unethical conduct. The current case volume is approximately 100–150 cases per year. Because complaints have both factual and emotional aspects, concerned members may be disappointed when the Committee fails to act swiftly against "obvious" wrongdoing. Because of the importance of being fair to all involved, administrative procedures often appear time-consuming, cumbersome, and occasionally expensive. Experience has shown that this system works best if the language of the Code is interpreted and applied quite literally, with analysis of evidence from all sides of a complaint analogous to a legal proceeding. Occasionally, a "dispute resolution" approach is more effective than an adversarial approach. Although it can be frustrating, the Committee cannot take action in response to certain kinds of complaints (such as those relating to distasteful advertising) that may offend aesthetics, but not ethics, as specifically defined in the Code.

If, after careful case review and a hearing, a member is found to be in violation of a specific provision of the Code, a Committee recommendation for sanctions is referred to the Board of Trustees. The maximal sanction is permanent dismissal from the Academy, with lesser sanctions such as suspension or letters of reprimand also possible. In some cases, ethics investigations will parallel civil or criminal state or federal legal proceedings. Although findings of the Academy can be made public at the discretion of the Board, a case record is otherwise confidential and protected as a peer review action under California law.

The Ethics Education Lecture Program

The Academy's Ethics Committee offers a complimentary ethics lecture designed as an educational tool. This lecture program is made possible in part by sponsorship from Alcon Laboratories, Inc. The individual lectures focus on topics selected by residents and program directors, such as the basic tenets of medical ethics, professionalism, co-management, government regulation, and the development of various codes of ethics. The lecture program also uses case studies to stimulate practice problem solving and to promote awareness on the part of those participating in the learning process.

Making Submissions to the Ethics Committee

Inquiries (general questions) may be considered without regard to their means or form of submission. *Challenges* (complaints about member ophthalmologists) relating to information not in the public domain are not considered unless they are submitted in writing and signed by the submitter(s). Challenges unrelated to a Fellow or Member of the Academy are not within the Ethics Committee's purview. Inquiries or challenges may be submitted by ophthalmologists (whether or not they are Fellows or Members of the Academy), other physicians, health care institutions, health care reimbursers, allied health professionals, patients, patients' families, or organizations representing any of these. Send submissions to: The Ethics Committee, American Academy of Ophthalmology, P.O. Box 7424, San Francisco, CA 94120.

Summary

The Ethics Committee, through education, policy development, and enforcement of a carefully crafted Code of Ethics, works toward the goal of rendering investigations and sanctions unnecessary. In the meantime, all of these activities, including the investigation of ethics violations, remain a focus for the dedicated volunteer members of the Academy's Ethics Committee. The box "Making Submissions to the Ethics Committee" describes the procedure for reporting potential ethical violations and requesting an investigation by the Committee.

The Code of Ethics

The Academy's Code of Ethics is applicable to all Academy Fellows and Members (see the box "The Code of Ethics"). However, the Academy's Code is only one set of ethical standards. Violations of the Code should not give rise to a legal cause of action, nor should they create a presumption that any legal duty has been breached. The Code of Ethics, and the Advisory Opinions and Policy Statements issued under it, are designed to provide ethical guidance, not to define legal liability. Moreover, in considering what constitutes appropriate conduct, ophthalmologists should consider not only the Code of Ethics, but also applicable laws, institutional rules, and their own sense of conscience and good medical practice. The ultimate goal of the ophthalmologist's practice—and of the Code of Ethics—is to advance the best interests of the patient.

The Code of Ethics consists of three parts: (1) the *Principles of Ethics,* which are aspirational norms toward which all Academy members are encouraged to strive; (2) the *Rules of Ethics,* which are mandatory and require compliance by all Academy Fellows and

✓ The Code of Ethics

The Code of Ethics of the American Academy of Ophthalmology applies to the American Academy of Ophthalmology and to its Fellows and Members, and is enforceable by the American Academy of Ophthalmology. (Source: The Preamble of the Code of Ethics.)

Members; and (3) the *Administrative Procedures,* which govern the functioning of the Academy's Ethics Committee and the handling of submissions to the Committee related to the Code of Ethics. The Code of Ethics is reproduced here to enable easy reference for students and practitioners alike. The entire Code is also available online at the Academy's web site (www.aao.org).

A. Principles of Ethics

The Principles of Ethics form the first part of this Code of Ethics. They are aspirational and inspirational model standards of exemplary professional conduct for all Fellows or Members of the Academy in any class of membership. They serve as goals for which Academy Fellows and Members should constantly strive. The Principles of Ethics are not enforceable.

1. Ethics in Ophthalmology. Ethics address conduct and relate to what behavior is appropriate or inappropriate, as reasonably determined by the entity setting the ethical standards. An issue of ethics in ophthalmology is resolved by the determination that the best interests of patients are served.

2. Providing Ophthalmological Services. Ophthalmological services must be provided with compassion, respect for human dignity, honesty, and integrity.

3. Competence of the Ophthalmologist. An ophthalmologist must maintain competence. Competence can never be totally comprehensive, and therefore must be supplemented by other colleagues when indicated. Competence involves technical ability, cognitive knowledge, and ethical concerns for the patient. Competence includes having adequate and proper knowledge to make a professionally appropriate and acceptable decision regarding the patient's management.

4. Communication with the Patient. Open communication with the patient is essential. Patient confidences must be safeguarded within the constraints of the law.

5. Fees for Ophthalmological Services. Fees for ophthalmological services must not exploit patients or others who pay for the services.

6. Corrective Action. If a member has a reasonable basis for believing that another person has deviated from professionally accepted standards in a manner that adversely affects patient care or from the Rules of Ethics, the member should attempt to prevent the continuation of this conduct. This is best done by communicating directly with the other person. When that action is ineffective or is not feasible, the member has a responsibility to refer the matter to the appropriate authorities and to cooperate with those authorities in their professional and legal efforts to prevent the continuation of the conduct.

7. An Ophthalmologist's Responsibility. It is the responsibility of an ophthalmologist to act in the best interest of the patient.

B. Rules of Ethics

The Rules of Ethics form the second part of this Code of Ethics. They are mandatory and descriptive standards of minimally acceptable professional conduct for all Fellows or Members of the Academy in any class of membership. The Rules of Ethics are enforceable.

1. Competence. An ophthalmologist is a physician who is educated and trained to provide medical and surgical care of the eyes and related structures. An ophthalmologist should perform only those procedures in which the ophthalmologist is competent by virtue of specific training or experience or is assisted by one who is. An ophthalmologist must not misrepresent credentials, training, experience, ability, or results.

(cont.)

2. Informed Consent. The performance of medical or surgical procedures shall be preceded by appropriate informed consent.

3. Clinical Trials and Investigative Procedures. Use of clinical trials or investigative procedures shall be approved by adequate review mechanisms. Clinical trials and investigative procedures are those conducted to develop adequate information on which to base prognostic or therapeutic decisions or to determine etiology or pathogenesis, in circumstances in which insufficient information exists. Appropriate informed consent for these procedures must recognize their special nature and ramifications.

4. Other Opinions. The patient's request for additional opinion(s) shall be respected. Consultation(s) shall be obtained if required by the condition.

5. The Impaired Ophthalmologist. A physically, mentally, or emotionally impaired ophthalmologist should withdraw from those aspects of practice affected by the impairment. If an impaired ophthalmologist does not cease inappropriate behavior, it is the duty of other ophthalmologists who know of the impairment to take action to attempt to assure correction of the situation. This may involve a wide range of remedial actions.

6. Pretreatment Assessment. Treatment shall be recommended only after a careful consideration of the patient's physical, social, emotional, and occupational needs. The ophthalmologist must evaluate the patient and assure that the evaluation accurately documents the ophthalmic findings and the indications for treatment. Recommendation of unnecessary treatment or withholding of necessary treatment is unethical.

7. Delegation of Services. Delegation is the use of auxiliary health care personnel to provide eye care services for which the ophthalmologist is responsible. An ophthalmologist must not delegate to an auxiliary those aspects of eye care within the unique competence of the ophthalmologist (which do not include those permitted by law to be performed by auxiliaries). When other aspects of eye care for which the ophthalmologist is responsible are delegated to an auxiliary, the auxiliary must be qualified and adequately supervised. An ophthalmologist may make different arrangements for the delegation of eye care in special circumstances, so long as the patient's welfare and rights are the primary considerations.

8. Postoperative Care. The providing of postoperative eye care until the patient has recovered is integral to patient management. The operating ophthalmologist should provide those aspects of postoperative eye care within the unique competence of the ophthalmologist (which do not include those permitted by law to be performed by auxiliaries). Otherwise, the operating ophthalmologist must make arrangements before surgery for referral of the patient to another ophthalmologist, with the patient's approval and that of the other ophthalmologist. The operating ophthalmologist may make different arrangements for the provision of those aspects of postoperative eye care within the unique competence of the ophthalmologist in special circumstances, such as emergencies or when no ophthalmologist is available, so long as the patient's welfare and rights are the primary considerations. Fees should reflect postoperative eye care arrangements with advance disclosure to the patient.

9. Medical and Surgical Procedures. An ophthalmologist must not misrepresent the service that is performed or the charges made for that service.

(cont.)

(cont.)

10. Procedures and Materials. Ophthalmologists should order only those laboratory procedures, optical devices, or pharmacological agents that are in the best interest of the patient. Ordering unnecessary procedures or materials or withholding necessary procedures or materials is unethical.

11. Commercial Relationships. An ophthalmologist's clinical judgment and practice must not be affected by economic interest in, commitment to, or benefit from professionally related commercial enterprises.

12. Communications to Colleagues. Communications to colleagues must be accurate and truthful.

13. Communications to the Public. Communications to the public must be accurate. They must not convey false, untrue, deceptive, or misleading information through statements, testimonials, photographs, graphics, or other means. They must not omit material information without which the communications would be deceptive. Communications must not appeal to an individual's anxiety in an excessive or unfair way; and they must not create unjustified expectations of results. If communications refer to benefits or other attributes of ophthalmic procedures that involve significant risks, realistic assessments of their safety and efficacy must also be included, as well as the availability of alternatives and, where necessary to avoid deception, descriptions and/or assessments of the benefits or other attributes of those alternatives. Communications must not misrepresent an ophthalmologist's credentials, training, experience, or ability, and must not contain material claims of superiority that cannot be substantiated. If a communication results from payment by an ophthalmologist, this must be disclosed unless the nature, format, or medium makes it apparent.

14. Interrelations Between Ophthalmologists. Interrelations between ophthalmologists must be conducted in a manner that advances the best interests of the patient, including the sharing of relevant information.

15. Conflict of Interest. A conflict of interest exists when professional judgment concerning the well-being of the patient has a reasonable chance of being influenced by other interests of the provider. Disclosure of a conflict of interest is required in communications to patients, the public, and colleagues.

16. Expert Testimony. Expert testimony should be provided in an objective manner using medical knowledge to form expert medical opinions. Nonmedical factors (such as solicitation of business from attorneys, competition with other physicians, and personal bias unrelated to professional expertise) should not bias testimony. It is unethical for a physician to accept compensation that is contingent upon the outcome of litigation. False, deceptive, or misleading expert testimony is unethical.

C. Administrative Procedures *The Administrative Procedures of the Code of Ethics, which comprise the third part of the Code, are not reprinted here in full, but can be accessed on the Academy's web site (www.aao.org). Significant parts of the Administrative Procedures relating to sanctions that may be recommended by the Ethics Committee to the Board of Trustees and imposed by the Board upon members found to be in violation are printed here for reference.*

(c) Determination of Non-Observance. The Board of Trustees makes the determination whether a Fellow or Member of the Academy has failed to observe the Rules of Ethics in

(cont.)

this Code and imposes an appropriate sanction upon the recommendation of the Ethics Committee arising from a challenge and following an investigation. The Board of Trustees reviews the recommendation of the Committee based upon the record of the investigation. The Board of Trustees may accept, reject, or modify the Committee's recommendation, either with respect to the determination of non-observance or with respect to the sanction. If the Board of Trustees makes a determination of non-observance, this determination and the imposition of a sanction are promulgated by written notice to the affected Fellow or Member of the Academy and to the submitter of the challenge, if the submitter agrees in advance and in writing to maintain in confidence whatever portion of the information is not made public by the Board. Additional publication occurs only to the extent provided in the sanctions themselves. If the Board of Trustees does not make a determination of non-observance, the challenge is dismissed, with notice to the affected Fellow or Member and to the submitter of the challenge.

(d) Alternative Disposition. Before the Committee makes any recommendation to the Board of Trustees as to a determination that a Fellow or Member of the Academy has failed to observe the Rules of Ethics in this Code, the Committee may extend to the Fellow or Member an opportunity to submit a proposed alternative disposition of the matter in whole or in part upon terms and conditions suggested by the Ethics Committee. The terms and conditions may include sanctions and restrictions which are the same as, different from, or more or less restrictive than the sanctions contained in the following lettered paragraph, but shall in all cases include a written assurance by the Fellow or Member that the possible non-observance has been terminated and will not recur. The decision of the Ethics Committee on whether to extend such an opportunity is entirely within the Committee's own discretion, based upon its investigation of the challenge and upon its assessment of the nature and severity of the possible non-observance when viewed from the point of view of what is in the best interests of patients of the Fellow or Member of the Academy who is the subject of the challenge. If an opportunity to submit a proposed alternative disposition is extended by the Ethics Committee, an alternative disposition will be considered only if the Fellow or Member of the Academy submits to the Ethics Committee the proposed alternative disposition within thirty (30) days of the date of the Ethics Committee's notice to the Fellow or Member that it is extending such an opportunity. If the Fellow or Member timely submits a proposed alternative disposition that is accepted by the Board of Trustees and Ethics Committee, the matter shall be resolved on the basis of the alternative disposition, and notice shall be given to the submitter of the challenge, only if the submitter agrees in advance and in writing to maintain the information in confidence.

(e) Sanctions. Any of the following sanctions may be imposed by the Board of Trustees upon a Fellow or Member of the Academy who, the Board has determined, has failed to observe the Rules of Ethics in this Code, although the sanction applied must reasonably relate to the nature and severity of the non-observance, focusing upon reformation of the conduct of the Fellow or Member and deterrence of similar conduct by others:

(i) Reprimand to the Fellow or Member of the Academy, with publication of the determination and with or without publication (at the discretion of the Board of Trustees) of the Fellow's or Member's name;

(cont.)

(cont.)

(ii) Suspension of the Fellow or Member from the Academy for a designated period, with publication of the determination and with or without publication (at the discretion of the Board of Trustees) of the Fellow's or Member's name; or

(iii) Termination of the Fellow or Member from the Academy, with publication of the determination and of the Fellow's or Member's name.

In addition to and not in limitation of the foregoing, in any case in which the Board of Trustees determines that a Fellow or Member has failed to observe the Rules of Ethics, the Board of Trustees may impose the further sanction that the Fellow or Member shall not be entitled to sponsor, present, or participate in a lecture, poster, film, instruction course, panel, or exhibit booth at any meeting or program of or sponsored by the Academy (A) for a period of up to five (5) calendar years from and after the effective date a sanction described in clause (i) or (ii) of this paragraph 4(e) is imposed for the first time upon him or her, or (B) at any time from and after the effective date a sanction described in clause (i) or (ii) of this paragraph 4(e) is imposed for a second time upon him or her, or (C) at any time from and after the effective date a sanction described in clause (iii) of this paragraph 4(e) is imposed upon him or her.

Fellows or Members of the Academy who are suspended are deprived of all benefits and incidents of membership during the period of suspension, except continued participation in Academy insurance programs. If the Fellow or Member is suspended with publication of the Fellow's or Member's name or terminated, and the appeal (if any) sustains the determination on which the sanction is based, the Board of Trustees may authorize the Ethics Committee to communicate the determination and transfer a summary or the entire record of the proceeding on the challenge to an entity engaged in the administration of law or a governmental program or the regulation of the conduct of physicians, in a proceeding that relates to the subject matter of the challenge, provided, however, that the entity is a federal or state administrative department or agency, law enforcement agency, physician licensing authority, medical quality review board, professional peer review committee, or similar entity; and the Chairman of the Ethics Committee may appear if requested as a witness to that determination and record. Except in the instance of communication of the determination and transferal of the record, or in the instance of request of the record by the Fellow or Member of the Academy who was the subject of the challenge, the entire record, including the record of any appeal, is sealed by the Ethics Committee and the Board of Trustees and no part of it is communicated by the members of the Board of Trustees, the members of any appellate body, the members of the Ethics Committee, the staff or any others who assisted in the proceeding on the challenge, to any third parties. Fellows or Members of the Academy who are terminated may not reapply for membership in any class.

Lifelong Learning

The goal of continuing ethics education, and thus of this text, is to create self-awareness of our obligations and limitations that encourages a lifetime as a humane, caring physician. Ethics education does not guarantee a virtuous physician, though it can teach physicians to be intellectually capable of analyzing ethical dilemmas and capable of *acting* ethically when such dilemmas arise.

Practical Aspects of Lifelong Learning

The Accreditation Council for Graduate Medical Education (ACGME) mandates six competency areas, and individual training institutions define and provide the specific knowledge, skills, behaviors, and attitudes required to meet them. Specifically, residents must be able to demonstrate:

- *Patient care* that is compassionate, appropriate, and effective for the treatment of health problems and the promotion of health
- *Medical knowledge* about established and evolving biomedical, clinical, and cognate (eg, epidemiological and social-behavioral) sciences and the application of this knowledge to patient care
- *Practice-based learning and improvement* that involves investigation and evaluation of their own patient care, appraisal and assimilation of scientific evidence, and improvements in patient care
- *Interpersonal and communication skills* that result in effective information exchange and collaboration with patients, their families, and other health care professionals
- *Professionalism,* as manifested through commitment to carrying out professional responsibilities, *adherence to ethical principles,* and *sensitivity* to a diverse patient population
- *Systems-based practice,* as manifested by actions that demonstrate an awareness of and responsiveness to the larger context and system of health care and the ability to effectively call on system resources to provide care that is of optimal value

The American Board of Ophthalmology (ABO) is an independent, nonprofit organization responsible for certifying ophthalmologists. The certifying evaluation is designed to assess the knowledge, skills, and experience requisite for the delivery of high standards of patient care in ophthalmology. The ABO also administers the maintenance of certification (MOC) program. By the end of each decade of certification, ophthalmologists again must qualify by supplying the following:

- Evidence of professional standing
- Evaluation of practice performance
- Evidence of commitment to lifelong learning and self-assessment
- Evidence of cognitive expertise

The ACGME program competencies and the ABO MOC competencies stress the paramount need for specialists such as ophthalmologists to participate in lifelong continuing medical education (CME) activities and self-assessment as part of their ethical responsibilities as physicians. CME consists of educational activities that serve to maintain, develop, or increase the knowledge, skills, and professional performance and relationships that a physician uses to provide services to patients, the public, and the profession.

See the box "Standards and Resources for Continued Learning" for selected online sources of information.

Standards and Resources for Continued Learning

The following organizations are sources of information about continuing medical education for ophthalmologists:

- Accreditation Council for Graduate Medical Education, www.acgme.org
- American Board of Ophthalmology, www.abop.org
- American Academy of Ophthalmology, www.aao.org

CHAPTER 15

Practical Case Studies

The case studies in this chapter present real-life dilemmas that you, as either a trainee or a practicing ophthalmologist, may face during routine patient care. Although the situations are hypothetical and the names of the participants are fictitious, the central ethical issues in each of these cases have been culled from one or more actual submissions to the Academy Ethics Committee.

These cases discuss the nuances of ethical behavior in the context of the Academy's Code of Ethics (reproduced in Chapter 14). However, the cases should not be construed as determining definitively what constitutes proper conduct in any particular case and should not be used to define legal liability. Moreover, ophthalmologists should consider not only the Code of Ethics, but also applicable laws, institutional rules, and their own sense of conscience and good medical practice when confronted with ethical dilemmas.

Case Study 1

Informed Consent

Abstract

The process of informed consent involves the interplay of four elements: (1) disclosure, (2) comprehension, (3) competence, and (4) voluntary choice on the part of the patient. The following case considers these elements in detail.

Case Study

Mr. Bluder, a 63-year-old laborer with little education and only a fair command of English, visited Dr. Miles for an exam. When asked the reason for his visit, he explained to the doctor that over the previous 6 months he had noted his vision becoming a little less clear at distance, although he had no problem with the little reading he did. Television viewing gave him no problem either, and he reported being able to drive without difficulty.

Dr. Miles found the patient's best-corrected visual acuity to be 20/40 in the right eye and 20/30 in the left eye, with one line of improvement in each eye with a small change in prescription. He also found bilateral nuclear sclerosis that was consistent with the patient's vision. The remainder of the examination revealed no other ocular problems.

Dr. Miles told the patient he would see much better if the cataracts were removed and mentioned that the surgery was a brief, safe procedure ("nothing to worry about") and that the longer he postponed the surgery, the more difficult and risky it would be. With his limited command of English, the patient didn't understand some of the terms the doctor was using, but believed the doctor knew what was best for him. He was uneasy questioning the authority of the learned physician, so he said "yes" when the doctor asked if he would like to have the surgery, even though he didn't feel significantly affected by the cataracts.

Mr. Bluder met with the surgical coordinator, who carried out a consent discussion, during which Mr. Bluder said very little. After that, an office technician performed the biometric studies. The coordinator gave Mr. Bluder some literature and a consent form to take home, read, and sign and asked him to bring the latter to the surgical facility the day of his procedure.

Discussion

The medical and surgical care of patients with cataracts has become a large part of many ophthalmic practices. With improvements in the surgical procedure, many patients with visual complaints from cataract can be treated earlier than in the past, and success rates are high. However, modern cataract surgery still involves significant risk, and not all cataracts have to be removed.

In the case presented, the patient did not complain of any disability due to his vision and came in for only minor symptoms. He was able to carry out his activities of daily living well. When and how to suggest surgical or medical remediation should depend on the medical condition and how it affects the patient, and on whether treating it will have some beneficial effect for the patient.

Physicians are trained to do what they can to make their patients better; ophthalmologists constantly try to improve and retain their patients' vision. However, when patients see adequately for their needs, the ophthalmologist must consider whether or not to recommend and perform a procedure solely because it might improve vision further.

The term "informed consent" has been used since the 1950s, when the duty to inform the patient about the procedure became a legal requirement. It is based on the principle that the patient should know what a "reasonable" patient would want to know before proceeding with a treatment.

✓ Rule of Ethics 2. Informed Consent

The performance of medical or surgical procedures shall be preceded by appropriate informed consent.

Informed consent is not merely a document signed by the patient and the doctor listing the risks and benefits of a planned procedure. Even a brief explanation that the planned treatment will likely improve or maintain vision is inadequate; without a discussion of alternatives and of risks and benefits, and without the certainty that the patient understands the issues involved, the basic requirements of informed consent have not been met.

There is a consensus that the surgeon should be the person to present the basic information needed for informed consent for a procedure. In this view, the ophthalmologist must personally conduct and evaluate the informed consent discussion, to be certain the patient has received and understood the needed information before deciding whether or not to proceed with treatment.

Informed consent has both informational and consent components. The informational part comprises *disclosure* and *comprehension*. Disclosure involves informing the patient of what is to be done, and of anticipated benefits, possible risks, and reasonable alternatives to what is being suggested. Comprehension refers to the patient's ability to understand the implications of what has been disclosed.

Comprehension further involves *competence* and *voluntary choice*. Competence relates to the physician's determination that the patient is able to process the information well enough to make an informed decision. Without patient competence, the physician must consider involving an appropriate surrogate to aid in the process. The informed consent process is not complete until the patient, on the basis of the information given, voluntarily chooses how to proceed.

Case Study 2

Patient Care and Delegated Services

Abstract

Appropriate delegation of medical services allows for the efficient delivery of information and technology. However, there is a limit to appropriate delegation, which ensures that the physician–patient relationship and traditional practices, and their respective ethical values, are maintained and nurtured.

Case Study

Dr. McDonagh, an Academy Fellow, has developed a large practice over the years. In order to see more patients, he has worked hard at organizing his office efficiently and has developed what he calls "staged competence." By this he means that a patient entering the practice will meet a series of people with increasing levels of competence until the patient's problem is resolved. He employs technicians, optometrists, and fellows to manage the flow of patients. He is always available to answer questions, but he routinely sees patients only after the history and visual acuity have been taken, the refraction has been performed, the pupils have been evaluated, and the eyes are dilated. After Dr. McDonagh sees the patient, an assistant writes out any prescriptions or instructions and escorts the patient from the examining room.

Dr. McDonagh is particularly proud of two aspects of his practice. First, he has a collection of high-tech screening equipment, such as automated refractors, computerized guides to diagnosis, automated perimeters, and instruments for electronically evaluated testing of various other eye functions. He feels that these tools enhance the expertise of his practice and make it less likely that any mistakes will be made. The second cause of

Dr. McDonagh's pride is a personnel innovation: he has moved one of his senior ophthalmic assistants to the reception/telephone area to manage incoming calls, questions, and new patients so that they are seen in the most efficient and logical manner. In this way, emergency patients can be evaluated and seen immediately, while other patients are worked into the schedule as time and conditions allow.

Dr. McDonagh believes that his practice makes optimal use of his time, while giving maximum attention to the particular problems and concerns of his patients. He is deeply involved in developing a similar system for his surgical practice, but those plans are not yet ready for implementation. In preliminary meetings with the hospital's surgical review committee, Dr. McDonagh has met a great deal of resistance to these plans.

Discussion

The overriding concern in this case study is whether the welfare of the individual patient is being served by Dr. McDonagh's practice arrangement. Whether Dr. McDonagh's system of staged competence is an advance in the provision of services or is ethically questionable must be measured in terms of its effect on patient care and expectations both in the individual case and in the broader public sense of the public's perception of professional services.

This case study poses dilemmas for individual patients and the public, as well as questions of ethical responsibility for the physician and his profession. If medicine is perceived only as the efficient delivery of information and technology, then traditional practices, and the ethical values they respect, may be seen as inefficient. As ethical physicians, our goals are to understand and define that part of medicine that is neglected in the scenario above.

In recent years, society has accepted a role for nonphysician practitioners in health care; it is now rare for a physician to perform all of the tasks that may be required. The assumption is that physicians delegate certain aspects of care to nonphysician practitioners and technicians in the interest of efficiency. Although efficiency is increasingly essential for the economic viability of health care delivery, inappropriate delegation has the capacity to affect the traditional ethical underpinnings of health care.

Rule 7 of the Academy's Code of Ethics states that those aspects of eye care within the "unique competence of the ophthalmologist" may not be delegated. But how do we identify those aspects requiring unique competence? Without question, Dr. McDonagh is ultimately responsible for the quality of the care provided by his practice. Nor is there doubt that he is uniquely qualified within that facility to determine what is competent in terms of ophthalmic practice, since he is the only ophthalmologist involved. This managerial approach to medicine may be viewed as an attempt to increase the output of the ophthalmologist purely for monetary gain, or it may be seen as the most efficient use of the ophthalmologist's precious training and talent. The ultimate test, again, is patient welfare and acceptance.

In brief, Dr. McDonagh may have breached the canons of professional ethics if he has delegated aspects of eye care that fall within the unique competence of the ophthalmologist, or if his manner of practice compromises the quality of service offered to the patient. Another ethical issue involves Dr. McDonagh's motivation for introducing "staged competence." Was personal gain placed ahead of the patients' best interests? Dr.

McDonagh must examine his motives for his atypical behavior, and we must examine our motives in questioning his motives.

With respect to Dr. McDonagh's planned efficiencies for his surgical practice, the same ethical tenets hold true as noted above regarding his in-office patient management. Dr. McDonagh may not delegate aspects of eye care that fall within the unique competence of the ophthalmologist that are not permitted by law to be performed by others. His manner of practice may not compromise the quality of service offered to the patient.

✓ Rule of Ethics 7. Delegation of Services

Delegation is the use of auxiliary health care personnel to provide eye care services for which the ophthalmologist is responsible. An ophthalmologist must not delegate to an auxiliary those aspects of eye care within the unique competence of the ophthalmologist (which do not include those permitted by law to be performed by auxiliaries). When other aspects of eye care for which the ophthalmologist is responsible are delegated to an auxiliary, the auxiliary must be qualified and adequately supervised. An ophthalmologist may make different arrangements for the delegation of eye care in special circumstances, so long as the patient's welfare and rights are the primary considerations.

Delegation of authority is not only efficient, but often mandatory. It would be impossible for a single person to perform all the diagnostic and therapeutic tasks required in the care of a patient, even if the physician devoted the entire practice to the needs of one individual. In the strictest sense, delegation of authority is implicit in the very information on the basis of which diagnostic and therapeutic decisions are made, because this information comes largely from outside the physician. Whether one chooses to diagnose and treat using traditional allopathic principles or using unconventional therapies, the patient is being managed according to guidelines probably not original with the physician. Nonetheless, the physician is still responsible for picking and choosing among competing theories, paradigms, and schools of thought for the good of the patient. Another example: the physician or surgeon routinely uses drugs and devices, such as intraocular lens implants, that would be impossible to manufacture within the practice. In a sense, manufacture of the drug or device has been delegated to an outsider, but the physician is still responsible for the choice of the producer and the product.

On a different scale are the daily problems of a private practice. It would be highly impractical for a busy physician to answer every phone call, although one could argue that the most competent person in a practice should do the telephone triage. In addition to handling public relations, the telephone receptionist performs an important medical function; it is this person who generally determines when and how the patient will be seen by the physician, possibly affecting the outcome of the physician's therapy. These considerations are so obvious as to be almost invisible. Without doubt, the physician delegates a great deal of authority to the telephone receptionist, but the physician must be responsible for the actions of that individual.

Any practice will have occasion to send patients and specimens to a technician or laboratory for information or services that cannot be provided on site. In these instances the physician is, in effect, delegating the authority to perform the tasks necessary to obtain the desired information or accomplish the requested service. The outside laboratory or service no doubt has its own professional and ethical obligations to the patient, but the physician still carries the ongoing responsibility for the referral and for the welfare of the patient.

When a physician refers a patient to obtain the expertise of a medical consultant, the physician's responsibility probably ends with due diligence in the referral; the physician's expertise cannot extend to all matters. On the other hand, when the physician refers to a party not under her or his personal control whose competence level is below that of the physician, responsibilities may shift. For example, a physician may arrange for a patient from a distant town to be seen by a local family practitioner or optometrist for the limited purpose of determining the intraocular pressure or the presence of a deep anterior chamber after glaucoma surgery. If the medical service is provided with competence and is the best or only means of caring for the patient, there should be little complaint. However, the referring physician still bears responsibility—certainly for the decision to refer and for the referral itself.

Case Study 3

Ophthalmic Co-Management

Abstract

The co-management of ophthalmic surgical patients is defined as the sharing of postoperative responsibilities between the operating surgeon and another health care provider. What are appropriate guidelines as to when this practice is ethical and proper and when it is unethical or even illegal?

Case Study

You are a young ophthalmologist who is starting a new practice in a large city in which you have never lived. In order to become more involved with the community you join a local religious group. At the first meeting you are introduced, and several individuals approach you for your professional card. One person asks to speak with you privately and you agree to meet. That person presents the opportunity to align yourself with several optometrists who also belong to the same religious group and who would like to help you get started in the community.

You meet with the optometrists to discuss the details of the co-management relationship. They would agree to send you all of their surgical cases and, where appropriate, would be allowed to bill for the pertinent pre- and postoperative care.

Discussion

Before entering into a co-management relationship it is important for the ophthalmologist to understand the ethical and legal considerations. Co-management can be defined as delegation of patient care services related to surgery: the surgeon arranges for certain aspects of pre- and/or postoperative care to be delivered by another health care provider (typically another ophthalmologist or an optometrist). These arrangements are not unethical per se; however, ethical and legal concerns arise when fees are divided between providers and/or when referral networks are established. Rule 7, Delegation of Services, of the Code of Ethics allows for the sharing of eye care when the competence of those providing the services is appropriate. An essential point in such sharing of patient care is that all providers of care must be competent in the aspects of care they provide. This sharing of patient care remains the responsibility of the operating surgeon, and therefore the surgeon must supervise all aspects of care and be the "captain of the ship."

✓ Rule of Ethics 7. Delegation of Services

Delegation is the use of auxiliary health care personnel to provide eye care services for which the ophthalmologist is responsible. An ophthalmologist must not delegate to an auxiliary those aspects of eye care within the unique competence of the ophthalmologist (which do not include those permitted by law to be performed by auxiliaries). When other aspects of eye care for which the ophthalmologist is responsible are delegated to an auxiliary, the auxiliary must be qualified and adequately supervised. An ophthalmologist may make different arrangements for the delegation of eye care in special circumstances, so long as the patient's welfare and rights are the primary considerations.

Some of the ethical tenets that relate specifically to co-management arrangements are autonomy, justice, benevolence, and agency.

Autonomy

Autonomy can be defined as the patient's ability to choose without coercion and in an informed manner. It is essential to a philosophic and legal basis for informed consent. Autonomy can be circumvented in co-management either by physician manipulation of the patient (ie, not telling the truth) or by not doing what is in the patient's best interest. Co-management has always existed in medicine; in fact, it is a basic tenet of medical ethics to seek the help of a colleague. Physicians often ask colleagues to help with a case, but there is no systematic transfer of money that relates to this assistance. What may be unique with some of the new co-management arrangements is the blatant "commodification" (turning patients into commodities) that disturbs and distorts the patient–doctor relationship with money. The exchange of money does change behavior, and it is doubtful that establishing referral networks based on an economic relationship will improve a clinician's ethical judgment or encourage the clinician to act in the patient's best interest. Instead, it creates a conflict of interest. Respect for patient and physician autonomy must be preserved for the integrity of the profession.

Justice

Justice can be defined rather simply as fairness. It is hard to imagine that any patient would want care rendered by a less-qualified provider. It is more likely that if the patient were given the choice, he or she would prefer to have the necessary postoperative care provided by the operating surgeon. "Even the veiled attempts to persuade patients that they would have to travel less or that the referring health care provider knows the patient better, frequently fail an ethical examination. Although the patient may be deceived by the apparent common sense or logic of a referral that has an undisclosed economic basis, the ethics required for the doctor–patient relationship is violated" (Packer S, Lynch J. Ethics of co-management. *Arch Ophthalmol.* 2002;120:71–76).

Benevolence

Benevolence can be defined as acting in the patient's best interests. Our covenant with society mandates that we, as professionals, must be trustworthy and self-effacing, that is, we must do what is best for the patient. If it is clear that patients are being manipulated for financial gain, the physician(s) and health care provider(s) involved are not acting with benevolence and are not acting as professionals.

Agency

The "agent" can be defined as the role the physician plays in helping the patient through the complex medical environment. A patient seeks medical care with the understanding that the physician will act as the agent. Patients are vulnerable because they do not have all the knowledge needed to make informed decisions about their medical care. The physician has an obligation to act as the patient's agent and to obtain the most appropriate care. This obligation would be interfered with if there were a conflict of interest. Co-management that is financially motivated induces a conflict of interest and eliminates the trust that is required because of the patient's vulnerability and that serves as the foundation for the doctor–patient relationship. The mere disclosure of a conflict of interest is often inadequate because the patient is in a vulnerable position and therefore expects that a physician can be trusted.

Summary

It is important to recognize those circumstances where co-management is both legal and ethical. These include the following:

- When the operating surgeon is going on a leave of absence immediately after the surgery and the patient's postoperative care has to be managed by another physician
- When the beneficiary is unable to travel the distance to the surgeon's office for postoperative care visits
- When the patient voluntarily wishes to be followed postoperatively by another provider
- When the care is provided in a health professional shortage area (HPSA) and the beneficiary is unable to travel to the surgeon's office

The Joint Position Paper of the American Academy of Ophthalmology and the American Society of Cataract and Refractive Surgery that examines the role of co-management of ophthalmic surgical patients states that ". . . the AMA and the American College of

Surgeons have [also] issued guidelines addressing this issue, agreeing that the operating surgeon has the responsibility for the postoperative care and disapproving if economic considerations drive the decision to transfer the care of a patient following surgery." (American Academy of Ophthalmology and American Society for Cataract and Refractive Surgery. Joint Position Paper. Ophthalmic Postoperative Care. 2002.) An additional concern is that perioperative care will be assigned to the "least-qualified" provider and that the surgeon (as a technician) will be limited to the operating room, thus further diminishing the profession in the minds of patients.

✓ Rule of Ethics 6. Pretreatment Assessment

Treatment shall be recommended only after a careful consideration of the patient's physical, social, emotional, and occupational needs. The ophthalmologist must evaluate the patient and assure that the evaluation accurately documents the ophthalmic findings and the indications for treatment. Recommendation of unnecessary treatment or withholding of necessary treatment is unethical.

✓ Rule of Ethics 8. Postoperative Care

The providing of postoperative eye care until the patient has recovered is integral to patient management. The operating ophthalmologist should provide those aspects of postoperative eye care within the unique competence of the ophthalmologist (which do not include those permitted by law to be performed by auxiliaries). Otherwise, the operating ophthalmologist must make arrangements before surgery for referral of the patient to another ophthalmologist, with the patient's approval and that of the other ophthalmologist. The operating ophthalmologist may make different arrangements for the provision of those aspects of postoperative eye care within the unique competence of the ophthalmologist in special circumstances, such as emergencies or when no ophthalmologist is available, so long as the patient's welfare and rights are the primary considerations. Fees should reflect postoperative eye care arrangements with advance disclosure to the patient.

What model does the profession of medicine and our society want? Do we want an entrepreneurial model, or an aspirational model that incorporates the classic triad of covenants (patient, society, and colleagues) and a promise of a fiduciary relationship? Our society is pluralistic, and there is a contrast between a society that is values based and one that is economically based. Co-management is a word for several different practices that now exist in ophthalmology. The consequence of our ethical position on co-management may have significant consequences that affect our relationship with patients, colleagues, and society. The recent iterations of co-management present several ethical dilemmas to which there may be several right answers. In analyzing this case, one must attempt to arrive at answers that are clear and consistent and that are good for the patient, for the ophthalmologist, for the profession of ophthalmology, and for our society.

Case Study 4

Gifts from Industry

Abstract

The pharmaceutical, device, and medical equipment industries serve society by funding research and development for new drugs and devices and by sponsoring medical education seminars and conferences. However, some of this largesse comes in the form of gifts directly to the physician, a practice that may not always be consistent with the accepted standards of medical ethics.

Case Study

A drug company representative approaches you to attend a weekend meeting at a local resort. There will be a 2-hour seminar on a new antibiotic that the company has just released. Speakers will be nationally recognized experts in the field of infectious diseases of the eye. All of the related expenses for you and your spouse, including coach airfare, transfers, meals, room, and a free spa treatment or a free round of golf, will be provided at the expense of the pharmaceutical company.

Discussion

The relationship between physicians and industry introduces ethical dilemmas that affect patient care and the role of a physician as a professional. Some questions to be considered before accepting such a generous offer include: Should I accept this gift? Is this a gift or merely a business transaction in which I will be expected to increase the sales of the new medication through changes in my prescribing habits? Why is this company so generous? Is it appropriate for me to take my spouse on this trip? Am I incurring an obligation to the drug company? Is this trip going to benefit my ability to care for my patients? Should I ask about the speakers' message and their financial relationship to the company? Rule 11 of the Academy's Code of Ethics addresses commercial relationships.

> ### ✓ Rule of Ethics 11. Commercial Relationships
>
> **An ophthalmologist's clinical judgment and practice must not be affected by economic interest in, commitment to, or benefit from professionally related commercial enterprises.**

It seems that this drug company's offer will result in substantial benefit to the doctor, in that the doctor and spouse will receive a free vacation. The ethical question to ask is: will this offer affect his or her clinical judgment, relationship with patients, and ability to act in patients' best interest?

Pharmaceutical companies have a recognized need to promote their products to both physicians and patients so that the company produces a profit. A public company has a primary fiduciary responsibility to its stockholders. There is a parallel duty for physicians to obtain information concerning medications, especially new medications, so as to be better able to care for their patients. The critical issue is the value and accuracy of the information that comes directly from the drug companies.

The rising cost of health care is in part due to the increasing cost of medications. Accordingly, the federal government and several medical organizations have tried to educate and regulate the marketing of medications. The government, through the Office of the Inspector General; industry, through the new PhRMA Code (available at PhRMA's web site, www.phrma.org); and medical organizations such as the American Medical Association and the American Board of Internal Medicine have all endeavored to foster a relationship between physicians and industry that allows industry to make a profit, and therefore to continue to be of benefit to society, while still allowing physicians to act in the best interests of their patients by avoiding conflicts of interest.

✓ Rule of Ethics 15. Conflict of Interest

A conflict of interest exists when professional judgment concerning the well-being of the patient has a reasonable chance of being influenced by other interests of the provider. Disclosure of a conflict of interest is required in communications to patients, the public, and colleagues.

The need for the physician to act as the patient's health care agent is critical to maintaining a trusting relationship with the patient. Patients enter the physician–patient relationship in a vulnerable state and do not expect to encounter conflicts of interests that may interfere with the provision of their medical eye care.

The commercialization of medicine has brought with it more financial interactions between physicians and industry. In communicating with physicians, drug company representatives are seeking to improve the corporation's financial status. It is this positive financial status that allows for funding for research and development of new medicines that will be of benefit to society.

The ability of a physician to interact with the pharmaceutical industry and not be influenced to act as an agent of the industry has been questioned by the medical profession. The egregious abuse of providing personal gifts to physicians as inducements has resulted in the need for both physicians and industry to abide by new regulations and guidelines. It remains to be seen whether these efforts will prove effective in protecting patients, society, and the profession.

A basic ethical concern in the relationship between physicians and industry is the maintenance of the doctor–patient relationship, that is, making sure that the vulnerability of the patient is not jeopardized by the financial influence of a drug company. The core value in the doctor–patient relationship is trust, and this trust is violated when a physician acts as the agent (overtly or covertly, consciously or unconsciously) of industry. Since most physicians are unaware of the influence that drug companies have on their behavior, it is necessary to educate physicians about preserving the relationships that serve as the foundation of the profession—our relationships with patients, colleagues, and society.

In order to place the issue of gifts from industry into perspective for the training or practicing ophthalmologist, the box reproduces an excerpt of the AMA's Policy Statement on "Gifts to Physicians from Industry," delineating recently approved guidelines.

Policy Statement: Gifts to Physicians from Industry (Excerpt)

To avoid the acceptance of inappropriate gifts, physicians should observe the following guidelines:

- Any gifts accepted by physicians individually should primarily entail a benefit to patients and should not be of substantial value. Accordingly, textbooks, modest meals, and other gifts are appropriate if they serve a genuine educational function. Cash payments should not be accepted. The use of drug samples for personal or family use is acceptable as long as these practices do not interfere with patient access to drug samples. It would not be acceptable for non-retired physicians to request free pharmaceuticals for personal use or use by family members.

- Individual gifts of minimal value are permissible as long as the gifts are related to the physician's work (e.g., pens and notepads).

- The Council on Ethical and Judicial Affairs defines a legitimate "conference" or "meeting" as any activity, held at an appropriate location, where (a) the gathering is primarily dedicated, in both time and effort, to promoting objective scientific and educational activities and discourse (one or more educational presentation(s) should be the highlight of the gathering), and (b) the main incentive for bringing attendees together is to further their knowledge on the topics being presented. An appropriate disclosure of financial support or conflict of interest should be made.

- Subsidies to underwrite the costs of continuing medical education conferences or professional meetings can contribute to the improvement of patient care and therefore are permissible. Since the giving of a subsidy directly to a physician by a company's representative may create a relationship that could influence the use of the company's products, any subsidy should be accepted by the conference's sponsor, who in turn can use the money to reduce the conference's registration fee. Payments to defray the costs of a conference should not be accepted directly from the company by the physicians attending the conference.

- Subsidies from industry should not be accepted directly or indirectly to pay for the costs of travel, lodging, or other personal expenses of physicians attending conferences or meetings, nor should subsidies be accepted to compensate for the physician's time. Subsidies for hospitality should not be accepted outside of modest meals or social events held as part of a conference or meeting. It is appropriate for faculty at conferences or meetings to accept reasonable honoraria and to accept reimbursement for reasonable travel, lodging, and meal expenses. It is also appropriate for consultants who provide genuine services to receive reasonable compensation and to accept reimbursement for reasonable travel, lodging, and meal expenses. Token consulting or advisory arrangements cannot be used to justify the compensation of physicians for their time or their travel, lodging, and other out-of-pocket expenses.

- Scholarship or other special funds to permit medical students, residents, and fellows to attend carefully selected educational conferences may be permissible as long as the selection of students, residents, or fellows who will receive the funds is made by the academic or training institution. Carefully selected educational conferences are generally defined as the major educational, scientific, or policymaking meetings of national, regional, or specialty medical associations.

(cont.)

(cont.)

- No gifts should be accepted if there are strings attached. For example, physicians should not accept gifts if they are given in relation to the physician's prescribing practices. In addition, when companies underwrite medical conferences or lectures other than their own, responsibility for and control over the selection of content, faculty, educational methods, and materials should belong to the organizers of the conference or lectures.

Source: from the Council on Ethical and Judicial Affairs (CEJA), American Medical Association, Chicago, IL. Issued as an opinion by the Council on Ethical and Judicial Affairs of the American Medical Association, December 3, 1990, and updated in 1996 and 1998. After CEJA published its guidelines on gifts to physicians from industry in a 1991 issue of the *Journal of the American Medical Association*, it followed up with detailed answers to a number of requests for clarification (Addendum II). These clarifications are presented in question and answer format and are intended to help users of the guidelines better understand how they are to be applied. Send reprint requests to the American Medical Association, 515 N. State St., Chicago, IL 60610 or on the web (www.ama-assn.org).

Case Study 5

Expert Witness Testimony

Abstract

Physicians have an obligation to offer expert testimony in court on behalf of the plaintiff or the defendant. The testimony should be provided in an objective manner using medical knowledge to form expert medical opinions.

Case Study

Ms. Jones is a 44-year-old with high myopic astigmatism. She seeks a laser in situ keratomileusis (LASIK) consultation from Dr. Via, a busy anterior segment surgeon in the desert southwest. Ms. Jones is found to be a suitable candidate for the refractive procedure and has LASIK performed on the left eye first. Although state of the art at the time of surgery, the laser used does not have the tracking technology common in more recent machines. During the procedure, the patient admits to losing fixation, and a decentered ablation and poor acuity result. An enhancement procedure is performed several days later. Although the best-corrected visual acuity (BCVA) is 20/15, the final refraction is $+0.75 + 3.50 \times 101$ in the left eye compared with $-6.00 + 1.75 \times 74$ in the unoperated right eye.

The patient complains of headaches, diplopia, and loss of depth perception and seeks a second opinion from Dr. Bernard, a competing ophthalmologist on the other side of town. Dr. Bernard's office records later show that he successfully fitted the patient with a contact lens in the left eye and made plans to perform LASIK in the right eye.

In the meantime, Ms. Jones also seeks the advice of an attorney and decides to file a lawsuit seeking $1.5 million in punitive damages against Dr. Via, who performed the LASIK and enhancement procedures in the left eye. The law firm retains two expert witnesses: (1) Dr. Reed, a refractive surgeon who has testified on behalf of the firm against several doctors in previous malpractice suits; and (2) Dr. Bernard, the subsequent treating physician.

In testimony, Dr. Reed asserts that poor visual acuity from irregular astigmatism cannot be corrected even with a rigid contact lens and that the patient would only be able to see clearly if she wore two pairs of glasses simultaneously. Dr. Reed also claims to have read articles on treating decentered ablations in "throwaway" journals, but these articles are subsequently found not to exist.

Dr. Bernard claims in a deposition that he could not successfully fit the patient with a contact lens and that he did not schedule the patient for LASIK. This is contradicted by the office records that clearly document, "VA good with CLs . . . well-centered, minimal debris, good tear layer," and "Scheduled surgery: LASIK OD, goal: distance OD, OS."

At trial, Dr. Via is exonerated of all punitive charges. Based on her standard pre-operative contract promising satisfaction or your money back, Dr. Via is ordered to refund Ms. Jones the $2200 cost of surgery.

Despite the trial's favorable outcome for her, Dr. Via (who has practiced 15 years without a lawsuit) files a challenge with the Ethics Committee against both Drs. Bernard and Reed, accusing them of providing false and misleading expert witness testimony.

✓ Rule of Ethics 16. Expert Testimony

Expert testimony should be provided in an objective manner using medical knowledge to form expert medical opinions. Nonmedical factors (such as solicitation of business from attorneys, competition with other physicians, and personal bias unrelated to professional expertise) should not bias testimony. It is unethical for a physician to accept compensation that is contingent upon the outcome of litigation. False, deceptive, or misleading expert testimony is unethical.

Discussion

This case highlights two areas of problematic expert witness testimony. Dr. Reed is a "hired gun" who regularly testifies for this particular law firm despite not being uniquely qualified to testify against Dr. Via. She, in fact, gave inaccurate testimony when she stated that irregular astigmatism cannot be corrected with a rigid contact lens. She ignored peer-reviewed literature and textbook ophthalmologic teaching in making this assertion.

Dr. Bernard's testimony was inherently tainted because of his role as a subsequent provider of care (witness of fact). As an expert witness, he was, in effect, expected to review his own treatment of the plaintiff. This represented a direct and glaring conflict of interest.

Rule 16 is the most recent amendment to the Academy's Code of Ethics. It became effective January 1, 2004, and establishes the following:

- Expert testimony should be objective and based on medical knowledge.
- Nonmedical factors (solicitations from attorneys, competition with other physicians, and personal bias) should not influence testimony.
- It is unethical to accept compensation that is contingent on the outcome of a lawsuit.
- False, deceptive, or misleading expert witness testimony is unethical.

The interests of the public and the medical profession are best served when scientifically sound and unbiased expert witness testimony is readily available to plaintiffs and defendants in medical negligence suits. Without the experts' explanation of issues such as standard of care, causation, and physical disability, juries would not be able to distinguish malpractice (poor care) from maloccurrence (poor outcome).

Providing expert witness testimony is becoming increasingly common. Historically, expert witnesses enjoyed immunity from civil liability for anything they said on the witness stand. There is a growing perception, however, that this immunity has created an atmosphere in which physician experts are not being held accountable for what they say.

The original purpose of the use of expert witnesses was to provide accurate, unbiased testimony. In theory, this testimony would be so objective that it could be used by either party involved in the lawsuit. However, because an expert witness is compensated either by the plaintiff or by the defendant, the role of the expert witness is evolving from being an objective third party to being more of an advocate for the side that is paying the bill. This financial arrangement can create an inherent conflict of interest when the testimony given is presumed to be unbiased.

In an effort to curb irresponsible expert witness testimony, numerous physician organizations have adopted new ethical rules and established formal grievance procedures. Some have formed peer review boards and established tribunals to adjudicate expert witness allegations. It is important for physicians who provide expert witness services to understand the proper procedures and relevant legal issues and requirements before undertaking such work.

Case Study 6

Professional Marketing

Abstract

Fundamental principles of medical advertising require that communications to the public not be false, deceptive, or misleading, but there is more here than meets the eye. Ophthalmologists must be aware of the inherent pitfalls in advertising.

Case Study

Dr. Bennet is a well-respected cataract surgeon, with an expanding practice in a small southwestern city. On several occasions he has offered his services to a charitable organization, which transports him and other eye care professionals to less-developed countries to perform eye surgery for periods of a week at a time. Dr. Bennet has not published any papers in major journals, but he has lectured at CME seminars on three separate occasions. Generally, he lectures on his success with a particular brand of intraocular lens in cataract surgery, noting his low rate of postoperative complications. Although his practice is largely local, he occasionally operates on visitors from abroad, particularly from Latin America.

In order to build his practice, Dr. Bennet places advertisements in local newspapers each Sunday. The ads state, in part: "If you need cataract surgery, don't you want a top surgeon? Call Dr. Bennet, a surgeon who is famous around the United States and in many other countries. Dr. Bennet has pioneered certain advances in cataract surgery and has participated in several developments in the field. He has lectured on his accomplishments to medical groups across the country. You'll be in experienced hands." Another ophthalmologist in the same city has inquired whether this advertisement contravenes Rule 13, Communications to the Public, of the Academy's Code of Ethics.

✓ Rule of Ethics 13. Communications to the Public

Communications to the public must be accurate. They must not convey false, untrue, deceptive, or misleading information through statements, testimonials, photographs, graphics, or other means. They must not omit material information without which the communications would be deceptive. Communications must not appeal to an individual's anxiety in an excessive or unfair way; and they must not create unjustified expectations of results. If communications refer to benefits or other attributes of ophthalmic procedures that involve significant risks, realistic assessments of their safety and efficacy must also be included, as well as the availability of alternatives and, where necessary to avoid deception, descriptions and/or assessments of the benefits or other attributes of those alternatives. Communications must not misrepresent an ophthalmologist's credentials, training, experience, or ability, and must not contain material claims of superiority that cannot be substantiated. If a communication results from payment by an ophthalmologist, this must be disclosed unless the nature, format, or medium makes it apparent.

Discussion

This advertisement is misleading in several respects. Merely traveling extensively, presenting addresses at professional meetings, or treating patients from abroad does not mean that a physician has an international reputation. To so indicate is to use the inherent imprecision of the concept of fame to mislead patients. There can be little question that such claims are employed to give patients the impression that the surgeon meets some objective, high level of competence, skill, or recognition—which probably does not apply to this advertiser. The same is true of Dr. Bennet's claim to be a "top surgeon."

Saying that one has "pioneered advances in cataract surgery" is also deceptive in this case. Such a phrase clearly connotes a major breakthrough, not a minor alteration or refinement of a conventional procedure. Simply being one of many investigators for one type of IOL, or using a slightly refined surgical procedure, does not justify a hyperbolic term such as "pioneer." Since all surgery requires some degree of innovation, a surgeon cannot meaningfully claim to be an originator or developer of a technique or product simply because he or she has modified in some minor way what previously existed.

Use of the phrase "participated in several developments in the field" suffers from a different flaw. Read literally, it means almost nothing; its only purpose is to suggest an accomplishment where none exists. Obviously, every surgeon, by performing surgery and maintaining patient records, "participates in" the accumulation of information on which advances in surgical techniques are based—just as every human being contributes to the "evolution of mankind toward wisdom and progress." To advertise such phrases is misleading unless the ophthalmologist has personally contributed specific advances that have been adopted by colleagues. This does not appear to be true of Dr. Bennet. Thus, Dr. Bennet appears to have acted unethically by engaging in advertising that is designed to, and might well, deceive potential patients.

The threshold principle in medical advertising is that communications to the public must be accurate. This principle does not hold ophthalmologists or other professionals to an unrealistic standard, that they must never be wrong. The principle simply requires that communications to the public not be false, deceptive, or misleading.

Advertising informs the public about a product or service, disseminates information, and differentiates products and services and can in general be categorized as informational, educational, or laudatory. The dissemination of information is consistent with the aims of medicine; indeed, in many instances, it is the health care provider's responsibility to inform the public about the availability of particular services. On the other hand, advertising that is laudatory—that is designed to promote a product's superiority—often poses problems. Claims of superiority, uniqueness, or exclusivity may create conflicts between the physician's business interests and the best interests of patients.

The term *marketing* includes all business activity involved in the moving of goods from the producer to the consumer. Advertising in the broad sense is a part of the activity of marketing. Physicians must maintain constant vigilance that the ethical guidelines are being adhered to when determining the best way to market their medical practice. The way we advertise affects the public perception of us as professionals.

Standards of ethical medical practice established prior to the twentieth century prohibited advertising. In 1847, the AMA's code of medical ethics stated the following (with punctuation as shown in the original edition):

> It is derogatory to the dignity of the profession, to resort to public advertisements or private cards or handbills, inviting the attention of individuals affected with particular diseases, –publicly offering advice and medicine to the poor gratis, or promising radical cures or to publish cases and operations in the daily prints or suffer such publications to be made; -to invite, laymen to be present at operations,-to boast of cures and remedies,- to adduce certificates of skill and success, or to perform any other similar acts. These are the ordinary practices of empirics, and are highly reprehensible in a regular physician.

Advertising was not considered a highly respected undertaking for professionals even as recently as 1949, as illustrated by the World Medical Association Declaration of Geneva (see Chapter 16), which states, in part, that:

> A doctor must not allow himself to be influenced merely by motives of profit. The following practices are deemed unethical: . . . any self-advertisement except such as expressly authorized by the national code of medical ethics.
>   A doctor is advised to use great caution in publishing discoveries. The same applies to methods of treatment whose value is not recognized by the profession.

By 1957, strict opposition to advertising by medical professionals appeared to be weakening. In that year, the American Medical Association merely noted that physicians should not solicit patients. No direct reference to advertising was made.

The premise for advertising by medical professionals was provided by the Sherman Antitrust Act of 1890. This law led the way to allowing and even encouraging professionals to advertise. The Sherman Antitrust Act was designed to promote competition by discouraging monopolistic practices. Pellegrino noted that the Supreme Court's decisions "reflect and reinforce the growing antielitism, distrust of privileged groups and moral pluralism characteristic of American society" (Pellegrino ED. What is a profession? The ethical implications of the FTC order and some Supreme Court decisions. *Surv Ophthalmol.* 1984;29:221–225). In 1975, the Federal Trade Commission successfully sued the American Medical Association over the issue of restricting advertising through its code of ethics, and in 1977, it became unlawful for physicians to restrict advertising.

There is much useful information that may be included in an ethical professional marketing plan. Advertisements can communicate the physician's type of practice, professional society memberships, specialty board certification, office hours and location, and a description of services provided by the physician. Endorsements and patient testimonials should represent an average patient's experience, and any claims of safety and expected amount of pain require scientific evidence. Any representations made in an advertisement should be able to be substantiated to be included in an ethical marketing plan. Figure 15-1 shows inappropriately worded advertisements, then and now. The boxed directives on page 214 give specific guidance to keep in mind when writing advertising materials.

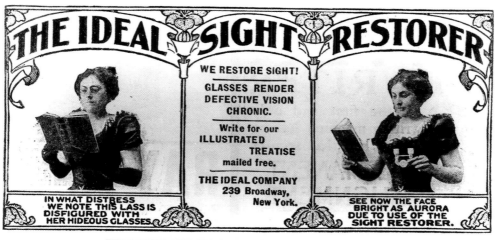

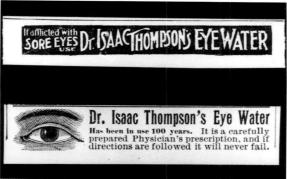

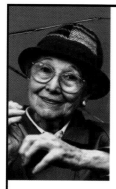

Miracle Eye Cure!

Getting older and going blind is not your only recourse!

Attend our **FREE** seminar to learn:

- How this new treatment reverses macular degeneration
- How your vision dramatically improves in 4 DAYS!
- Why your eye doctor doesn't know about this **miracle** eye cure
- That over 70% of patients have visual improvement

Call 123-678-0000

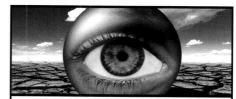

Our Gifts To You!

The Clear Natural Vision of LASIK and a Cashable Voucher Worth Up To $2,000!

- **LASIK is the preferred method for laser vision correction**
- **Lasers correct nearsightedness, farsightedness, and astigmatism**
- **Your vision can be corrected painlessly in just seconds at an affordable cost**

The Board-Certified ophthalmologists at the Midwest Regional Eye Institute are the most experienced and only eye doctors in the tri-state area with a VISX Star S3 "eye-tracking" laser.

Call 123-678-0000

Figure 15-1 Inappropriately worded advertisements, then and now.

Advertising Directives of the American Academy of Ophthalmology

- Communications must be accurate.
- Communications must not be deceptive.
- Communications should avoid appeals to anxieties and vulnerabilities of patients.
- Communications should not create unjustified expectations.
- Communications should provide a realistic assessment of risks, benefits, and alternatives.
- Communications should never misrepresent credentials.
- Communications should not make claims of superiority that cannot be objectively substantiated.
- All paid communications must be acknowledged.

Sources: American Academy of Ophthalmology: Code of Ethics, Rule of Ethics 13; Communications to the Public [Advisory Opinion], 1992 p. 3; *Ethics in Ophthalmology. A Practical Guide,* 1986; and Advertising Claims Containing Certain Potentially Misleading Phrases [Advisory Opinion] 1992, pp. 2–4.

Advertising Directives of the American Medical Association

Principles:

- Advertisements should not contain material false claims or misrepresentations of material fact. (Something is material if it would affect the behavior of the ordinary patient.)
- Advertisements should not contain material implied false claims or implied misrepresentations of material fact.
- There should not be omissions of material fact from advertisements.
- Physicians should be able to substantiate material claims and representations made in an advertisement.

Source: American Medical Association. Guidelines for Truthful Advertising of Physician Services. Issued April 1977, updated June 1996.

Case Study 7

Communications with Patients and Colleagues

Abstract

Physicians have a responsibility to one another and to their profession, but their first and foremost responsibility is to their patients. Constructive interactions help define and maintain performance standards, thus ensuring the provision of high-quality medical care.

Case Study

Dr. Welch refers a patient to Dr. Ruiz for help in the management of a postoperative surgical complication. The patient is a 40-year-old man who had a trabeculectomy performed 1 week earlier. According to a note from Dr. Welch, the patient's anterior chamber was very shallow on the first postoperative day, but no other problems were apparent. The day before the referral, the anterior chamber became even shallower, and now the chamber angle appears to be completely occluded and vision has declined. Dr. Welch's note requests Dr. Ruiz's evaluation of the patient to assist Dr. Welch in determining how she should proceed with the patient.

Dr. Ruiz examines the patient and concludes that surgery was properly performed. The anterior chamber is completely flat, and Dr. Ruiz believes that re-formation of the anterior chamber is the next appropriate step. He advises the patient in this regard and turns to pick up the phone to convey this information to Dr. Welch. At that point, the patient says, "Doctor Ruiz, I know you said that Doctor Welch didn't make any mistakes, but she did send me to you for your opinion, and that shows that you must know more and be more experienced in these cases than she is. I would like you to do the next surgery." Dr. Ruiz is concerned because Dr. Welch's note specifically requests a consultation and makes no mention of Dr. Ruiz's proceeding with surgery or any other treatment.

Discussion

This case describes a common dilemma for a consulting physician. The referring physician, Dr. Welch, has provided the patient with appropriate care and believes that it is in the patient's best interest to return to her for continuing treatment. The patient complicates the picture by stating that he wants the consulting physician, Dr. Ruiz, to continue his care in place of the referring physician.

Dr. Ruiz's primary responsibility is to the patient, but he also has obligations to himself, to the community, to the referring physician, and to the medical profession. If he simply accedes to the patient's request, he will no doubt alienate Dr. Welch, who will be reluctant to send patients to him for consultation and/or management in the future. This action may also dissuade other colleagues from referring patients to Dr. Ruiz.

✓ Rule of Ethics 4. Other Opinions

The patient's request for additional opinion(s) shall be respected. Consultation(s) shall be obtained if required by the condition.

An appropriate next step is for Dr. Ruiz to explain to the patient in more detail that he found no indication that Dr. Welch's treatment was improper and that referral was not an unfavorable comment on Dr. Welch's competence; rather, the request for a consultation was an appropriate action that he, Dr. Ruiz, frequently took himself. Also, the operating surgeon, Dr. Welch, knew the details of the surgical procedure as performed in this specific case better than he as a consulting physician and was in a better position to perform the re-operation. Therefore it would be in the patient's best interest to return to the referring doctor, Dr. Welch, for continuing care.

> ### ✓ Rule of Ethics 14. Interrelations Between Ophthalmologists
>
> **Interrelations between ophthalmologists must be conducted in a manner that advances the best interests of the patient, including the sharing of relevant information.**

If, at the end of the discussion, the patient still insists on having the next surgery performed by Dr. Ruiz because of lost confidence in Dr. Welch's abilities, Dr. Ruiz must proceed very carefully. One approach would be for Dr. Ruiz to explain that, although sympathetic to the patient's concerns, he did not believe them justified; that, for the patient's best interests he considered Dr. Welch to be the most appropriate surgeon to continue treatment; and that he (Dr. Ruiz) was not willing to perform the surgery.

The dilemma facing Dr. Ruiz is the balancing of the patient's right to autonomy against his own ethical obligation to do what is in the best interests of the patient. Although a competent patient has the right to decline recommended treatment, so, too, a physician has the right to decline compliance with a patient's request that he or she does not believe to be in the patient's best interests—particularly when other ethical obligations are involved, as in this case. The consulting physician may believe that the appropriate resolution in the present situation requires placing a greater weight on the principle of collegiality than on the principle of autonomy. In most cases, when a consulting physician reassures an anxious patient that the referring doctor has in fact performed competently and insists that it is in the patient's best interest to return to the referring doctor, the patient accepts the recommendation.

How could the uncomfortable situation described above have been avoided? One way would have been for Dr. Welch to discuss clearly with the patient why he was being referred and what she expected from Dr. Ruiz. The patient was being referred for a second opinion. Dr. Welch planned to proceed herself with the surgery that she believed Dr. Ruiz would recommend. If at that point the patient had told Dr. Welch that he really was quite discouraged and would prefer to have Dr. Ruiz perform any additional surgery, Dr. Welch could then reconsider whether Dr. Ruiz was the ideal person to perform the consultation. If she thought he was, she should have altered her referral note to indicate to Dr. Ruiz that if any further surgery was appropriate, she wished him to proceed.

Remarkably, most patients are *not* well informed as to why they are being referred. A comment such as "I want you to see Doctor Ruiz" is often all the patient is told. Frequently, the patient arrives at the consultant's office without a prior call or even an explanatory note. Not surprisingly, this type of referral leads to confusion and sometimes resentment. It does not respect either the autonomy of the patient or collegiality with fellow physicians. It does not promote good patient care or good relationships.

Collegiality is built on tradition and trust. One of the great traditions of medicine has been the passage of information from teacher to student and from colleague to colleague. When collegiality is subverted so that its purpose becomes the promotion of the power of the colleague, then collegiality becomes at least partially the enemy of the basic purpose of the profession. The tradition to be cherished, then, is not the exclusiveness with which the knowledge of the profession is maintained and passed from one generation to the next or from colleague to colleague, but rather the sharing of knowledge that will make it possible for colleagues to do a better job, that is, to take care of patients more competently.

A second aspect of relationships with colleagues that must be stressed has to do with honesty. Meaningful communication demands honesty. Where communications are not honest, they do not serve their primary purpose, which is to transmit and receive information in a way that allows both parties to understand each other better. With less than honest communication, it is certain that the best interest of the patient will not be served. Also, to work together effectively, colleagues must respect each other. If one physician believes that another is lying or withholding information, there can be no sense of mutual respect, and the collegial relationship breaks down.

Both professional ethics and professional etiquette are essential to the proper practice of medicine. Ethics (especially as it relates to collegiality) and etiquette, although easily confused with each other, are not the same thing. Both ethics and etiquette may incorrectly be considered to be methods used to promote the profession or the professional, sometimes at the cost of other people. Both do concern themselves with the integrity of the profession. Ethics, however, is a far more global term, relating to the fundamental, ongoing purpose of the medical profession, whereas etiquette describes more local and changeable codes of behavior.

Professional etiquette refers to the manners considered proper for a member of a professional group. The term may carry with it connotations of apparent superficiality, but professional etiquette is not unimportant. Even the relatively superficial aspects of behavior profoundly affect relationships. It is no mystery that the niceties of behavior are a consequential aspect of every group, including physicians. Etiquette is what makes day-to-day living pleasant and workable.

While ethics is also concerned with norms of behavior, at the basis of professional ethics is the question, "Is the behavior in the best interest of the patient?" Collegiality, as an aspect of professional ethics, is important because the profession as a group is usually a surer guide to what is in the best interest of the patient than the individual physician, who of necessity will be limited more severely by his or her own biases. The measure of professional etiquette is whether it enhances the well-being of the practitioner and the profession. The measure of professional ethics is whether it enhances the well-being of the patient.

Collegiality does not have to do with methods of protecting individual referrals or professional turf. Collegiality refers to the manner in which physicians relate to each other so as to ensure that patients will be cared for properly. Proper care requires that physicians work with each other, educate each other, and pass on to the new generation of physicians the knowledge and values, the science and the art, that they have found requisite to being of service to patients.

Collegiality is sometimes considered a matter of professional etiquette rather than a fundamental part of medical ethics and is often trivialized. When professional relationships are not characterized by collegiality, however, the patient suffers. Collegiality works not only to the benefit of the patient, the profession, and society; it also works to the benefit of the individual physician.

One tragic aspect of modern medical care is that physicians and physician groups are encouraged to compete with each other. It is now routine for physicians to refer to their fellow physicians as "competitors." Competitors are not likely to be colleagues; competitors try to promote themselves at the expense of the "opponent." Efforts are made to "beat" the competition by a variety of means: by providing a unique service, by presenting oneself as "the best," by calling oneself "a pioneer," by downgrading the competence of the competitor, or by making the offered service seem less expensive, such as by offering "free cataract extraction."

Competition among physicians can sometimes work in the best interest of the patient. When physicians know they will not be paid unless they provide care for patients, they will make efforts to make themselves available. When a system exists that remunerates physicians on the basis of the *quality of care* provided (measured in terms of outcomes such as patient satisfaction and incidence of surgical successes and failures), physicians will compete to provide the highest quality of care.

Thus it is not competition per se that is the villain, but rather the self-promotion, the deception, the ruses used to prey on vulnerable patients, and the gimmicks that divert attention from the proper purpose of medical care. These aspects of competition have become so routine that they are often not seen to be what they really are, that is, behavior that is primarily in the best interest of the provider rather than of the patient. The acceptance of self-promoting competition—rationalized and made acceptable by the now widely used term marketing—as the modus operandi of medical care is one of the great tragedies of medical history.

A major change in the medical profession has occurred. Regardless of the myth that advertising is supposed to provide information to help customers select the goods or services they want, the fact is that the purpose of almost all advertising is to create demand. The essence of advertising is competition. The antitrust laws, to which physicians are now subject, assume competitive behavior. Yet competition, as ordinarily defined, is the antithesis of collegiality. Behavior that has traditionally been considered proper for physicians may now actually be illegal. For example, it is necessary from an ethical point of view for the medical profession to try to modify the behavior of doctors that is considered inappropriate, such as setting excessive fees, but to do so might violate antitrust law. In today's environment, the physician may be required to choose between obeying federal law or professional canon, because they may now may be incompatible.

Case Study 8

The Learning Curve

Abstract

There are both ethical and practical aspects of learning new techniques. Ophthalmologists have responsibilities to patients, colleagues, and themselves with respect to learning new techniques or assimilating new modifications of familiar techniques.

Case Study

Dr. Flap is an experienced ophthalmologist who has been in an active surgical practice for approximately 10 years. Although he had some experience in corneal and refractive surgery when radial keratotomy was the best refractive surgical technique available, he has never done LASIK, and he wishes to add this procedure to the services he offers. He has read some consumer journal articles on LASIK technique, and he asks a colleague if he might use his laser facility to treat a patient. On surgery day, Dr. Flap has the patient sign a form attesting to her understanding of LASIK, and Dr. Flap, the patient, and a technician proceed to the operating room. The technician helps Dr. Flap through the procedure step by step, and although the preparations and intraoperative explanations are lengthy, both surgeon and patient manage well, and Dr. Flap's first LASIK is concluded without complication.

Discussion

The technology available to ophthalmologists continues to develop rapidly. It is usually not difficult for experienced ophthalmologists to assimilate new modifications of familiar techniques. Occasionally, however, new techniques require the development of skills that differ significantly from prior experience, and formal study, rather than a self-styled or haphazard approach, should be undertaken to achieve competence. Although recent literature addresses the learning curve in resident surgical experience, there has been less discussion about the established practitioner who wishes to learn a new technique. When a new technique is introduced, and especially if it is shown to be superior to an older one, its benefits should be available to patients. This creates a dilemma for the experienced ophthalmologist who is not facile with the newer technique. Since optimal care of the patient must be the foremost consideration, the ophthalmologist must decide whether to incorporate the new technique into his or her practice or to refer patients who would benefit from the new technique to colleagues who are already proficient. Ophthalmologists seldom elect to continue to offer only those procedures they learned in formal training. More likely, the ophthalmologist will want to learn new techniques. Ophthalmologists must also reflect upon their own careers, however, deciding whether the additional stress and disruption of learning a new technique is in their professional interest.

When the ophthalmologist decides to incorporate a new technique or technology into her or his practice, a commitment to formal study is strongly recommended. The extent of the formal study depends on the degree to which the new technique varies from previously learned skills. Suggested resources may include skills transfer courses, slide scripts, videotapes, self-assessment materials, the assistance of a skilled mentor, and the review of the first cases with a mentor. Appropriate patient selection is a particularly important factor in ensuring success with early cases, in building confidence in performing the technique, and in reducing the likelihood of complications. Patient selection should initially be made on the basis of anticipated technical difficulty. Patient personality should also be considered; patients who exert additional pressures through anxiety, impatience, or demanding personality style may not be suitable candidates.

> ✓ **Rule of Ethics 6. Pretreatment Assessment**
>
> **Treatment shall be recommended only after a careful consideration of the patient's physical, social, emotional, and occupational needs. The ophthalmologist must evaluate the patient and assure that the evaluation accurately documents the ophthalmic findings and the indications for treatment. Recommendation of unnecessary treatment or withholding of necessary treatment is unethical.**

Of special consideration is the process of providing appropriate informed consent. The ophthalmologist should disclose his or her level of experience both as a surgeon generally and with the new technique specifically. For incremental changes (eg, the transition from extracapsular cataract technique to phacoemulsification), an experienced surgeon can appropriately inform the patient that the learning involves modifying or improving a portion of an otherwise familiar procedure. For more comprehensive changes in technique, full disclosure, in the context of rapport with a trusting patient, is recommended. When discussing success rates for a given procedure, it may be appropriate to provide data from more experienced surgeons, provided, however, that the less-experienced surgeon does not imply that these success rates are necessarily his or her own. The patient should be made aware of the mentor's role, if any, as part of the surgical team.

> ✓ **Rule of Ethics 2. Informed Consent**
>
> **The performance of medical or surgical procedures shall be preceded by appropriate informed consent.**

The operating surgeon should carefully evaluate patients postoperatively during the learning period. In the event of a serious complication, appropriate disclosure to the patient is an ethical imperative, as is prompt management. A second opinion about management of the complication might be obtained from the mentor, or if complications are severe, referral for subspecialist care may be necessary depending on the problem and the desires of the patient. Dispassionate assessment and understanding of how a complication arose will help avoid future complications.

> ✓ **Rule of Ethics 8. Postoperative Care**
>
> **The providing of postoperative eye care until the patient has recovered is integral to patient management. The operating ophthalmologist should provide those aspects of postoperative eye care within the unique competence of the ophthalmologist (which do not include those permitted by law to be performed by auxiliaries). Otherwise, the operating ophthalmologist must make arrangements before surgery for referral of the patient to another ophthalmologist, with the patient's approval and that of the other ophthalmologist. The operating ophthalmologist may make**

different arrangements for the provision of those aspects of postoperative eye care within the unique competence of the ophthalmologist in special circumstances, such as emergencies or when no ophthalmologist is available, so long as the patient's welfare and rights are the primary considerations. Fees should reflect postoperative eye care arrangements with advance disclosure to the patient.

The ophthalmologist is ready to perform a new technique alone when sufficiently proficient. Typically, hospitals or ambulatory surgery centers have stringent guidelines governing the physician's qualification to perform new procedures; qualification is usually accomplished under the supervision of the department chief or medical director. For covered services, managed care entities may have their own guidelines, and these should be reviewed carefully.

A learning curve is an integral part of the acquisition of new skills, and all ophthalmologists work through this process at various stages in their careers. A careful, honest, and ethical approach will distinguish the competent ophthalmologist who is learning a new technique. The suggestions given here will help place the patient first, minimize the risk of complications, and allow the ophthalmologist to gain technical expertise with confidence.

Case Study 9

New Technology

Abstract

By definition, innovative therapies may not represent the standard of practice, and practitioners using a novel procedure must be careful to remain objective in their assessment of the procedure's safety and efficacy.

Case Study

Dr. Sand has practiced refractive surgery for some time, but for various reasons he has been frustrated by shortcomings of conventional refractive surgery procedures. Being innovative and imaginative, he has combined his knowledge of corneal surgery with his experience in contact lens manufacture to invent an alternative technology of his own invention, a rotating concave diamond burr that can reshape the cornea.

To develop his invention, Dr. Sand tests a prototype on experimental animals, in conjunction with a university animal laboratory. His data are promising, and he subsequently submits a proposal to the hospital institutional review board to proceed with clinical trials. With board approval, he then recruits patients who are monocularly blind from retinal disease, and after a detailed description of the research he has the patients sign a special informed consent that discloses the unconventional nature of the treatment. After performing his procedure in a small series, he becomes convinced that his instrument is not only equivalent, but superior to, current methods, and he submits his findings to a peer-reviewed journal. The journal expresses some interest but has some reservations that delay publication. While his manuscript is in review, the local newspaper and television news hear of his invention and interview him in the media about his device. Patients begin to ask about his procedure as an alternative to conventional surgery, believing the assertions that it offers advantages over current methods. Colleagues show interest as well, so Dr. Sand schedules informal classes for training in the procedure.

Discussion

The limitations of current therapies lead imaginative practitioners to develop new therapies with which to help patients. By definition, however, innovative therapies do not represent the standard of practice, and practitioners using novel procedures must be careful to remain objective in the investigation of their safety and efficacy. In evaluating Dr. Sand's activities, consider the following:

- How should a physician manage situations in which conventional therapies appear inadequate?
- Should a physician continue with a standard treatment, while believing that another approach is better or safer?
- If a physician believes that a standard therapy is outdated or harmful, should that assertion be taken directly to the public if professional channels resist?
- Is there a duty to protect the public from a new therapy, when a physician has doubts about its safety or efficacy?
- Should a new therapy be used for marketing?
- How should one respond when patients ask about unconventional therapies or ask to be referred for such therapy?

Dr. Sand, as well as his critics, may find guidance in the Academy Code of Ethics. The first concern is always patient welfare. This implies competent delivery of services to those desiring those services, after full disclosure of their nature. The profession must ensure that the services its members render are within these limits, which implies evaluation and control of aberrant practitioners to determine what is truly competent, effective, and in the best interest of each patient. Dr. Sand's work may be promising, but all clinical theories, therapies, and procedures must be considered experimental until validated. The conventional progression from theory to animal models to regulated clinical trials must be respected. Until such studies are complete and evaluated, patients and the public must be informed of the special nature and tentative status of any innovation. Therapies might be classified in a spectrum that includes "experimental," "investigational," "new standard," "established," and finally "outdated."

For investigational modalities, communications to the public should honestly portray the innovation as unproven or controversial. Marketing of an unproven therapy is dangerous to the public and to the profession, regardless of its popularity or the proponent's heartfelt conviction of its value. Mere assertions of value, or acceptance in the market, should never substitute for scientific evaluation.

Dr. Sand's refractive surgery concept may be sound, but it must be evaluated. He begins appropriately, although he soon strays from ethical principles as he shortcuts delays in peer review; as he begins to communicate directly to the public through the media; and especially when he trains colleagues in his procedure. Instructional courses would not be illegal, but there could be serious questions regarding the liability for instructing colleagues to do such a procedure, especially if a course is marketed and sold. In the event of another surgeon's subsequent complication, both the operating surgeon and the instructor may be found liable if the procedure was performed as taught. The instrument itself would need approval from the Food and Drug Administration (FDA).

It can be said that every great idea "begins as heresy and ends as superstition." The objective evaluation of current and new therapies is an integral part of medicine, although there will always be practitioners who inappropriately embrace the new, and those who blindly defend the old. Objective scrutiny of the value of innovation is both an individual and a collective professional responsibility. The license physicians have, both literally as a legal privilege and figuratively in the sense of the public's trust in us, is based on an understanding that the therapies we offer meet certain consensus standards. This functions much like a franchise: a customer of a particular franchise has expectations based on knowledge of that franchise. If the franchisee has idiosyncratic practices that depart too greatly from those of the franchise, expectations are not met, and both the franchise at large and the individual customer are dissatisfied. The physician is in a similar position: success in a medical practice is based to a large degree on the public perception of the profession, rather than exclusively on the personal acquaintance of the patient with the practitioner. It is therefore beneficial to both the profession and the patient that the physician does not damage the reputation of the profession by straying too far from consensus practice. The public assumes that it will receive services that reflect the image and beliefs of the profession. In addition, the public expects other physicians to exert pressure on the practitioner, who is privileged with the imprimatur of the profession, to maintain some reasonable level of quality control.

The physician who has an unorthodox idea must inform his patients of the established ideas concerning their clinical problem.

✓ Rule of Ethics 2. Informed Consent

The performance of medical or surgical procedures shall be preceded by appropriate informed consent.

If the benefit/risk profile of a major innovation is significantly different than established treatments, or even if less data are available, the innovation should never be misrepresented as an inconsequential variation of established technique. The collective profession also has an obligation to its members and the public to ensure that its practitioners truly represent established standards. This activity is both pragmatic and ethical. It is pragmatic in the sense that aberrant activities of one practitioner can damage the prospects of other members. It is ethical in that the public is depending on the reputation of the profession for the effectiveness and safety of treatment, rather than exclusively on the reputation of the individual practitioner.

The disadvantage of the above is that physicians may feel disinclined to stray from tradition or to allow other colleagues to stray. While innovation may be an opportunity for the imaginative practitioner, it may be perceived as a threat to those in competition. Because it is the common duty of all practitioners to put the interests of the public ahead of their own, the profession is obligated to evaluate new ideas with unbiased objectivity in order to clarify what is best for the patient. Medical history shows numerous examples of successful new ideas, as well as disasters. For example, Ignaz Semmelweis attempted to convince his colleagues to wash their hands between autopsies and deliveries in order to stem an epidemic of puerperal sepsis. He was driven out of his profession by those unwilling to consider his new idea. On the other hand, Egas Moniz developed prefrontal lobotomy in the 1930s as a treatment for psychiatric disorders, and although the idea was temporarily accepted, as evidenced by his Nobel Prize, the results were tragic. Without objective evaluation, no person can presume to know intuitively whether an old or a new therapy is better.

The foregoing concepts are codified in the Academy's Code of Ethics in Rule 3, governing clinical experimentation, and Rules 12 and 13, governing communications to colleagues and the public.

✓ Rule of Ethics 3. Clinical Trials and Investigative Procedures

Use of clinical trials or investigative procedures shall be approved by adequate review mechanisms. Clinical trials and investigative procedures are those conducted to develop adequate information on which to base prognostic or therapeutic decisions or to determine etiology or pathogenesis, in circumstances in which insufficient information exists. Appropriate informed consent for these procedures must recognize their special nature and ramifications.

✓ Rule of Ethics 12. Communications to Colleagues

Communications to colleagues must be accurate and truthful.

✓ Rule of Ethics 13. Communications to the Public

Communications to the public must be accurate. They must not convey false, untrue, deceptive, or misleading information through statements, testimonials, photographs, graphics, or other means. They must not omit material information without which the communications would be deceptive. Communications must not appeal to an individual's anxiety in an excessive or unfair way; and they must not create unjustified expectations of results. If communications refer to benefits or other attributes of ophthalmic procedures that involve significant risks, realistic assessments of their safety and efficacy must also be included, as well as the availability of alternatives and, where necessary to avoid deception, descriptions and/or assessments of the benefits or other attributes of those alternatives. Communications must not misrepresent an ophthal-

mologist's credentials, training, experience, or ability, and must not contain material claims of superiority that cannot be substantiated. If a communication results from payment by an ophthalmologist, this must be disclosed unless the nature, format, or medium makes it apparent.

These rules require potential beneficiaries of new therapies to understand that the value of the innovation is under investigation. Under these rules, one might ethically advertise for subjects in a study to evaluate efficacy, but the requirements of informed consent would be rigorous.

The colleagues of an innovative practitioner have an obligation to evaluate the therapy: scientific progress demands that nontraditional ideas be challenged and tested. In doing so, the profession is best positioned to exclude poor ideas and embrace good ones. The patient who asks about an innovative therapy deserves unbiased, honest communication from the physician about the extent of current knowledge. Throughout the entire process of scientific innovation, the primary controlling interest of all involved in the profession is the welfare of the individual patient. Individual physicians and groups of physicians who truly keep this principle foremost will come to the best decisions for the individual patient, the public, and the profession.

Case Study 10

Research: Conflicts of Interest and Commercial Relationships

Abstract

Ethical dilemmas arise when the physician has commercial and financial relationships while being involved in related clinical trials and/or investigational procedures.

Case Study

An elderly woman presents to the University Eye Clinic with a chief complaint of deteriorating vision. She states that she is eager to undergo any treatment if it offers hope of improving her vision.

She is examined by a second-year resident who diagnoses exudative age-related macular degeneration in both eyes. Visual acuity is 20/200 in both eyes. The patient does not fit any current treatment guidelines, but the resident remembers a recent grand rounds presentation in which a staff ophthalmologist recommended very high doses of a specific oral medication for such patients. The resident calls the ophthalmologist for more information and learns of an ongoing study, approved by the institutional review board, that is being led by the ophthalmologist.

The staff ophthalmologist has been very encouraged by results obtained in several patients treated with the medication. In fact, one of the patients was so pleased that, through her business connections, she secured a mention of the treatment in a local news release. The ophthalmologist delights in the resident's interest and offers the opportunity to participate in his clinical research project, which is designed to evaluate the efficacy of specific treatment protocols. The resident, who has already begun to pursue a vitreo-retinal fellowship, readily accepts the offer.

The resident discusses what is known about the new treatment with the patient, who enthusiastically volunteers to participate in the research program. The resident and the patient agree in a signed consent document that she will be enrolled in a study involving a variety of treatments and will return monthly for visual acuity testing. As a research subject she will receive free medical care.

The resident soon learns that interest in this oral medication has grown to the extent that the pharmaceutical company's stock price is rising. Although he is not in the habit of investing in equities, he takes some of his savings and buys a significant number of shares.

Discussion

This case illustrates the major force that drives many research endeavors: the patient with a problem for which present solutions are limited or nonexistent. Unfortunately, this status makes this patient vulnerable, as she is desperately afraid of losing more vision and is searching for any hope. In such a situation it is imperative that the physician act as the agent for the patient and act in the patient's best interest.

One could argue that the appropriate role of a supportive ophthalmologist is to acknowledge the disease entity and to help the patient adjust realistically to the limitations placed on her by the disease. Further assistance should be offered, such as a comprehensive low-vision examination, resources for patients with low vision, and referral for appropriate visual rehabilitative services.

While commendable, the optimism and enthusiasm expressed by the resident in this case pose a potential problem in the accurate evaluation of the patient and the accurate evaluation of the proposed treatment. In particular, the resident may lack the skills needed to design and conduct a controlled study of the oral medication. Without such skills, the resident may not recognize the biases of both the patient and the investigators.

> ✓ **Rule of Ethics 3. Clinical Trials and Investigative Procedures**
>
> **Use of clinical trials or investigative procedures shall be approved by adequate review mechanisms. Clinical trials and investigative procedures are those conducted to develop adequate information on which to base prognostic or therapeutic decisions or to determine etiology or pathogenesis, in circumstances in which insufficient information exists. Appropriate informed consent for these procedures must recognize their special nature and ramifications.**

For peripheral reasons, the resident and the senior ophthalmologist have a vested interest in the success of the experimental medication, an interest that may influence the accuracy of their observations and the interpretation of results. The ophthalmologist has already obtained "encouraging" results in other patients, and the publicity over apparent success is "validation" that is difficult to ignore, particularly if the senior ophthalmologist's practice has noticeably increased in volume. The resident, of course, is eager to please the senior ophthalmologist, as a recommendation to a good fellowship may depend on the success of this research project. In addition, the resident now has a significant conflict of interest with his financial interest in the success of this research, given his recent purchase of the manufacturer's stock.

> ✓ **Rule of Ethics 15. Conflict of Interest**
>
> **A conflict of interest exists when professional judgment concerning the well-being of the patient has a reasonable chance of being influenced by other interests of the provider. Disclosure of a conflict of interest is required in communications to patients, the public, and colleagues.**

The patient's hopes of regaining any part of her vision could result in a subjective improvement in function following treatment with the experimental medication, even though her measured visual acuity may not have changed. The free care provided to the patient may also influence her subjective report of the outcome.

Summary

In summary, the reported outcome of the experimental treatment in this case, successful or not, will be suspect because the resident and the senior ophthalmologist have failed to control for the biases of both patient and investigators and have disregarded the rigorous requirements of a research study. A basic ophthalmic examination and measurement of visual acuity before and periodically after treatment are not sufficient observation to evaluate the efficacy of the medication. Research studies are generally collaborative efforts that require the expertise of professionals in diverse disciplines to design and conduct a meaningful protocol and to evaluate the results. In this instance, the resident and the senior ophthalmologist erred in not consulting with others more experienced in research before undertaking even a limited trial of the experimental medication. Were this done, the resident, no doubt, would have been advised to perform a more intensive initial assessment of the patient's status and to schedule repeated examinations according to a specific, predetermined protocol during and following the course of treatments. Evaluations by two different physicians would have been recommended to control for inter-observer variation. The patient would have been counseled that the medication at such high doses was experimental, with only a small amount of preliminary evidence to suggest that it might help. She should have been informed of all possible outcomes, including the possibility that she might experience no change in her condition or the possibility that she might experience unforeseen systemic complications from the oral medication. Finally, the resident would have been well advised to read all available information on the safety of the medication and to monitor the patient during treatment to reduce the risk of adverse reactions. Ideally, the objectives and protocol for the research project would have undergone the rigorous review of an affiliated institutional review board prior to its initiation.

To obtain a truly meaningful evaluation of the medication, multiple patients with similar retinal involvement would have to be included in the study, half to receive the experimental preparation and half to receive a placebo, to control for both patient and physician bias. Ideally, the study would be double-masked; that is, neither the patient nor the ophthalmologist would know which of the two, medication or placebo, was being given.

Conducting clinical research involving human subjects requires rigorous ethical scrutiny. It requires recognizing the unique ethical responsibility placed on the physician when using patients to advance medical treatment and science as a whole. Personal interests, bias, and enthusiasm must be held in check while ethical obligations to the patient and the scientific community are honored.

The Ethics of Research on Human Subjects

The purpose of ophthalmologic research is to prevent the onset of ocular disease, to improve treatment methods, and to gain a better understanding of the function of the visual system. Each of these goals implies a gap in our knowledge that remains to be filled. Thus, patients participating in a research study are treated by physicians who acknowledge that the optimal form of treatment is still unknown. Some would argue that this practice is in itself unethical, since the treatment may not benefit the patient.

The fact is, of course, that there often is no optimal form of treatment for every single patient, and there is no guarantee that every treatment or procedure will produce a successful result. In this sense, an element of trial and error is implicit in the management of every patient. For this reason, even with treatment by recommended procedures and with medications known to be safe and effective, the prudent physician monitors the patient and is prepared with backup alternative measures in case of nonresponsiveness or untoward incidents.

The same approach is applicable in research studies, but here the requirements for protection of participating patients are more rigorous and stringent than those for treatment recognized as standard of care. In the case of medications, laboratory studies and animal testing precede human investigation to obtain a preliminary measure of activity and safety. Analogous studies in normal human volunteers generally follow to confirm preliminary findings. Only then is the experimental preparation tested in patients to determine its efficacy and safety in the treatment of a specific condition.

Initial clinical trials often compare experimental preparations with the currently recommended treatment, and the study is usually "open-label"—both the physician and the patient know which treatment is being used. If, after an appropriate period, response to the experimental medication is not equivalent or superior to more widely accepted management, the study is terminated, and the patients on the experimental treatment are switched to the standard treatment. In placebo-controlled, double-masked studies, where neither the physician nor the patient knows whether the active drug is being used, the study may be interrupted and the code broken if patients fail to show a positive response. Nonresponding patients who are found to have received placebo are immediately started on treatment with the experimental or recommended medication.

For the validity of the study and the protection of participating subjects, each patient requires an intensive and comprehensive evaluation before treatment begins. Thereafter, throughout and following the study, careful monitoring is employed to determine the response to treatment and to detect any adverse events.

In reference to the ethics of clinical trials, Friedman and colleagues take the view that "... properly designed and conducted clinical trials are ethical. A well-designed trial can answer important public health questions without impairing the welfare of individuals. There may, at times, be conflicts between a physician's perception of what is good for his patient, and the needs of the trial. In such instances, the needs of the subject must predominate" (Friedman LM, Furberg CD, DeMets DL. *Fundamentals of Clinical Trials.* 2nd ed. Littleton, Mass: PSG Publishing Co; 1985:6).

Informed Consent

Participation in a research project requires the patient to sign a *special* informed consent statement. The purpose of the document, which is based on principles established as a result of the Nuremberg trials following World War II, is to ensure that the subject fully understands the purpose of the study, the medical procedures to be performed, and the attendant risks of the procedures. In many instances, the consent form will even describe in great detail concerns relating to medications or procedures that are part of a "routine" eye examination (eg, dilating drops).

The document also confirms that the patient has volunteered to participate freely and without coercion and that the patient is aware that he or she may elect to withdraw from further participation at any time. If the treatments are to be randomized or administered in a double-masked manner, the patient must understand the purpose of the experimental design. Finally, any financial interests of the investigators must be disclosed. (See "The Belmont Report" in Appendix II.)

✓ Rule of Ethics 2. Informed Consent

The performance of medical or surgical procedures shall be preceded by appropriate informed consent.

Who Pays?

Funding for research projects is provided by a variety of government, public, and private sources. When federal and institutional funds are involved, research protocols and personnel commonly receive careful peer review before support is granted. Thereafter, the investigator is generally permitted to pursue the research without interference, so long as the study is performed in accord with the agreed-upon protocols.

Similar procedures may be followed when commercial or private funding is being considered, but the prudent investigator must take added precautions to ensure that, in the case of a potential conflict of interest, such funding does not interfere with the scientific process or with reporting of results. The investigator must also be prepared to resist outside efforts to influence the research program and must be willing to acknowledge the source of the financial support in subsequent publications.

Concern has been raised about the effect of evolving health care delivery systems on the research process. In large part, this concerns payors of health care being unwilling to participate in research projects due to added expense. Another concern is that the goal of such funded research is not so much the discovery of better treatments as the definition of the most cost-effective therapy.

A patient who participates in a research project may be treated at a reduced charge or for no fee. In some cases, the patient may receive a stipend or travel expenses. The investigator must acknowledge such financial considerations, particularly if the study involves subjective measurements.

In summary, ethical issues relating to the conduct of research place new burdens on the ophthalmologist. In addition to caring for the patient, the ophthalmologist involved in research must honor an obligation to the scientific process, the scientific community, and the future of medicine itself. The vulnerable status of patients participating in clinical research requires that the researcher be aware of the potential for paternalistic behavior and of patients' lack of understanding about research in general. Most patient volunteers believe that clinical researchers will act in their best interests, and they are likely to have little concept of the potential conflicts of interest involved.

Case Study 11

Racial Disparities and Gender Issues

Abstract

Studies have shown that in the emotionally charged environment of a health care facility, compounded by complex explanations of medical treatments and devices, patients often do not adequately assimilate information they are given, and they may be hesitant to ask appropriate questions. This is especially true when the patient is of a different gender or race than the physician. In turn, physicians may erroneously assume that they understand the patient's social, emotional, and occupational needs without being sensitive to racial and gender disparities and inequalities.

Case Study

Ms. Lee is a 43-year-old international hedge fund manager who is also politically active in her Korean community. She has noticed increased fullness of her upper eyelids, and she complains of the sensation of "heaviness" after prolonged near work. Her mother, with whom she lives, has significant hooding of the upper eyelids, to the point where they look closed all the time, but has never sought surgical intervention. At the recommendation of a co-worker, Ms. Lee makes an appointment with Dr. Woodson, a prominent oculoplastic surgeon in the community.

Ms. Lee reports to the office on the day of her appointment, and while waiting to be examined, looks at a number of before and after photo albums highlighting various facial plastic surgical procedures. As she is escorted to the exam room she passes by several autographed, glossy portrait photographs of prominent local athletic and entertainment celebrities.

Presently, Dr. Woodson breezes into the examination room and cordially introduces himself. Ms. Lee feels immediately at ease with his reassuring and charming demeanor. Dr. Woodson takes a thorough history and performs a complete exam. He discusses his findings with the patient and, based on her complaints, recommends bilateral upper eyelid blepharoplasty as a surgical option and recommends alternatives for management. He explains the potential benefit of the procedure, which includes relief of heaviness by removal of excess skin, and mentions well-known risks, which include asymmetry, scarring, dry eyes, and the unlikely possibility of postoperative hemorrhage and blindness. Ms. Lee asks a few questions about recuperation and about postoperative activity restrictions. After all her questions are answered, she is photographed and signs the consent for surgery.

On the day of surgery, Dr. Woodson performs his customary aggressive skin and fat excision. He performs a deep eyelid crease formation prior to wound closure, and Ms. Lee is discharged in excellent condition. She is swollen but otherwise comfortable at her 1-week postoperative visit.

When the patient returns for her 1-month postoperative visit, Dr. Woodson's staff is effusive in their comments on her attractive and improved appearance. Indeed, Ms. Lee has had several co-workers inquire whether she'd been away on vacation and express their observation that she looks "more rested."

When Dr. Woodson enters the exam room, his face lights up as he admires Ms. Lee's excellent surgical results. As he shakes her hand and pulls up a chair, the patient breaks down and through her tears manages to whisper, "I don't look like myself anymore. . . . My mother says I have brought shame on her and our family by trying to look 'white'." Dr. Woodson is speechless with surprise as Ms. Lee continues to struggle with her words. "I wanted to get rid of my tired eyes . . . not my Korean eyes."

Discussion

It is well accepted that "beauty is in the eye of the beholder." The same axiom can be applied to certain aspects of medicine where a "successful" surgical outcome is also in the eye of the beholder. Dr. Woodson, a gifted surgeon with thousands of happy and satisfied patients, failed Ms. Lee by neglecting to consider her cultural and racial identity. His technical expertise in the preoperative work-up and in the performance of surgery cannot be disputed. He was also thorough in describing alternatives, benefits, and risks of blepharoplasty to Ms. Lee. However, Dr. Woodson failed to account for the anatomic differences and cultural needs of his patient and erred in his presumption that Ms. Lee wanted a Western ideal of beautiful eyes.

Failure to respect a patient's cultural and racial identity may constitute a lack of proper informed consent.

✓ Rule of Ethics 2. Informed Consent

The performance of medical or surgical procedures shall be preceded by appropriate informed consent.

An Asian patient considering upper eyelid surgery would be reasonably expected to understand what, if any, changes in anatomic appearance might result from a proposed procedure.

As stated in Rule 6 of the Academy's Code of Ethics, "Treatment shall be recommended only after a careful consideration of the patient's physical, social, emotional, and occupational needs." Patient dissatisfaction may be created even with a successful surgical outcome, if psychosocial and racial/cultural factors are not taken into account. A surgeon may perform technically flawless surgery, but may still have failed in his duty to respect what is in the best interest of the patient.

> **✓ Rule of Ethics 6. Pretreatment Assessment**
>
> **Treatment shall be recommended only after a careful consideration of the patient's physical, social, emotional, and occupational needs. The ophthalmologist must evaluate the patient and assure that the evaluation accurately documents the ophthalmic findings and the indications for treatment. Recommendation of unnecessary treatment or withholding of necessary treatment is unethical.**

Case Study 12

The Impaired Ophthalmologist

Abstract

Impaired physicians are, by definition, not fully competent to practice their craft. Impaired physicians also frequently fail to recognize their impairment, or they may deny its significance.

Case Study

Dr. Hale is a 47-year-old ophthalmologist who performs a wide variety of kinds of anterior segment surgery. He has had extensive training and has been on the faculty of a major urban medical school since finishing his fellowship. He also has a practice in a suburb of the city. Dr. Hale is intent on maintaining a respectable practice that produces income sufficient to sustain the lifestyle to which he and his family have become accustomed. Dr. Hale knows that he has not managed his finances well; the large debt he incurred during his training has been augmented by the expense of a large mortgage on his home and the education of his children.

Dr. Hale therefore feels compelled to increase his productivity, and soon his surgical volume begins to grow exponentially. He now starts his workday at 5:00 in the morning and finishes his charts after midnight. Before long, Dr. Hale begins to take Ritalin, which he obtains by writing prescriptions in other people's names, so that he can continue working after a few short hours of sleep each night, and can continue to perform as many surgeries as possible. He takes the drug more than once a day, depending on his surgical schedule. Late at night, he takes a barbiturate obtained in the same manner to help him settle down for a few hours of rest. The operating room staff soon note that the frequency of Dr. Hale's intraoperative complications has become unusually high and that he appears to be driven constantly by time considerations. His chart notes and patient orders are incomplete and erratic, he is often late for meetings and other appointments, and he will occasionally make inappropriate comments in front of patients. His behavior becomes the talk of the hospital. On one especially busy day, Dr. Hale performs a corneal transplant in the wrong eye of a patient with bilateral corneal disease. The residents and nurses are disturbed and express concern. On hearing of the event, Dr. Hale's partner is especially concerned and is trying to decide what to do.

Discussion

This case study describes a technically competent surgeon who becomes incompetent because of external pressure, compulsive behavior, and a dependence on drugs. While his willingness to work hard and continuously may be commendable, the quality of his efforts has suffered through overextending himself and the related reliance on drugs. He is at extreme risk for harming, rather than helping, his patients.

Such instances of compulsive behavior, whether in the drive to work or the use of drugs, are especially tragic because the development of the "impairment" is frequently insidious and unrecognized by the physician. Often a major error, such as operating on the wrong eye, is required to make the physician recognize that something has gone seriously awry. The ophthalmologist described in this case study is incompetent because he has not looked at himself realistically and has become impaired.

The first rule of the Academy's Code of Ethics stipulates that the physician must be competent.

> ### ✓ Rule of Ethics 1. Competence
>
> **An ophthalmologist is a physician who is educated and trained to provide medical and surgical care of the eyes and related structures. An ophthalmologist should perform only those procedures in which the ophthalmologist is competent by virtue of specific training or experience or is assisted by one who is. An ophthalmologist must not misrepresent credentials, training, experience, ability, or results.**

Impaired physicians are at risk for violating this important ethical principle because, by definition, they are not fully competent to practice their craft. In such cases, the burden for addressing the problem frequently falls to colleagues because the impaired physician frequently fails to recognize the impairment and may deny its significance. Ethical issues regarding the impaired physician therefore concern the profession's obligations in coming to the aid of members whose competence is in question, as well as the impaired physicians' own responsibility to patients, themselves, their families, and their colleagues. The profession's responsibility to act can extend to the physician's peers or peer groups, such as medical societies. Although recognized causes for physician impairment include aging, substance abuse, and illness, this case study does not explore impairment in this broad sense but focuses instead on one example—the ophthalmologist impaired by drug abuse.

Problems with drug abuse are typically difficult to identify. According to statistics, impaired physicians are often first identified by their spouses. If the spouse is unable to effect a change in behavior, the impairment will most likely become more severe and will interfere with the physician's professional life. Early detection and appropriate treatment are important to reducing the risks to patients and returning the affected physician to a healthy lifestyle.

The essential role that denial plays in impairment cannot be overemphasized. Denial makes it hard, if not impossible, for people to understand that they need healing. In cases where a physician refuses to acknowledge a problem, or where inappropriate behavior continues, it is necessary to exert more coercive group authority. Most hospitals and national professional organizations now have ethics committees designed to consider, among other issues, matters of impairment.

The primary objective in addressing physician impairment is to protect patients from harm. This is accomplished by removing the physician at the earliest opportunity from direct responsibility for patient care. Secondary, but still important, objectives include protection of the profession and the remediation of the physician.

Another major consideration regarding the impaired physician concerns the responsibility of other members of the profession: when the profession does not address the problem of impaired physicians who continue to practice, the trust of the public is quickly lost. The impression is left that ensuring appropriate patient care is no longer the primary interest of the profession as a group. This obligation is expressed in Rule 5 of the Academy's Code of Ethics.

✓ Rule of Ethics 5. The Impaired Ophthalmologist

A physically, mentally, or emotionally impaired ophthalmologist should withdraw from those aspects of practice affected by the impairment. If an impaired ophthalmologist does not cease inappropriate behavior, it is the duty of other ophthalmologists who know of the impairment to take action to attempt to assure correction of the situation. This may involve a wide range of remedial actions.

Recognition by the profession that it has a responsibility to deal with impaired physicians acknowledges that the profession has a collective responsibility to its physician members, impaired and whole, as well as to the public. Efforts by the profession to resolve problems related to an impaired physician are not only in the interest of patients and of the particular impaired physician but are also ultimately in the profession's best interest.

The first approach to solving the problem of the impaired physician is attempted remediation. The concerned colleague who notices the impairment and brings it to the attention of appropriate authorities may not, for several reasons, be the best person to initiate a discussion with the physician who is accused of being impaired. These reasons may include past noncollegial interactions with the affected physician (potentially influ-

Sources of Information about Impairment

The following organizations can provide additional information on addictive behavior and/or on impaired-physician programs:

- Alcoholics Anonymous, www.alcoholics-anonymous.org
- American Society of Addiction Medicine, Inc., www.asam.org
- California Diversion Program for Impaired Physicians, www.physicianassistant.ca.gov/diversion.htm
- Talbott Recovery Center, www.talbottcampus.com
- American College of Surgeons, www.facs.org

encing others' reactions to the reporting), a potential liability risk to his or her own professional career, practice competition, and other professional conflicts of interest. Such discussions are more likely to be effective and to change behavior when they occur between the impaired physician and a person he or she respects and to whom he or she is most likely to listen.

The issue of competence is at the heart of this case study. Medical competence requires at least two components, the first composed of knowledge and skills, and the second of judgment and ethical behavior. These two components have traditionally been called "the science" and "the art" of medical practice. It has been recognized for centuries that both science and art must be present in full measure for physicians and surgeons to practice their craft properly. The impaired physician cannot be considered competent because of the impairment. An ethical approach to issues of impairment will distinguish the roles of the individual physician, his or her colleagues, and the profession. Further sources of help and information are listed in the box "Sources of Information about Impairment."

Case Study 13

Alternative and Complementary Therapies

Abstract

The dissatisfaction with traditional medicine, or with an insufficient "cure," has led some patients to seek alternative sources of care. Sensitivity to the relationship between beneficial as opposed to harmful, and between traditional as opposed to alternative or complementary, therapies is essential for the practicing ophthalmologist. As in all physician–patient relationships, physicians must uphold the trust placed in them by patients, who are in a vulnerable position regarding their health, and offer only those procedures, devices, or pharmacological agents that are in the patients' best interest.

Case Study

An elderly gentleman shows his retina specialist a magazine article that describes a method to "reverse macular degeneration" using "microcurrent stimulation." The article advertises equipment, for use in the home setting, to provide electrical stimulation to the eye. This equipment sells for $800. The ophthalmologist promoting the new treatment states that over 70% of patients with macular degeneration who use this treatment have visual improvement. The patient, who is slowly losing vision because of age-related macular degeneration, calls for more information and learns that the equipment really costs $1500. He asks his retina specialist if he should pursue this therapy.

Discussion

Alternative or complementary therapies arise out of nonallopathic schools of medicine and are generally not validated treatments. Most of the "proof" of efficacy exists in homeopathic health journals or in advertising sections in the lay press. Often the "clinical studies" are done without control subjects or objective endpoints. Sometimes the cited "evidence" is nothing more than single case reports or patient testimonials. Occasionally, physicians will promote these therapies and thereby grant "MD approval" of the treatment. Nevertheless, complementary therapies are attractive to patients. In the United States the use of complementary therapies is at an all-time high and visits to practitioners of alternative medicine exceed visits to doctors of evidence-based medicine. In addition, many patients now expect their physicians to understand and comment on these complementary therapies. For these reasons and more, complementary therapies create unique ethical circumstances that cannot be ignored by the practicing ophthalmologist.

In this particular example an elderly gentleman is losing vision because of age-related macular degeneration. Evidence-based medicine has had little to offer him, and he is understandably drawn to promises of visual improvement with a new treatment. This patient is vulnerable to any new treatment making the right promises. Some of these treatments, at best, may be expensive and a waste of money. Others, at worst, may be harmful or dangerous. In this situation, the ophthalmologist must act as the patient's agent or advocate, approaching him with understanding, compassion, honesty, and respect for human dignity. Good communication with the patient is essential, and it takes time.

> ✓ **Rule of Ethics 2. Informed Consent**
>
> **The performance of medical or surgical procedures shall be preceded by appropriate informed consent.**

In addition, the ophthalmologist must be knowledgeable. A full discussion of the advertisement and its implications for the patient requires the ophthalmologist's full understanding of this new treatment. This presupposes continuing medical education, even outside the halls of universities, on the part of the physician. To ignore information about this therapy simply because the therapy wasn't taught during residency training would not be good medicine.

The advertisement itself is ethically troubling. It makes claims for "reversing" macular degeneration. The lay public would have little notion of whether that was true or even possible. In the advertisement, the physician promoting the new treatment states that over 70% of patients have visual improvement, but a more inquisitive reader would want to know what kind of visual improvement—for example, visual acuity, reading speed, visual field. The advertised cost of $800 rises to $1500 once an interested reader calls for more information. Several statements in this advertisement are misleading to the public and raise the issue of truth in advertising.

> ### ✓ Rule of Ethics 13. Communications to the Public
>
> **Communications to the public must be accurate. They must not convey false, untrue, deceptive, or misleading information through statements, testimonials, photographs, graphics, or other means. They must not omit material information without which the communications would be deceptive. Communications must not appeal to an individual's anxiety in an excessive or unfair way; and they must not create unjustified expectations of results. If communications refer to benefits or other attributes of ophthalmic procedures that involve significant risks, realistic assessments of their safety and efficacy must also be included, as well as the availability of alternatives and, where necessary to avoid deception, descriptions and/or assessments of the benefits or other attributes of those alternatives. Communications must not misrepresent an ophthalmologist's credentials, training, experience, or ability, and must not contain material claims of superiority that cannot be substantiated. If a communication results from payment by an ophthalmologist, this must be disclosed unless the nature, format, or medium makes it apparent.**

One may speculate about the physician's motive for promoting the complementary therapy in this advertisement. The physician could truly believe in the success of the therapy, or he could have an academic, career-building interest in it. Both attitudes would represent bias and require the physician to pursue traditional methods of validating the therapy before publicizing it in the lay press. Even more likely, a commercial relationship or related financial conflict of interest exists. The physician is charging high sums of money for an unproven therapy directed toward a vulnerable population of patients.

The Scientific Process

The fundamental ethical issue in promoting new treatments is the obligation to fulfill the requirements of evidence-based medicine. Failure to do so returns medicine to the early part of the last century when our profession was plagued by charlatans and quacks (see Chapter 13). Today the public assumes that persons with an "MD" behind their names are committed to the scientific process in which treatments are validated. Thus, physicians could potentially offer a great service to the field of complementary medicine by examining potential nonallopathic treatments in a rigorous manner free of bias. According to the Belmont Report (see Chapter 16 and Appendix II), "When a clinician departs in a significant way from standard or accepted practice, the innovation does not, in and of itself, constitute research. The fact that a procedure is 'experimental' in the sense of new, untested, or different, does not automatically place it in the category of research. Radically new procedures of this description should, however, be made the object of formal research at an early stage, in order to determine whether they are safe and effective."

Communication and Reporting

Another ethical issue associated with complementary therapies relates to communication. On concluding an investigation of an alternative or complementary therapy, the ophthalmologist bears an ethical responsibility to report the data and results, using the appropriate avenues of communication. Although the temptation exists to contact the public media first with promising preliminary results, the more correct and responsible approach is to present such information at recognized meetings of peers, or to publish the results in a scientific journal refereed by other knowledgeable physicians in the field. By following this peer review process, the ophthalmologist maintains his or her own identity as the originator of the information or the idea and effectively protects the public from the misuse of a new therapy. When the findings on new therapies are eventually communicated to the public, they must be truthful. The promulgation of flawed data and conclusions or of promised benefits where there are none must be avoided.

Conflict of Interest

Ophthalmologists must be continually alert to the inevitable pressure generated when undue financial benefit may result as a consequence of offering a new alternative or complementary therapy. While we all acknowledge the ethical mandate to rise above the conflict of interest present in everyday fee-for-service medicine and to offer only those therapies in the best interest of the patient, the bar is even higher for nonvalidated, unproven therapies. Any alternative or complementary therapy offered to the patient should have a high likelihood of benefiting the patient, and the remuneration for that treatment should be reasonable and commensurate with similar treatments. To reap undue financial profit from the use of nonvalidated complementary therapies is unethical.

> ✓ **Rule of Ethics 15. Conflict of Interest**
>
> **A conflict of interest exists when professional judgment concerning the well-being of the patient has a reasonable chance of being influenced by other interests of the provider. Disclosure of a conflict of interest is required in communications to patients, the public, and colleagues.**

Commercial Relationships

Until relatively recently, the complexity of new commercial relationships was not of great concern to most physicians. Traditional codes of ethics forbade alliances that would result in financial gain from other than professional services. In the past, morally responsible physicians would shun relationships that had even the appearance of a commercial enterprise. But what was unthinkable 25 years ago (eg, dispensing glasses) is now considered an acceptable option by many physicians and, in some cases, a matter of survival. How do we ethically deal with these new pressures to engage in commercial relationships?

Some answers to these questions have been proposed in a thoughtful and provocative article by Arnold S. Relman, MD, former editor-in-chief of the *New England Journal of Medicine*. As an editorial comment preceding the article observes, "[Dr. Relman] fears that his profession has lost its ethical way. Doctors, he argues, are not and should not be businessmen, and yet financial and technological pressures are forcing more and more of them to act like businessmen, with deleterious consequences for patients and for society as a whole." In the article itself, Dr. Relman reviews the historical ethical position of physicians. From its beginnings, medicine has "steadfastly held that physicians' responsibility to their patients takes precedence over their own economic interests" (Relman AS. What market values are doing to medicine. *The Atlantic Monthly.* March 1992;03:96–106).

The Hippocratic Oath and the International Code of Medical Ethics of the World Medical Organization emphasize this principle (see Chapter 16). In its 1957 Principles of Medical Ethics, the American Medical Association stated that "the principal objective of the medical profession is to render service to humanity. . . . In the practice of medicine a physician should limit the source of his professional income to medical services actually rendered by him, or under his supervision, to his patients." (See Chapter 14 for the contemporary preamble to the AMA's Principles of Medical Ethics.)

Because of its pledge to comply with these fundamental admonitions, the medical profession has enjoyed a privileged position in society, and society, in return, expects ethical behavior.

✓ Rule of Ethics 1. Competence

An ophthalmologist is a physician who is educated and trained to provide medical and surgical care of the eyes and related structures. An ophthalmologist should perform only those procedures in which the ophthalmologist is competent by virtue of specific training or experience or is assisted by one who is. An ophthalmologist must not misrepresent credentials, training, experience, ability, or results.

General References for Case Studies

American Academy of Pediatrics. *Guidelines for Expert Witness Testimony in Medical Malpractice Litigation.* Policy Statement. May 2002.

American Medical Association. Council on Ethical and Judicial Affairs Opinion E-9.011. *Continuing Medical Education.* Issued December 1993, updated June 1996. Also Opinion E-8.061. *Gifts to Physicians from Industry.* Adopted December 1990, updated June 1996 and June 1998.

Angell M. The pharmaceutical industry—to whom is it accountable? *N Engl J Med.* 2000;342:1902–1904.

Bates v Virginia State Bar, 433 US 350 (1977).

Bell JD, Fay M. The medical profession and changing attitudes towards advertising and competition. *NZ Med J.* 1991;104:69–71.

Bettman JW. The role and way of the expert witness. *Argus.* February 1995.

Coyle SL. Physician-industry relations. Part 1: Individual physicians. *Ann Intern Med.* 2002;136:396–402.

DeAngelis CD. Conflicts of interest and the public trust. *JAMA.* 2000;284:2237–2238.

Dyer AR. Ethics, advertising, and the definition of a profession. *Med Ethics.* 1985;11:72–78.

Goldfarb v Virginia State Bar, 421 US 773 (1975).

Gorney M. Expert witnesses: caught in a moral and ethical dilemma. *Bull Am Coll Surg.* 2003;88:11–14.

Hoskins HD Jr. Co-management: does the "Co" stand for "cooperation" or "coercion"? *EyeNet.* 1999;3:8:14-15.

Friedman LM, Furberg CD, DeMets DL. *Fundamentals of Clinical Trials.* 2nd ed. Littleton, Mass: PSG Publishing Co; 1985:6.

Hyde GAOL. How to recognize and help an impaired surgeon. *Bull Am Coll Surg.* 1989;73:4–10.

Milunsky A. Lies, damned lies, and medical experts: the abrogation of responsibility by specialty organizations and a call for action. *J Child Neurol.* 2003;18:413–419.

Nelson LJ, Clark HW, Goldman RL, et al. Taking the train to a world of strangers: health care marketing and ethics. *Hastings Center Report.* 1989;19:5:36-43.

Reiser SJ, Dyck AJ, Curran WJ, eds. *Ethics in Medicine, Historical Perspectives, and Contemporary Concerns.* Cambridge, Mass: MIT Press; 1982.

Relman AS, Lindberg GD. Business and professionalism in medicine at the American Medical Association. *JAMA.* 1998:270:169–170.

Revicki DA, Brown RE, Adler MA. Patient outcomes with co-managed postoperative care after cataract surgery. *J Clin Epidemiol.* 1993;46(1):5–15.

Rodning CB, Dasco CC. A physician/advertiser ethics. *Am J Med.* 1987; 82:1209–1214.

Vaillant GE. Path to recovery. *Arch Gen Psych.* 1982;39:127–133.

Wazana A. Physicians and the pharmaceutical industry. Is a gift ever just a gift? *JAMA.* 2000;283:373–380.

Wittchow K. Forensic consulting: from immunity to liability. *OMIC Digest.* 2003;13:1,4–5.

CHAPTER 16

Foundation Documents of Medical Ethics

This chapter includes the texts of several of the fundamental documents on which medical ethics is based:

- Hippocratic Oath (Classical Version)
- Hippocratic Oath (Modern Version)
- Islamic Code of Medical Ethics
- International Code of Medical Ethics of the World Medical Association
- Declaration of Geneva
- American Medical Association Principles of Medical Ethics
- Belmont Report (Protection of Human Subjects) (summary)

These documents have helped shape the development of medicine and continue to have an effect on the field today. Of course, many other documents exist that are important to medical ethics. Those included here relate to ethical issues raised in this text.

Several documents in this chapter, including the Declaration of Geneva and the Belmont Report, were written to clarify for society the goals of medicine in general. In addition, several of these documents strive to ensure that research and study subjects fully understand the purposes of the studies, the medical procedures to be performed, and the attendant risks of the procedures. Another equally important purpose is to ensure that the patient who volunteers to participate in a study is doing so freely and without coercion. Whether written for this purpose, for general professional guidance, or for any other reason, these foundation documents have much to teach us, and it is well worth our while as physicians to review them regularly throughout the course of our careers.

Hippocratic Oath, *Classical Version*

I swear by Apollo Physician and Asclepius and Hygieia and Panaceia and all the gods and goddesses, making them my witnesses, that I will fulfill according to my ability and judgment this oath and this covenant:

To hold him who has taught me this art as equal to my parents and to live my life in partnership with him, and if he is in need of money to give him a share of mine, and to regard his offspring as equal to my brothers in male lineage and to teach them this art— if they desire to learn it—without fee and covenant; to give a share of precepts and oral instruction and all the other learning to my sons and to the sons of him who has instructed me and to pupils who have signed the covenant and have taken an oath according to the medical law, but no one else.

I will apply dietetic measures for the benefit of the sick according to my ability and judgment; I will keep them from harm and injustice.

I will neither give a deadly drug to anybody who asked for it, nor will I make a suggestion to this effect. Similarly I will not give to a woman an abortive remedy. In purity and holiness I will guard my life and my art.

I will not use the knife, not even on sufferers from stone, but will withdraw in favor of such men as are engaged in this work.

Whatever houses I may visit, I will come for the benefit of the sick, remaining free of all intentional injustice, of all mischief and in particular of sexual relations with both female and male persons, be they free or slaves.

What I may see or hear in the course of the treatment or even outside of the treatment in regard to the life of men, which on no account one must spread abroad, I will keep to myself, holding such things shameful to be spoken about.

If I fulfill this oath and do not violate it, may it be granted to me to enjoy life and art, being honored with fame among all men for all time to come; if I transgress it and swear falsely, may the opposite of all this be my lot.

Source: Translation from the Greek by Ludwig Edelstein. (From Edelstein L. *The Hippocratic Oath: Text, Translation, and Interpretation.* Baltimore, Md: Johns Hopkins Press; 1943.)

Note: Numerous versions of the Hippocratic Oath with various omissions are in print.

Hippocratic Oath, *Modern Version*

I swear to fulfill, to the best of my ability and judgment, this covenant:

I will respect the hard-won scientific gains of those physicians in whose steps I walk, and gladly share such knowledge as is mine with those who are to follow.

I will apply, for the benefit of the sick, all measures which are required, avoiding those twin traps of overtreatment and therapeutic nihilism.

I will remember that there is art to medicine as well as science, and that warmth, sympathy, and understanding may outweigh the surgeon's knife or the chemist's drug.

I will not be ashamed to say "I know not," nor will I fail to call in my colleagues when the skills of another are needed for a patient's recovery.

I will respect the privacy of my patients, for their problems are not disclosed to me that the world may know. Most especially must I tread with care in matters of life and death. If it is given me to save a life, all thanks. But it may also be within my power to take a life; this awesome responsibility must be faced with great humbleness and awareness of my own frailty. Above all, I must not play at God.

I will remember that I do not treat a fever chart, a cancerous growth, but a sick human being, whose illness may affect the person's family and economic stability. My responsibility includes these related problems, if I am to care adequately for the sick.

I will prevent disease whenever I can, for prevention is preferable to cure.

I will remember that I remain a member of society, with special obligations to all my fellow human beings, those sound of mind and body as well as the infirm.

If I do not violate this oath, may I enjoy life and art, respected while I live and remembered with affection thereafter. May I always act so as to preserve the finest traditions of my calling and may I long experience the joy of healing those who seek my help.

Source: Written in 1964 by Louis Lasagna, Academic Dean of the School of Medicine at Tufts University, and used in many medical schools today.

Islamic Code of Medical Ethics

The Oath of the Doctor

I swear by God, The Great;

To regard God in carrying out my profession;

To protect human life in all stages and under all circumstances, doing my utmost to rescue it from death, malady, pain, and anxiety;

To keep people's dignity, cover their privacies, and lock up their secrets;

To be, all the way, an instrument of God's mercy, extending my medical care to near and far, virtuous and sinner and friend and enemy;

To strive in the pursuit of knowledge and harnessing it for the benefit but not the harm of mankind;

To revere my teacher, teach my junior, and be brother to members of the medical profession joined in piety and charity;

To live my Faith in private and in public, avoiding whatever blemishes me in the eyes of God, His apostle, and my fellow Faithful;

And may God be witness to this Oath.

Source: Sachedina A. Islam. In: Reich WT, ed. *Encyclopedia of Bioethics.* Rev ed. New York, NY: Simon and Schuster/Prentice Hall International; 1995. p. 2705.

International Code of Medical Ethics of the World Medical Association

DUTIES OF PHYSICIANS IN GENERAL

A PHYSICIAN SHALL always maintain the highest standards of professional conduct.

A PHYSICIAN SHALL not permit motives of profit to influence the free and independent exercise of professional judgment on behalf of patients.

A PHYSICIAN SHALL, in all types of medical practice, be dedicated to providing competent medical service in full technical and moral independence, with compassion and respect for human dignity.

A PHYSICIAN SHALL deal honestly with patients and colleagues, and strive to expose those physicians deficient in character or competence, or who engage in fraud or deception.

The following practices are deemed to be unethical conduct:

a) Self advertising by physicians, unless permitted by the laws of the country and the Code of Ethics of the National Medical Association.

b) Paying or receiving any fee or any other consideration solely to procure the referral of a patient or for prescribing or referring a patient to any source.

A PHYSICIAN SHALL respect the rights of patients, of colleagues, and of other health professionals and shall safeguard patient confidences.

A PHYSICIAN SHALL act only in the patient's interest when providing medical care which might have the effect of weakening the physical and mental condition of the patient.

A PHYSICIAN SHALL use great caution in divulging discoveries or new techniques or treatment through nonprofessional channels.

A PHYSICIAN SHALL certify only that which he has personally verified.

DUTIES OF PHYSICIANS TO THE SICK

A PHYSICIAN SHALL always bear in mind the obligation of preserving human life.

A PHYSICIAN SHALL owe his patients complete loyalty and all the resources of his science. Whenever an examination or treatment is beyond the physician's capacity he should summon another physician who has the necessary ability.

A PHYSICIAN SHALL preserve absolute confidentiality on all he knows about his patient even after the patient has died.

A PHYSICIAN SHALL give emergency care as a humanitarian duty unless he is assured that others are willing and able to give such care.

DUTIES OF PHYSICIANS TO EACH OTHER

A PHYSICIAN SHALL behave towards his colleagues as he would have them behave towards him.

A PHYSICIAN SHALL NOT entice patients from his colleagues.

A PHYSICIAN SHALL observe the principles of the "Declaration of Geneva" approved by the World Medical Association.

Adopted by the 3rd General Assembly of the World Medical Association (WMA), London, England, October 1949; amended by the 22nd WMA General Assembly, Sydney, Australia, August 1968, and again by the 35th WMA General Assembly, Venice, Italy, October 1983.

Declaration of Geneva

AT THE TIME OF BEING ADMITTED AS A MEMBER OF THE MEDICAL PROFESSION:

I SOLEMNLY PLEDGE myself to consecrate my life to the service of humanity;

I WILL GIVE to my teachers the respect and gratitude which is their due;

I WILL PRACTICE my profession with conscience and dignity;

THE HEALTH OF MY PATIENT will be my first consideration;

I WILL RESPECT the secrets which are confided in me, even after the patient has died;

I WILL MAINTAIN by all the means in my power, the honor and the noble traditions of the medical profession;

MY COLLEAGUES will be my sisters and brothers;

I WILL NOT PERMIT considerations of age, disease or disability, creed, ethnic origin, gender, nationality, political affiliation, race, sexual orientation, or social standing to intervene between my duty and my patient;

I WILL MAINTAIN the utmost respect for human life from its beginning even under threat and I will not use my medical knowledge contrary to the laws of humanity;

I MAKE THESE PROMISES solemnly, freely and upon my honor.

Adopted by the 2nd General Assembly of the World Medical Association, Geneva, Switzerland, September 1948; amended by the 22nd WMA General Assembly, Sydney, Australia, August 1968, by the 35th WMA General Assembly, Venice, Italy, October 1983, and by the 46th WMA General Assembly, Stockholm, Sweden, September 1994.

American Medical Association Principles of Medical Ethics

Preamble

The medical profession has long subscribed to a body of ethical statements developed primarily for the benefit of the patient. As a member of this profession, a physician must recognize responsibility to patients first and foremost, as well as to society, to other health professionals, and to self. The following Principles adopted by the American Medical Association are not laws, but standards of conduct which define the essentials of honorable behavior for the physician.

I. A physician shall be dedicated to providing competent medical care, with compassion and respect for human dignity and rights.

II. A physician shall uphold the standards of professionalism, be honest in all professional interactions, and strive to report physicians deficient in character or competence, or engaging in fraud or deception, to appropriate entities.

III. A physician shall respect the law and also recognize a responsibility to seek changes in those requirements which are contrary to the best interests of the patient.

IV. A physician shall respect the rights of patients, colleagues, and other health professionals, and shall safeguard patient confidences and privacy within the constraints of the law.

V. A physician shall continue to study, apply, and advance scientific knowledge, maintain a commitment to medical education, make relevant information available to patients, colleagues, and the public, obtain consultation, and use the talents of other health professionals when indicated.

VI. A physician shall, in the provision of appropriate patient care, except in emergencies, be free to choose whom to serve, with whom to associate, and the environment in which to provide medical care.

VII. A physician shall recognize a responsibility to participate in activities contributing to the improvement of the community and the betterment of public health.

VIII. A physician shall, while caring for a patient, regard responsibility to the patient as paramount.

IX. A physician shall support access to medical care for all people.

Adopted by the AMA's House of Delegates on June 17, 2001.

The Belmont Report

The Belmont Report (1979), commissioned by the Department of Health Education and Welfare, is the major ethical statement guiding human research in the United States. In summary:

> On July 12, 1974, the National Research Act (Public Law 93348) was signed into law, thereby creating the National Commission for the Protection of Human Subjects of Biomedical and Behavioral Research. One of the charges to the Commission was to identify the basic ethical principles that should underlie the conduct of biomedical and behavioral research involving human subjects, and to develop guidelines, which should be followed to assure that such research is conducted in accordance with those principles. In carrying out the above, the Commission was directed to consider: (i) the boundaries between biomedical and behavioral research and the accepted and routine practice of medicine, (ii) the role of assessment of risk-benefit criteria in the determination of the appropriateness of research involving human subjects, (iii) appropriate guidelines for the selection of human subjects for participation in such research, and (iv) the nature and definition of informed consent in various research settings.
>
> The Belmont Report attempts to summarize the basic ethical principles identified by the Commission in the course of its deliberations. It is the outgrowth of an intensive four-day period of discussions that were held in February 1976 at the Smithsonian Institution's Belmont Conference Center, supplemented by the monthly deliberations of the Commission that were held over a period of nearly four years. It is a statement of basic ethical principles and guidelines that should assist in resolving the ethical problems that surround the conduct of research with human subjects.
>
> By publishing the Report in the Federal Register, and providing reprints upon request, the Secretary intends that it may be made readily available to scientists, members of in-

stitutional review boards, and Federal employees. The two-volume Appendix, containing the lengthy reports of experts and specialists, who assisted the Commission in fulfilling this part of its charge, is available as DHEW Publication No. (OS) 78-0013 and No. (OS) 78-0014, for sale by the Superintendent of Documents, U.S. Government Printing Office, Washington, D.C. 20402.

Unlike most other reports of the Commission, the Belmont Report does not make specific recommendations for administrative action by the Secretary of Health, Education, and Welfare. Rather, the Commission recommended that the Belmont Report be adopted in its entirety, as a statement of the Department's policy. The Department requests public comment on this recommendation.

For the full text of the report, refer to Appendix II.

PART III

Advocacy for Ophthalmology

Advocate *(v.):* to champion a cause, to seek support for a position, to defend, to protect.

As this definition suggests, physician advocacy is much more than a casual commitment or a philosophically agreeable concept. Ever-increasing clinical complexity and socioeconomic pressure, as well as the influence of government and industry on the practice of medicine, have added to physicians' obligations the requirement of being an aggressive advocate for their patients and their profession. Today more than ever before, advocacy is a physician's duty.

Your commitment to advocacy empowers you to directly affect legislation, regulation, policy, and even public and professional opinion on matters as diverse as patient care, patients' rights, access to health care, research funding, device and medication development, nonphysicians' scope of practice, and medical practice liability insurance. Without your commitment, the power to make decisions is effectively granted to others, whose interests may not match those of your patients or your profession.

The many partners and players in health care today—from physicians to allied health personnel to legislators to corporate executives—need to work together to ensure that America has the best patient care and the most competent care givers. In doing so, physicians need to position themselves as part of the solution, rather than letting themselves be cast as part of the problem. The advocacy efforts of individual ophthalmologists on the federal, state, local, and corporate levels are crucial to both patients' eye health and the health of the profession.

The chapters that follow discuss how advocacy has developed over the centuries, where and how decisions affecting the practice of medicine and ophthalmology are made, and how every ophthalmologist—whether new or experienced, practicing or retired, generalist or subspecialist—can make a difference. Most important, these chapters are meant to inspire you to become active in the continuing effort to advocate for and improve the profession to which you have dedicated your training, skill, and effort.

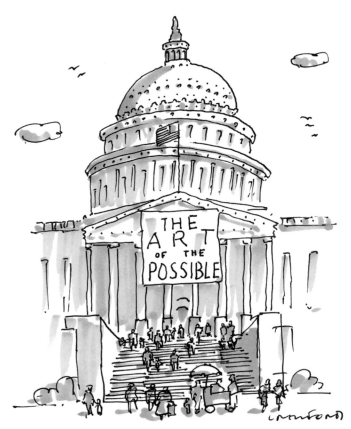

THE
ART
OF THE
POSSIBLE

CHAPTER 17

The History of Advocacy

In his *History of Ophthalmology*, Dr. George Gorin quotes the English surgeon Edward Treacher Collins: "The chief object of raking over the ashes of the past should be to acquire inspiration for the future." If we are to become effective advocates for the medical profession, and for ophthalmology itself, the history of advocacy must be appreciated and cannot be ignored. This chapter briefly describes the early history of medical organizations with regard to advocacy and summarizes the principal recent political events and social influences that you need to understand before becoming an effective advocate for ophthalmology.

Medical Societies and the Growth of Modern Organized Medicine

As with many other kinds of professionals in thirteenth-century Europe, groups of local physicians and surgeons organized themselves into guilds. Besides setting standards of professional behavior (see "Medical Ethics and the Guilds" in Chapter 13), these guilds regulated many aspects of practice, including medical training, certification, and treatments. Guilds, including those based on the practice of medicine, received their legitimacy from "letters patent" or other legal warrants issued by a ruler, which guaranteed certain business rights to guild members, as well as protections to those receiving guild members' services or goods. The petitioning of a monarch and others in positions of power to grant these letters patent and other privileges might be thought of as the origin of advocacy for the medical profession.

Medical guilds benefited patients by enabling them to expect a specific level of care from a qualified practitioner, often regardless of their ability to pay. As with all guilds, they also offered their members professional prestige and security, in this case partially by excluding untrained and "quack" healers, thereby controlling local physician-to-patient ratios and ensuring ample work for all within the guild. As exploration and trade increased over the centuries, so did urban populations, inevitably accompanied by unsanitary living conditions and disease. Governments came to rely on physicians to help control public health, thus increasing large-scale governmental interest in medical certification, licensure, and practice.

As the centuries passed, the medical profession itself experienced pendulum swings from disorganization and disagreement back to unity and solidarity. Governmental influence in medicine waxed and waned according to political events, social upheaval, technological advances, fads, and fashions. Through it all the profession continued to exercise self-regulation as a means of ensuring quality care and professional security.

The establishment in 1847 of the American Medical Association (AMA) resulted from a convention of physicians in New York concerned about poor medical training and quackery in the United States. Within a few decades the AMA became the preeminent physicians' "guild" in America.

Meanwhile, the growth of medical knowledge helped lead to physician specialization and, in turn, specialty societies. In Europe, the development of the ophthalmoscope, and Donders's work *On the Anomalies of Accommodation and Refraction of the Eye*, published in 1864, contributed to the demarcation of ophthalmology as a unique specialty. That same year, the American Ophthalmological Society (AOS) was established as this nation's first medical specialty organization. In 1896, the Western Ophthalmological, Otological, Laryngological, and Rhinological Association emerged as a true professional organization (Figure 17-1) and, in 1903, was renamed the American Academy of Ophthalmology and Otolaryngology, later to become the American Academy of Ophthalmology. The American Board of Ophthalmology, formed in 1916 as the American Board for Ophthalmic Examinations and renamed in 1933 as the first American specialty medical board, was an outgrowth of an AMA joint committee of eye, ear, and throat specialists originating as far back as 1914.

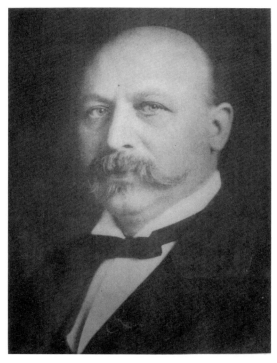

Figure 17-1 Adolph Alt, MD (1851–1920). Dr. Alt was the first President of the Academy of Ophthalmology and Otolaryngology in 1897. *(Photograph, 1897. Courtesy of Museum of Vision & Ophthalmic Heritage.)*

Organized Medicine Begins to Employ Advocacy

With the rise of corporations and the trade union movement in the late 1800s, all types of independent American professionals recognized the need to protect their economic and business interests by influencing governmental policies. Pharmacists, embalmers, and accountants, as well as physicians, sent advocates to state and local legislatures requesting licensing laws to regulate everything from professional standards of practice to fees, training, and criteria for entry into the profession. Concerned with the proliferation of schools offering substandard medical training, organized medicine was particularly anxious to set educational standards and to regulate medical schools. Because of successful physician advocacy, by 1901 all states, except two, had legislation requiring that new practitioners pass a state licensing exam and hold a diploma from an approved institution.

In that same year, the AMA established a House of Delegates consisting of proportional representation from each state's medical society. Belonging to a state society in effect became a requirement for AMA membership, and membership in state societies increased rapidly as a consequence. Because the individual states then, as now, held most of the nation's regulatory and licensing powers, physician members of these well-organized state societies were better positioned than ever to advocate for their patients and their profession.

Advocacy in medicine was not limited to just the legislative arena. In 1905, the AMA joined with reform-minded journalists in an effort to inform the public directly about the many ineffective and dangerous patent medicines then widely being advertised and to expose as quacks practitioners promising cure-alls using such remedies. This effort, as well as the publication the next year of *The Jungle,* Upton Sinclair's indictment of the meat-packing industry, caused a public outcry. On June 30, 1906, Congress passed into law the Food and Drugs Act, prohibiting interstate commerce in misbranded and adulterated foods, drinks, and drugs, and the Meat Inspection Act, outlawing poisonous food additives and regulating meat processing. With these new and far-reaching laws, the role of the medical profession as an authority in the development, efficacy, use, and distribution of pharmaceuticals was on its way to becoming established.

Advocacy and Federal Health Care Legislation

Governments worldwide exert considerable influence on health care delivery and policy. The United States federal program known as Medicare is so intertwined with patient care, medical practice, and medical advocacy that an understanding of its origins is necessary for every ophthalmologist who intends to serve as an effective advocate for medicine in the future.

National health insurance was one of the goals of the New Deal reforms under President Roosevelt in the 1930s. However, in 1934 Roosevelt decided not to include health insurance because of cost implications when he proposed the Social Security Act. In 1945, President Truman supported a national health insurance product and endorsed a bill, which did not pass Congress. In 1952 he proposed Medicare as a scaled-down version of national health insurance that would cover Social Security beneficiaries (the elderly, orphans, and widows). This bill failed to pass and was not submitted again until the early 1960s, when it again died in Congress.

Health insurance for the elderly and the poor, known respectively as Medicare and Medicaid, was finally approved by Congress in 1964 and signed into law by President Johnson on July 30, 1965, as Title XVIII of the Social Security Act (Figure 17-2). Medicare was initially a limited health insurance benefit covering 50% of the actual cost of services. Based on the Blue Cross–Blue Shield health insurance model in existence at that time, it did not include prescription drugs, preventive services, hearing aids, or glasses. Medicaid was a program to fund medical assistance for certain individuals and families with low incomes and resources.

Medicare was initially administered by the Social Security Administration (SSA), while the federal part of Medicaid was the responsibility of the federal Social and Rehabilitation Service (SRS). Both of these agencies were a part of the Department of Health, Education and Welfare (HEW), which has since been renamed the Department of Health and Human Services (HHS). In 1977, the Health Care Financing Administration (HCFA) was created within HEW to run the Medicare and Medicaid programs. In 2001, HCFA was renamed the Centers for Medicare and Medicaid Services (CMS).

A year after the legislation passed, when Medicare became operational in July of 1966, it had 19 million beneficiaries. In 1972, Congress extended Medicare to include people with end-stage renal disease who were on dialysis or awaiting a kidney transplant and the disabled on Social Security Disability Insurance (SSDI). By 2004, coverage had expanded to 42 million people, primarily as a result of aging. This figure is expected to nearly double to 77 million by 2030 primarily as a result of an aging population.

Medicare Matures and Grows

Understandably, Medicare program costs have increased over the years, because of inflationary pressures, market changes, medical technology innovations and pharmaceutical

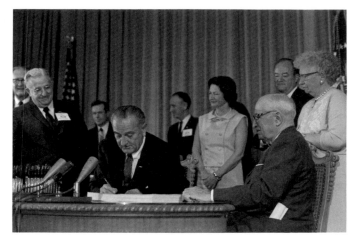

Figure 17-2 Signing of the Medicare Bill, July 30, 1965. *(Courtesy the Lyndon Baines Johnson Library and Museum.)*

advances. In addition, Congress has adopted numerous initiatives intended to hold spending in check and to ensure optimal patient care, with the goal of safeguarding the program.

In 2003, Congress passed the Medicare Prescription Drug, Improvement, and Modernization Act. Intended to modernize Medicare, this legislation allows for the expansion of preventive benefits, the coverage of an outpatient prescription drug benefit, and a change in the payment methodology for drugs administered in a physician's office (moving from paying average wholesale price to paying the average sales price and group purchasing rather than physician purchasing). Other features include support for new managed care options, including both health maintenance organizations (HMOs) and preferred provider organizations (PPOs), called Medicare Advantage under Part C.

Currently 95% of the elderly in America receive health care services from Medicare. Because of the many ophthalmic conditions that develop with age, the elderly make up the majority of most ophthalmologists' patient base. In 2003, the specialty of ophthalmology ranked first in the percentage of revenues from Medicare by specialty, fourth in absolute dollars ($4.4 billion), and first in the percentage of participating physicians. In 2004, Medicare accounted for 55% of a typical ophthalmologist's revenue. With its increasing scope of services, Medicare clearly has an enormous effect on the quality of care that ophthalmologists can give their patients, as well as on the practice of ophthalmology itself. For this reason, federal health care legislation and, particularly, issues surrounding Medicare are an intense focus of ophthalmology advocacy today.

The box "Medicare Milestones" details important legislative actions that have shaped the program into its present form, and it is fair to expect program changes to continue as fiscal, political, social, and technological forces affect the nature of patient care and the practice of medicine. See Chapters 5 and 6 in Part I for more specific information about the structure of Medicare and Medicaid and the practicalities of fee schedules and reimbursement. In Chapter 21, the case study examining reimbursement issues provides an interesting and instructive real-world look at this advocacy issue.

Medicare Milestones

1965: Authorized under Title XVIII of the Social Security Act, Medicare was enacted July 30, 1965, to cover the elderly. (Seniors were the population group most likely to be living in poverty; about half had insurance coverage.) Medicare was divided into two parts. Part A, hospital payments, is financed with payroll taxes that are placed in a trust fund. Under Part B, which is financed with current income tax revenues, Medicare pays physicians and ambulatory surgical centers for their services and for drugs administered in physicians' offices.

1966: Medicare was implemented and more than 19 million people were enrolled on July 1. **1970:** Over 20 million older Americans were enrolled in Medicare.

1972: Medicare coverage was extended to the disabled and to those with permanent kidney failure. Two million more people subsequently enrolled in the program.

1977: The Health Care Financing Administration (HCFA) was established to administer the Medicare and Medicaid programs.

1980: Coverage of home health services was broadened. Medicare supplemental insurance, also called "Medigap," was brought under federal oversight. More than 28 million people were enrolled in Medicare.

1982: While managed care plans could participate in the program since its inception, the Tax Equity and Fiscal Responsibility Act of 1982 (in provisions implemented in 1985) made it easier and more attractive for health maintenance organizations to contract with the Medicare program by introducing a risk-based option.

1983: A new prospective payment system (PPS) for hospitals was implemented to slow the growth of hospital spending and preserve the life of the Hospital Insurance Trust Fund. The PPS, in which a predetermined rate is based on the patient's diagnosis, was adopted to replace cost-based payments.

1988: The Medicare Catastrophic Coverage Act was enacted to include an outpatient prescription drug benefit and a cap on patient liability.

1989: The Medicare Catastrophic Coverage Act was repealed after higher-income elderly people protested the new premiums. A new fee schedule for physician services was enacted, to be based on resources rather than historical charges.

1996: A Social Security Act amendment mandated that Medicare practice expenses (PEs) be resource based.

1996: The Health Insurance Portability and Accountability Act of 1996 (HIPAA) was enacted to amend the Public Health Service Act, the Employee Retirement Income Security Act of 1974 (ERISA), and the Internal Revenue Code of 1986 to provide improved continuity or "portability" of group health plan coverage provided through employment or through the individual insurance market (ie, not connected with employment). HIPAA also allowed HCFA to regulate small and individual private health insurance markets. The act created the Medicare Integrity Program, which dedicated funding to program integrity activities and allowed HCFA to competitively contract for program integrity work. Furthermore, HIPAA enacted national administrative simplification standards for all electronic health care transactions.

(cont.)

(cont.)

1997: The Balanced Budget Act of 1997 included the most extensive legislative changes for Medicare since the program was enacted:

- Established a single conversion factor
- Established a new methodology for practice expenses
- Established, as Part C of the Medicare program, Medicare + Choice, creating an array of new managed care and other health plan choices for beneficiaries, with a coordinated open enrollment process
- Developed and implemented several new payment systems for Medicare services, to improve payment accuracy and to help further restrain the growth of health care spending
- Tested other innovative approaches to payment and service delivery through research and demonstrations
- Expanded preventive benefits

1998: The Internet site www.medicare.gov was launched to provide updated information about Medicare.

1999: The Balanced Budget Refinement Act (BBRA) made substantial investments to meet the needs of our nation's hospitals and their patients.

2000: Medicare served 39 million seniors and disabled Americans. Medicare trustees estimated that Medicare will be solvent through 2025. The Benefit Improvements and Protection Act of 2000 made additional investments for providers and expanded preventive benefits.

2004: Implementation of the Medicare Prescription Drug, Improvement, and Modernization Act of 2003 resulted in expanded preventive services, creation of Part D to administer a new prescription drug card and benefit plan, enhanced support of Medicare managed care through the creation of Medicare Advantage HMOs and regional PPOs, and creation of a competitive demonstration program pitting the Medicare fee-for-service plan against the Medicare Advantage plan.

Source: www.cms.hhs.gov/about/history/mcaremil.asp

CHAPTER 18

Advocacy and Ophthalmology-Specific Issues

The need for you to become an active advocate for "your patients and your profession" is increasingly apparent in virtually every aspect of your professional life. The external factors that have come to influence your "independent" decisions as a physician are dependent upon decision makers in government and industry who need your input on the formation of their policies and the impact of their actions. These factors range from the frequency and completeness of the exams that you perform, to the procedures that you do, the tests that you are allowed to order, the medications that you can prescribe and the reimbursement that you receive for your training and skills,

Beyond general concerns, several ophthalmology-specific issues have involved advocates in recent years. Such issues have included lobbying for the following:

- The Veterans Eye Treatment Safety Act to guarantee that veterans receive the same standard of care as all other individuals and have surgery performed by trained medical physicians and not by medical paraprofessionals
- The need for medical liability reform to slow the rise in malpractice insurance premiums and redefine the progressively adversarial doctor-patient relationship
- A mandated vision screening program for school-age children that does not involve full examinations
- The Children's Access to Vision Care Act providing state grants for eye examinations and follow-up treatment for uninsured youth identified through a screening process
- Reimbursement for routine ophthalmological examinations of diabetics
- Reimbursement for ophthalmological examinations of people at risk for developing glaucoma
- Medicare and third-party insurers payment for low vision rehabilitation
- The need for a fair Medicare reimbursement formula not linked to the sustainable growth rate (SGR) so that physicians can continue to participate in Medicare and patients have access to quality eye care (see "Medicare Matures and Grows" in Chapter 17)
- Statutory relief from complying with new Medicare policies including the publication of regulations on a monthly basis, allowing for a 30-day grace period for compliance, providing educational programs for coding and compliance, and reforming the audit process and manner in which overpayments are recouped

- Patient protections in a managed care world, including point-of-service options at the time of enrollment, independent appeals mechanisms of adverse decisions, a ban on financial incentives to reduce or deny care, a restriction on gag clauses limiting physician discussion of treatment options, and a full explanation of plan performance
- The ability of physicians to collectively negotiate contracts with managed care organizations
- Increases in the National Eye Institute (NEI) budget

Given the range, breadth, and depth of the issues facing ophthalmologists, it is clear that once you make a commitment to advocacy, you will have no trouble finding subjects that are personally significant to you. For additional discussion of key issues, see the next section as well as the case studies on reimbursement and tort reform in Chapter 21.

Ophthalmology and Optometry

The social history of medicine includes numerous instances of trained practitioners opposing untrained or inadequately trained individuals who were delivering health care, particularly opposing their attempts to perform procedures or administer treatments beyond their training. For example, medieval physicians sought to limit the practices of self-trained herbal healers. In late nineteenth-century America, highly trained physicians worried about patients being harmed by practitioners who received their education at substandard institutions. Since that time, legal action and legislative advocacy have been increasingly employed to protect both patients and practitioners. The relationship between ophthalmology and optometry serves as an example of an area that has involved strong advocacy efforts over the years.

Ophthalmology had begun to establish itself as one of medicine's first specialties by the early 1800s. Modeled on the London Eye Infirmary, which was established in 1805, the New York Eye and Ear Infirmary first employed ophthalmologists in 1820. Ophthalmologists increasingly distinguished themselves from general practitioners who provided some eye care but had no specialty training. At the beginning of the twentieth century, ophthalmic specialists, with their broad and increasing array of impressive new devices, surgical methods, and scientific knowledge, concentrated on eye pathology and surgery and paid little attention to refractive errors, despite the public's growing need for spectacle correction.

As providers of spectacles, opticians naturally took an interest in advances regarding the knowledge of physiological and physical optics in the mid to late 1800s. The dispensing of glasses by dispensing opticians as well as vision exams and spectacle prescribing by refracting opticians (who later renamed themselves "optometrists"), became an area in which substantial profits could be made. Ophthalmologists became more interested in refracting patients, which refracting opticians saw as a threat to their own businesses. Optometry eventually achieved the status of a legislated profession when Minnesota passed an optometry licensure bill in 1901, and by 1924 all existing states plus the District of Columbia had formally legislated optometric licensing. (See the box "The States' Impact on Scope of Practice.")

The States' Impact on Scope of Practice

In the United States, the first physician licensure laws appeared as early as the 1700s. State licensure of professions broadened in the nineteenth century to include nurses, dentists, and many of the allied health professions in existence today, with the purpose of protecting the public from unprofessional, improper, and incompetent professional practice. State laws stipulate a level of education and training required to obtain the license. State boards of the individual professions enforce those laws.

Because control of the health care professions has been significantly concentrated in the state governments, and because most controls are statutorily defined, state legislatures have been the major arena for defining scope of practice, both in limiting and expanding it. As ophthalmology and optometry continue to debate scope-of-practice issues today, advocacy at a state level remains an important activity.

Ophthalmology and optometry have since co-existed, sometimes easily and sometimes uneasily. With regard to early legislation, ophthalmology initially offered only weak or occasional opposition to optometric licensure. Describing a newly passed optometric practice bill in his state, a Connecticut physician delegate at an AMA conference in 1914 remarked that "since this bill was the least objectionable yet, the medical society let it go, providing it included a caveat against the title 'doctor' or its synonym being used by optometrists." As with other specialty physicians, ophthalmologists' practices traditionally have been concentrated in urban areas, leaving rural eye care largely to general practitioners. Optometrists have historically served the refractive needs of rural populations, as they require a smaller population base for a practice and do not need the resources of a hospital. They also frequently had knowledge and ophthalmic instruments that a rural physician lacked, thereby functioning by default as the local eye specialist. The result has been confusion that has continued for decades in the public's mind about the difference between an ophthalmologist and an optometrist.

Another issue concerns the fact that legislated payment rules permit ophthalmologists and optometrists to share a fee when the optometrist provides postoperative care. In the 1980s HCFA began to allow the splitting of the payment for an operation under Medicare from the postoperative care by the use of a 54/55 modifier on the submitted claim. This addressed the concern of nonpayment to a physician who was rendering postoperative services to a patient who was treated in another state while traveling, sometimes great distances, and who required follow up upon returning home. It also resolved compensation issues that arose when a specialist traveled to a small town and performed a complex procedure, and the postoperative care was assumed by the local doctor. By 2002, 65% of this co-management under Medicare was occurring between an ophthalmologist and an optometrist, and 15% of cataract procedures performed in the United States used this co-management modifier. In 2002, the American Academy of Ophthalmology and the American Society of Cataract and Refractive Surgery issued a joint position paper on the role of co-management of ophthalmic surgical patients and offered guidelines as to when this practice is ethical and proper and when it is unethical and even illegal. The position paper states that if the reason for sharing postoperative care with another provider (however well trained) is economic—specifically, as an inducement for surgical referrals or the result of coercion by the referring practitioner—it is patently unethical and, in many jurisdictions, illegal. The Office of the Inspector General of the U.S. Department of Health and Human Services has also expressed concern about co-management that is based on economic considerations rather than on clinical appropriateness and has refused to provide safe harbor protections for such arrangements, preferring to review cases on an individual basis. The joint position paper is available on the Academy's web site (www.aao.org/aaoesite/promo/compliance/joint_position.cfm).

Optometry Expands through State Advocacy

Professionals in ophthalmology and optometry work well together in most circumstances to benefit patients and provide quality care. However, issues of scope of practice have played a large role in the history of the two professions, and they continue to affect their relationship, especially when patient health and safety are at stake.

Beginning in the 1950s, organized optometry sought the introduction of state legislation to allow optometrists to use diagnostic eyedrops to identify ophthalmological abnormalities in the performance of "ocular health exams." Any abnormalities identified were to be referred immediately to a qualified medical practitioner for diagnosis and treatment. As time passed, the legislation introduced sought authorization for optometrists to diagnose certain eye pathologies and to use therapeutic drops, oral drugs, controlled substances, and injections.

At first these bills engendered little concern in the medical and ophthalmological communities and had only token opposition. By the mid 1980s, however, nearly every state in the country had enacted a bill permitting optometrists to use diagnostic pharmaceutical agents (DPAs), and more than half had statutes on their books permitting their use of some therapeutic pharmaceutical agents (TPAs).

In the 1990s, optometrists began to advocate for two new goals: the right to do surgery and the ability of the state board of optometry to determine what their profession can and cannot do. In 1998, optometrists were authorized by Oklahoma law to perform laser surgery, except for retinal procedures, laser in situ keratomileusis (LASIK), and cosmetic eyelid surgery. In 2004, Oklahoma law authorized optometrists to perform nonlaser surgery procedures, as determined by the Oklahoma Board of Examiners in Optometry. Attempts to pass laser surgery legislation in other states have followed, but as of 2004, none have been successful, primarily because of advocacy efforts by organized ophthalmology.

The regulation of these continuing expansions of the scope of optometric practice is vested in state boards of optometry, not state medical boards. Recently, optometrists have also supported legislation to place the authority to define the scope of optometric practice in the board of optometry, instead of in the state legislature (see the box "Limited-License Professions"). They argue that it will relieve legislators of the burden of dealing with scope-of-practice issues and that the judgment of the board of optometry would be sufficient. Organized medicine argues that this change will effectively deliver oversight of optometric scope of practice to optometrists without the opportunity for effective comment and review by organized medicine and the public.

Limited-License Professions

In general, states define the professions of medicine and osteopathy as unlimited-license professions under state law. This means that any and all means of diagnosis and treatment may be used, as the profession deems appropriate. Other health care professions are "limited license," because their scope of practice is restricted to that defined by the state statute. Professional boards such as the board of optometry may be set up for these professions, but the board's mandate is to ensure that licensure requirements and quality-of-care standards consistent with the profession's limited scope are met.

Antitrust Issues

Appropriate relationships with colleagues and organizations are central to the preservation and improvement of the medical profession. Guidelines from the American Academy of Ophthalmology note the kinds of discussions for members to avoid in formal or informal meetings of any other professional or governmental organization, and in all other contacts with actual or potential competitors. Such discussions include the following subjects:

- Discussions about, or that may have the effect of, fixing, raising, depressing, pegging, or stabilizing prices or fees, or any element of prices or fees, or establishing minimum or maximum prices or fees
- Discussions about, or that may have the effect of, either withholding patronage or services from or otherwise discouraging dealings with, or encouraging exclusive dealings with, any health care provider or group of health care providers, any supplier or purchaser or group of suppliers or purchasers of health care products or services, any actual or potential competitor or group of actual or potential competitors, or any patient, group of patients, or other segment of the public
- Discussions about, or that may have the effect of allocating or dividing geographic or service markets, customers, or patients
- Discussions about, or that may have the effect of, restricting, limiting, prohibiting, or sanctioning advertising, or soliciting which is not false, misleading, or deceptive
- Discussions about, or that may have the effect of, discouraging entry into or competition in any segment of the health care market
- Discussions about whether or not the practices of any member, actual or potential competitor, or other person are "unethical" or "anticompetitive"
- Discussions about the safety, quality or efficacy of the products or services of, or the prices or fees charged by, any health care provider or group of health care providers, any supplier or purchaser or group of suppliers or purchasers of health care products or services, or any actual or potential competitor or group of actual or potential competitors. This does not restrict or prohibit study and reasonable discussion and assessment of the safety or efficacy of technology, drugs, and devices.

For more information, see "Guidelines for the Avoidance of Inadvertent Anticompetitive Conduct" on the Academy's web site (www.aao.org/aao/member/policy). Also see Case Study 7 in Chapter 15.

Lobbying Activities

Certain activities of the Academy and its members are protected from antitrust laws under the First Amendment right to petition the government. The antitrust exemption for these activities, often referred to as the *Noerr-Pennington Doctrine,* protects ethical and proper actions or discussions by members designed to influence: (1) legislation at the national, state, or local level; (2) regulatory or policymaking activities (as opposed to commercial activities) of a governmental body; or (3) decisions of judicial bodies. However, the exemption does not protect actions constituting a "sham" to cover anticompetitive conduct. A member who makes knowing and willful false statements to the government likewise does not enjoy immunity.

Lobbying activities involving optometry or eye care for veterans are examples of areas where antitrust issues may come into play. To illustrate, as you choose to become involved in lobbying for your patients and profession, you should be aware that asking an individual Veterans Affairs facility to limit the performance of eye surgery to physicians does not constitute lobbying activity. Such discussion is not immune under the Noerr-Pennington Doctrine.

In addition, never threaten or imply any form of retaliation or the withholding of services if the VA facility fails to agree with the Academy's position (ie, emphasis on factual matters comparing the education, training and experience of ophthalmologists to that of optometrists and the strong preference of veterans to have their eye surgery performed by physicians). Strikes, "job actions," work slowdowns, and/or boycotts can constitute a group boycott that violates the antitrust laws and Section 5 of the Federal Trade Commission Act, 15 U.S.C. § 45. The fact that the target of the proposed strike or other activity is the government does not render the conduct immune from antitrust exposure.

Never disparage the individual optometrist who either has privileges or is seeking privileges; instead, keep the discussion in general terms (for example, the education, training and experience of the ophthalmologist).

The Future of Ophthalmology Advocacy

The safety of patients and the quality of ophthalmic care, particularly as manifested by scope of practice issues, will continue to drive the advocacy efforts of ophthalmology on both a state and a federal level. Medicare coverage and payment is another area where effective advocacy will be essential. Medical liability reform (tort reform) is also an important issue affecting all physicians. Working with state officials on state-level reimbursements for Medicaid and other state-controlled programs will be required to continue effective ophthalmic practice.

The American Academy of Ophthalmology has established a robust political advocacy presence in Washington, DC, and it encourages members' participation. In addition, each of the 50 states has a state ophthalmological society that depends on effective advocates in its efforts to ensure that legislation that is passed preserves quality eye care for every patient. Clearly, continued advocacy is essential for our patients and our profession.

Recommended Reading

Jacobs LR. *The Health of Nations. Public Opinion and the Making of American and British Health Policy.* Ithaca, NY: Cornell University Press; 1993.

Starr P. *The Social Transformation of American Medicine.* New York, NY: Basic Books, Inc.; 1982.

Wallace N, Wedding D. The battle for the use of drugs for therapeutic purposes in optometry: lessons for clinical psychology. *Prof Psychol Res Pr.* 2004;130:323–328.

CHAPTER 19

Advocacy Principles, Resources, and Methods

Government and politics greatly influence the practice of medicine in America today. Political engagement on behalf of your patients and your profession is, therefore, an extension of your medical practice. In twenty-first-century America, advocacy—the structured approach to achieving an organization's policy objectives—is crucial to the continued existence of our profession and our specialty.

This chapter introduces the principles and methods of advocacy—the activities encompassed and the structures and situations in which they take place. Through this introduction, the authors hope that you will come to appreciate the purpose and power of advocacy and make the decision to include advocacy for ophthalmology in your lifelong commitment to your chosen profession.

Advocacy: The Reality

Becoming an advocate for ophthalmology can be personally and professionally fulfilling. However, it is wise to approach advocacy with reasonable expectations. What can be accomplished frequently depends on a policymaker's philosophy, interest in your issues, and political party affiliation. As an advocate for medicine today, you will need the abilities to:

- Appreciate the complex historical, political, social, cultural, philosophical, and economic aspects of a given issue.
- Listen with sincere interest to the arguments and positions of other stakeholders.
- Recognize the levers that may be effective in getting them to support your position.
- Understand that the best you can do may be just to continue communicating your position and to never give up trying to influence legislation and policy.

As an example of this, consider the issue of medical liability and tort reform. Certain American civil laws—specifically, torts—permit patients to sue medical providers for virtually unlimited amounts when malpractice occurs in the course of treatment. As a result, the cost of medical liability insurance has become increasingly prohibitive, physicians are leaving the profession, and patient access to doctors, particularly in high-risk specialties, is in jeopardy.

Despite broad agreement that this part of the judicial system seems to be broken, positions differ widely on how best to solve the problem. Trial lawyers and some patient groups oppose any solution they feel would limit patients' rights and victimize them. Physicians, on the other hand, need protection from frivolous lawsuits and ruinous judgments. (For a description of this issue and specific methods of advocacy that may be applied to it, see Case Study 2 in Chapter 21.) Although a workable solution may take years to achieve, it will not take place at all unless practitioners of medicine advocate for changes to the laws. In fact, this example only underscores the need for more ophthalmologist advocates and more vigorous advocacy efforts. You can make a difference, but only if you integrate advocacy into your professional activities.

Advocacy: Principles

A few basic principles can help you to stay focused, build on your successes, learn from your failures, and, ultimately, make a difference through advocacy. These principles include the following:

- Know the issues.
- Know the decision makers and the decision-making process.
- Have a clear objective.
- Be committed to the process.

Knowing the Issues

As an advocate you will find dozens of issues worthy of your enthusiastic championing. You might be drawn to those affecting medicine as a profession, such as Medicare reimbursement or the need for research freedom and funding. Ophthalmology-specific issues, such as scope-of-practice concerns or public screening for glaucoma and diabetic eye disease, might attract your interest. Whatever issues you select for your own advocacy efforts, research them thoroughly—their clinical, economic, and social ramifications; their legislative and regulatory history; and their past and present supporters and opponents.

The Internet has made it easier and more convenient than ever before to get detailed historical information and up-to-date news on any issue you care to research. Resources for learning about issues appear later in this chapter.

Knowing the Decision Makers and the Decision-Making Process

An important technique of advocacy is to influence decision makers such as elected and appointed officials. The Internet has made it easy to identify your state and federal legislators—you can start with the listings available at the Academy's web site (www.aao.org).

If your chosen advocacy issue is not specifically legislative, your research into the issue itself will likely turn up the names or at least the titles of other decision makers who might be involved, such as hospital board members or medical directors, insurance company executives, public health officials, school board members, or Food and Drug

Administration (FDA) regulators. Again, as discussed throughout this chapter, the Academy and the Internet are excellent sources of information about who is in charge of what.

Having a Clear Objective

Once you have determined where you want to direct your advocacy efforts, consider the outcome you want and can reasonably expect. Is it the passage of a certain bill? Is it a change in policy, practice, or attitude? Having a specific objective gives you a concrete way to measure the success or failure of your advocacy efforts.

Do not forget about the smaller goals you'll need to set in order to achieve the larger objectives such as gaining the ear of a policymaker or educating patients and the public on an issue that affects their eye health or your ability to serve them. Ways to achieve these smaller, yet very important, goals are discussed later in this chapter.

Being Committed to the Process

Like anything else worth achieving, advocating for the medical profession and ophthalmology cannot be an occasional activity to be picked up and dropped again like a hobby. Relationships can take years to build, information years to disseminate, and legislation years to pass. The purpose of advocacy is positive change and progress, neither of which occurs swiftly or easily. If you decide to be an advocate, you will stand the best chance for success if you stay focused on the issues and on the processes by which you will affect the issues. The remainder of this chapter provides an overview of the various resources available to you and some basic processes of advocacy.

Advocacy: Resources

The most important concept to understand as you embark on your "career" in advocacy is that *you are not expected to go it alone.* An elaborate support structure exists that will welcome your participation in the process and prepare you to be a confident, informed, effective advocate for ophthalmology from the start. Through these resources, information is readily available about issues of importance, the points that need to be made, the people who affect policy, and the techniques for advocacy.

These supportive resources include the American Academy of Ophthalmology, state ophthalmological societies, and dozens, if not hundreds, of other organizations for medical professionals, patients, industry, and other special interests. These resources are introduced in the next section, and specific ways of working with them in your own advocacy efforts are described in "Advocacy: Methods" in this chapter.

American Academy of Ophthalmology

In addition to education, advocacy is a primary focus of the American Academy of Ophthalmology. Recognizing the importance of legislative advocacy, the Academy opened its Governmental Affairs Division in Washington, DC, within 1 year of its independent formation in the late 1970s. The Academy was also the first major medical specialty organization to start a political action committee (PAC). Realizing how much the political and legislative processes affect patient care and the practice of medicine, the Academy has devoted itself to advocacy in a way that has become a model for many specialty societies. Most significant, perhaps, is the effort the Academy makes to engage and inform its members as advocates for ophthalmology.

The Advocacy Action Center on the Academy's web site is a key resource for those just starting in advocacy as well as for seasoned ophthalmology advocates (see Appendix III for more information about the Academy's advocacy information online, its Governmental Affairs Division, OPHTHPAC and the Congressional Advocacy Committee, and state affairs activities.)

State Ophthalmological Societies

State ophthalmological societies represent the local backbone of political advocacy. Since scope-of-practice, insurance regulation, and patient access issues are primarily affected by state legislative and regulatory actions, effective representation in this venue is essential. State ophthalmological societies play a leadership role in political advocacy in state capitals. In addition to political activities, state societies are involved in public outreach programs, such as vision, glaucoma, and diabetes screenings. Partnering with patient coalitions in representing the interests of the citizens of a state and their right to receive competent and appropriate health care is a growing and important role for advocates working through state societies.

State ophthalmological societies provide their members with a wide range of services in addition to political representation. Such activities include affinity programs (eg, discount drugs, office supplies, phone services); help with insurance problems; ombudsman support; courses for physicians and their staffs on general, subspecialty, and socioeconomic issues; and help with day-to-day office economic issues and expenses. Just being available as an important source of advice makes membership in your state society essential and a great investment in your future. Last, but certainly not least, is the opportunity that the state ophthalmological societies can offer you for gaining your initial introduction to and training in advocacy.

Coalitions

Coalitions, or alliances based on common concerns, are created to advance specific goals that organizations share. National and state medical societies, specialty societies, patient advocacy groups, and many other organizations with a stake in health care and its delivery understand that they strengthen their advocacy efforts when they work together in a common interest, pooling people, resources, and influence.

Patient Coalitions

The most important, and therefore the most effective, coalition member is the patient. The public, lawmakers, and physicians are most interested in how issues affect patients. Patients participate in coalition building, often as individuals. Any person who writes to a congressperson or the local media, or who discusses issues with friends, can be a powerful advocate and an influential coalition partner.

A considerable number of patient advocacy groups exist in the United States, with the common goals of establishing and protecting the interests of patients. Senior citizen groups such as the American Association of Retired Persons (AARP) focus on issues of geriatric disorders, insurance, and affordable health services for low-income retirees. Public interest groups and service organizations, such as the Lions Club, Kiwanis, the National Association for the Visually Handicapped, Prevent Blindness America, and local low-vision and visual rehabilitation service groups, lobby on eye care issues. The approach of such groups is to influence policy and create a powerful voice through an organization representing large numbers of patients with common concerns. In the hundreds of patient advocacy groups that exist, you are likely to find one that aligns with your interests.

Coalitions of Professional Societies

Physicians in large, inclusive medical organizations such as the AMA come from all specialties. When working together to represent the interests of many physicians, such groups can potentially have substantial influence.

Because specialty societies represent alliances of physicians with common practice issues and educational needs, physicians commonly identify most strongly with these groups. Coalitions between general medical organizations such as the AMA or a state medical association and specialty societies are essential for effective advocacy. For example, the affiliation between the American Academy of Ophthalmology and the American Medical Association has allowed ophthalmology to introduce issues into the AMA House of Delegates (its representative body), to develop AMA positions, and to present a unified front, as well as to carry additional influence when we speak with federal and state legislators.

In addition, ophthalmology aligns naturally with other specialties that share our scope-of-practice concerns. Psychiatry, plastic surgery, obstetrics and gynecology, anesthesiology, orthopedics, and family practice look to ophthalmology for support in scope-of-practice issues and vice versa. For example, in 2001 eight national medical specialty societies, including the American Academy of Ophthalmology, collaborated to create a joint exhibit at the National Council of State Legislatures' annual meeting to educate legislators about important patient care and scope-of-practice issues and to demonstrate medicine's solidarity.

Coalitions of Other Organizations

Because a uniform, consistent message is more effective than many individual, inconsistent ones, organizations with shared interests routinely make informal and formal coalitions to lobby jointly for a specific political or social goal. At any given time in your career, you may find coalitions with organizations other than those strictly for physicians or patients to be useful.

For example, ophthalmologists might successfully join with others in the health care field, including hospital and health insurance executives, to work on clinical or practice issues such as glaucoma, cataract, and diabetes screenings for underserved hospital clinic populations and to achieve effective preventative medicine for those with health insurance. Becoming involved with your hospital medical staff leadership can demonstrate your commitment to medicine in general and can help you gain support from these respected community organizations for ophthalmology-specific issues when they arise.

Legislators will also feel much more of an effect when the same message is delivered by multiple groups. One example is that of the Veterans Eye Treatment Safety (VETS)

Coalition led by the Academy, which sent letters to every congressperson requesting co-sponsorship of a bill, ensuring that military veterans in Veterans Affairs hospitals receive eye surgery by trained surgeons rather than by nonphysicians. The letter was signed by 147 medical specialty and state societies and resulted in broad bipartisan support for the legislation.

The nature of American politics gives both local and national coalitions the potential for considerable influence. Forming coalitions among several organizations to coordinate grassroots advocacy is an effective way to get legislators' attention and to let them know that many constituents from different groups feel strongly about a given issue.

Although there is no specific list of organizations that should be considered in forming coalitions, the particular issue under consideration and common sense will dictate where you might look and whom you can consider approaching. The Academy has formed and continues to participate in a significant number of coalitions on issues such as patient protections, medical liability reform, and Medicare reimbursement policy, representing general medical, specialty-specific, and patient issues on a national basis. Depending on which issues concern you most, with a little thought you can find dozens of groups with whom you might profitably ally yourself, such as research scientists, pharmaceutical industry professionals, and ethnic-oriented interest groups. The essential point here is that coalitions of like-minded people increase individuals' voices not just linearly but exponentially.

Advocacy: Methods

Three basic methods of purely political advocacy are:

- Become a grassroots activist.
- Get involved in local politics.
- Offer financial and volunteer support to elected officials, political campaigns, and political action committees that represent the interests of ophthalmology.

Another highly effective method of advocacy is to communicate with your patients and the media. All of these approaches are described in this section.

Becoming a Grassroots Activist

Who you know, how well you know them, and the trust that you gradually develop with them are at the heart of influencing policy at any level. One of the most effective ways of becoming a grassroots activist is by building relationships with your elected officials, other policy and decision makers, and those who advise them.

Beginning this process is as simple as calling, writing, e-mailing, or faxing these people to let them know how an issue affects you and your patients. The Academy can provide you with talking points on the major issues affecting ophthalmology—check the Advocacy section of the Academy web site. The box "Tips on Writing to Congressional Representatives" describes ways to get in touch with your legislators and proper forms of address to use in correspondence.

Tips on Writing to Congressional Representatives

Here are some suggestions to ensure the effectiveness of your letter to a member of Congress:

- State your purpose for writing in the first paragraph of the letter. If your letter pertains to a specific piece of legislation, identify it; for example, House bill: H. R. ____, Senate bill: S. ____.

- Be courteous, keep to the point, and include key information, using examples to support your position.

- Address only one issue in each letter and, if possible, keep the letter to one page.

Addressing Correspondence to a Senator:

The Honorable (full name)
__ (Rm. #) __ (name of) Senate Office Building
United States Senate Washington, DC 20510

Dear Senator:

Addressing Correspondence to a Representative:

The Honorable (full name)
__ (Rm. #) __ (name of) House Office Building
United States House of Representatives Washington, DC 20515

Dear Representative:

Note: When writing to the chair of a committee or the Speaker of the House, the proper salutation would be Dear Mr. Chairman, Dear Madam Chairwoman, or Dear Mr. Speaker.

The Advocacy section of the Academy web site offers many tools to help in your advocacy efforts, including the ability to send a letter to your members of Congress on an important issue for which the Academy is lobbying. Form letters are available either to e-mail to your representatives directly from the Action Center or to download onto your practice letterhead and fax to members of Congress or other public officials. If you don't know who your representatives are, you can simply type in your ZIP code and the names will appear.

Organized Group Visits

Calling and writing legislators requires little financial outlay and can be extremely effective; however, a face-to-face meeting is an even more productive method of advocacy. Regardless of your enthusiasm for or expertise about an issue, reaching busy legislators in person is rarely easy, especially for those new to advocacy. Fortunately, numerous organizations and tools are available to facilitate this process. One of the most effective of these is the annual Congressional Advocacy Day sponsored by the American Academy of Ophthalmology. For this event, ophthalmologists from around the country meet in Washington, DC, to be briefed by Academy lobbyists on the issues. The next day, you have the opportunity to meet face to face with your own members of Congress to let them know how key governmental policies affect your practice and your patients. These face-to-face meetings are an effective and time-honored way of educating your federal representatives and a unique opportunity to begin personal relationships with your fed-

Attend an Academy Congressional Advocacy Day

Advocacy Day is each member's day to come to Washington, be part of the solution to the problems we face, and to promote positive change.

Any member of the Academy can attend Advocacy Day, which is held yearly in the spring. There is no fee. Registration information and forms can be found at www.aao.org/aao/member/myf/change_med.cfm, or call the Academy's Washington office at 202-737-6662. The Academy provides all necessary materials to educate participants on the issues, so no prior lobbying experience is necessary. The Academy gives participants appropriate talking points, provides tips on lobbying, and awards CME credits for participation.

eral legislators. The box "Attend an Academy Congressional Advocacy Day" provides details on how to participate.

Many state ophthalmological medical societies and special interest groups hold similar annual "Legislative Day" visits to state representatives' offices in the state capital. "Advocacy: Resources" earlier in this chapter and Appendix III discusses the Academy and other specific advocacy groups and types of opportunities.

Town hall meetings, often held by elected officials when they are home in their districts, offer another good opportunity to communicate face to face on issues that matter to you and your profession and to inform as well as ask what your elected official's position is and what he or she can do to help you. Call your congressperson's district office to find out when these meetings are scheduled, or work through your state ophthalmological society.

One-on-One Meetings

The single most significant instrument in your advocacy tool kit is your personal relationship with your legislators. Charles Hebner, former Speaker of the Delaware House of Delegates, has explained it this way: "The most effective lobbyist I will ever face is a registered voter from my district who comes to me with a well-documented explanation of how the legislation will affect him." Close relationships can only be built over time, based on face-to-face meetings. For those just embarking on advocacy activities, the first challenge will be making the initial appointment with the legislator.

Gaining access to a busy U.S. senator can be difficult, especially if you are new to advocacy and do not have an established relationship. On the other hand, congressional representatives, with their smaller and more local constituencies, are generally more available for appointments, particularly in their district offices. You can find the office numbers and addresses of your senators and congressional representative easily at the Advocacy section of the Academy web site (www.aao.org/aao/advocacy).

It may be easiest to schedule appointments with your representatives in the home district, as they are likely to be more available and less distracted, and your travel time is shorter.

Regardless of the meeting location, the approach to the meeting is the same:

- Be prepared.
- Be succinct.
- Be polite.

Do Your Homework

Elected officials have an obligation to listen to the constituents they represent, but they are not likely to be receptive to the causes of anyone who berates, cajoles, or harangues them. Be respectful of legislators' time and, most important, *know where they stand on a particular bill* before engaging them in the advocacy conversation. In other words, do your homework! The Academy can provide you with insights about your representative as well as talking points to keep your conversation focused on key issues.

- Do not assume that the person you are speaking with is ignorant of your issues and does not appreciate the nature of your concerns.
- Make a well-reasoned and well-organized presentation on just your most important few issues.
- Be ready for a discussion, at times a debate, but not a one-sided conversation.

The box "Do Your Homework" offers another perspective on your meetings with busy legislators.

In addition to personal visits to your elected officials' offices, invite your legislators to your office to see for themselves how your business operates and how particular issues affect you and your patients. For example, if the topic being discussed is regulatory reform, show your representatives the insurance-related paperwork that you and your staff must process to provide patient care. Legislators often welcome an invitation to tour a clinic or hospital because it increases their public visibility.

Meeting with Staff Aides

When you schedule office visits with your elected officials to discuss issues important to you and your profession, meet with their key staff if you can—they are the eyes and ears of the official, and they provide daily counsel to their bosses. The legislator looks to them for insight and information. Make them your allies.

Getting Involved in Local Politics

For the ophthalmology advocate, getting involved in politics at the local level can result in your establishing political relationships—even friendships—that can last a lifetime. A majority of members of Congress began their political careers at the local and state levels. Politicians welcome the help and counsel of physicians, who are seen as being among the most educated and responsible community members, with the ability to offer insights on a range of complex medical issues, both scientific and socioeconomic.

Getting involved in local politics can be as simple as voting. Other activities can include volunteering in an election campaign or serving on a candidate's health policy advisory committee. Committee work provides an excellent opportunity to share—and become known for—your special professional knowledge, insight, and advice. When the legislator or staff health aide has questions on medical issues, your ability to offer clear, impartial, unbiased information will give you credibility and make you a genuine asset. Being seen as a valuable resource because of your professional perspective and expertise in scientific and socioeconomic issues will foster a relationship of mutual respect with law makers.

Fundraisers combine volunteering with financial support. Attending a fundraiser often takes little more effort than participating in a community social event, with a nominal associated cost. By far the most effective statement you can make is to contribute funds, either personal or PAC supported, to physician-friendly candidates. In addition to making a contribution, sponsoring or organizing fundraisers elevates your profile even higher. The Academy can help you with the details of organizing an effective fundraiser.

Offering Financial and Volunteer Support

According to AMA statistics, in the 2002 elections the average House election campaign cost close to $900,000, and some campaigns cost as much as $10 million. That same year, the average Senate election campaign cost $4.8 million, with some running as high as $26.9 million. These costs are staggering and reinforce the message that money, and lots of it, is key to running a successful campaign.

As you become involved in the political process, it is essential to understand that when you make a contribution, you do not buy a vote. Nevertheless, your donations are a sign that you are serious about your political involvement, and they help build a relationship that ensures your calls to your elected officials' offices are taken and that your views are heard and seriously considered.

Contributions are generally made in one of two ways: private donations and donations to PACs. A private contribution may take the form of an unsolicited donation, which you can personally offer at a breakfast or other function, in a sealed envelope with a business card and a note. More likely, you might privately donate in response to a fundraising request by mailing a check to a campaign treasurer. If you respond early and at a sponsorship level, your name may appear in the final fundraiser announcement. Contributing at something above the lowest level, which is often not that much more expensive, does gain you attention. Always report your personal contributions to the Academy or your state ophthalmological society so that your contributions can be leveraged.

Donations to PACs that Represent Ophthalmology's Interest

OPHTHPAC is the Academy's voluntary, nonpartisan political action committee that helps elect "friends of ophthalmology." OPHTHPAC is a key reason the Academy earned a listing in *Fortune* magazine as one of the most influential trade associations in Washington. OPHTHPAC raised and donated more than $1 million in contributions during the 2003–2004 election cycle, allowing Academy involvement in more than 200 congressional races. Ninety percent of OPHTHPAC-supported candidates won in that cycle.

State ophthalmological societies and state medical societies often have PACs that make contributions to both state and federal legislators. They are always looking for well-informed and well-spoken advocates with personal relationships to deliver these checks.

One notch above making a campaign contribution or attending a fundraiser is actually hosting a fundraiser yourself, as noted above in "Getting Involved in Local Politics." This is an activity that quickly elevates you to a special status with your legislator and promotes your goal of establishing a productive working relationship with him or her.

The Value of Volunteer Work

Volunteering to work on a candidate's campaign is not limited to stuffing envelopes or making telemarketing calls. Contributing your time and energy to an election effort can take a variety of forms. For example, you can offer to sit on the campaign's finance (fundraising) or health policy committee, where your expertise will be respected and helpful.

Communicating with Patients and the Media

It has often been said that our patients are our best potential allies. As such, they are woefully underutilized. Physicians should not be shy about letting patients know what is going on in Washington or the state capital and about how their interests will be affected by proposed rules and laws. Your volunteer work for a candidate can be as simple as placing brochures or a sign in your office waiting room.

An important way you can influence public opinion is by regularly writing letters on issues of ophthalmic concern to the editor of your local newspaper, making succinct points and using personal anecdotes. Use the Academy's (or your state ophthalmological society's) talking points on the issue as a whole. To increase the effect of your efforts, copy your state or congressional legislators, or send clippings if the letter is published. If you have public speaking talent, consider becoming an expert commentator for local broadcast outlets or volunteer as a guest speaker at meetings of consumer groups and benevolent societies that may be affected by issues concerning eye health, cost of health care, patient access to quality care, and other issues important to ophthalmology.

It Is Never Too Late to Advocate

Your path to advocacy involvement is best summarized by the proverb, "The longest journey begins with the first step." The need to become involved is clear; ultimately, advocacy can add a rewarding new dimension to your personal and professional life. Both easy and more challenging approaches to advocacy have been described here. Be assured that you have the full support of the Academy and your state ophthalmological society through the many resources they can provide.

CHAPTER 20

Government and Other Policymaking Structures

Federal and state governments wield considerable control over matters dealing with the delivery of medical care. Private insurers also influence your practice and the way you care for your patients. Even with corporate vendors of medical supplies, you may find yourself needing to advocate for the benefit of your own practice. Understanding how these entities are organized, how they make policy, and who has decision-making authority is crucial to your effectiveness as an advocate for ophthalmology.

This chapter is intended to provide basic information to help you understand how these various organizations work. Remember that the Academy's Governmental Affairs Division is available to answer questions and to help you find your niche in ophthalmological advocacy. With their local and regional knowledge, state ophthalmological societies also provide valuable additional support, and you are encouraged to partner with them as you begin navigating the maze of state agencies and private corporations.

Policymaking and Lawmaking at the Federal Level

The executive branch (the president and the administration) has far-reaching effects on the profession of medicine and on ophthalmology. Two powerful agencies for policymaking and control within the administration are the Domestic Policy Council and the Office of Management and Budget (OMB). The Domestic Policy Council, which advises the president, ensures that domestic initiatives are coordinated and consistent throughout federal agencies. In addition, the Domestic Policy Council monitors the implementation of domestic policy and presents the president's priorities to other branches of government. Among the many domestic areas within the purview of the council, those of most interest to ophthalmologists are health care and veterans' affairs.

The OMB assists the president by overseeing the preparation of the federal budget (thereby influencing policy) and by supervising the dispensing of funding in executive branch agencies. The OMB evaluates the effectiveness of agency programs, policies, and procedures; assesses competing funding demands among agencies; sets funding priorities; and ensures that agency reports, rules, testimony, and proposed legislation are consistent with the president's budget and with administration policy.

Ideas for federal legislative proposals may come from a U.S. representative or senator, from the president and the executive departments of the government, from private organized groups or associations, or from any citizen. However, only senators and representatives can introduce legislation into their respective houses of Congress.

Bills to carry out the recommendations of the president are usually introduced by request by the chairs of the various committees or subcommittees that would have jurisdiction over the subject matter. Sometimes the committees themselves may submit and order a bill reported to the House or Senate. Members of Congress who introduce legislation are known as the bill's "sponsors." Bills and resolutions are numbered sequentially and designated H.R. in the House and S. in the Senate—for example, bill number 100 would be listed as H.R. 100 or S. 100.

Legislation in Congress goes through a specific series of steps before it becomes enacted into law (Table 20-1). This chapter briefly summarizes this complex and lengthy process. The box "Everything You Always Wanted to Know about the Federal Government" directs you to the informative House and Senate web sites, where you can find information not just about the legislative process but also about current legislation, committee action, and a wide variety of other relevant topics.

Table 20-1 The Federal Legislative Process

Step 1. A bill is introduced by a sponsoring senator or representative and referred to the relevant standing House or Senate committee or subcommittee.

Step 2. The committee "marks up" (amends) a bill, votes a recommendation ("orders a bill reported") to the House or Senate, or kills a bill by inaction.

Step 3. For bills ordered reported, the committee staff prepares a written report describing the intent and scope of the legislation, the effect of the bill on existing laws and programs, the position of the executive branch on the bill, and the views of dissenting members of the committee.

Step 4. The bill is reported back to the chamber where it originated and is placed on the legislative calendar.

Step 5. The bill is debated on the floor of the House or Senate; amendments may be proposed.

Step 6. The bill is passed or defeated by majority vote.

Step 7. A passed bill is sent to the other chamber to follow similar committee and floor action. A bill may be approved as received, rejected, ignored, or changed. Parallel bills are frequently introduced simultaneously.

Step 8. Bills accepted with minor changes are returned to the originating chamber for concurrence. If alterations are significant, a conference committee is formed to reconcile the differences between the House and Senate versions. If the conferees are unable to reach agreement, the legislation dies.

Step 9. Passed bills are sent to the president to sign into law or veto.

Step 10. If a bill is vetoed, Congress may attempt to override a veto by a two-thirds roll call vote of members, who must be present in sufficient numbers for a quorum.

Everything You Always Wanted to Know about the Federal Government

The House and the Senate web sites contain extensive information about their legislative processes, current legislation, names and members of committees, hearing schedules and outcomes, and other relevant topics. Consult www.house.gov and www.senate.gov. The web site for the office of the president, with information about the cabinet, the administration's policymaking, and regulatory agencies and commissions, is found at www.whitehouse.gov/government/.

Introduction of Legislation

At the federal level, legislation is drafted by a senator or representative who has an interest in a particular issue. It is common for a special-interest group to approach a member of Congress to introduce a piece of legislation and to play a role in developing the wording of the bill.

For example, in 2003 the Academy was interested in making sure that uninsured children receive eye exams and follow-up treatment when a problem is identified through a preschool vision screening. The Academy drafted a bill that would create a grant program for states to finance such services and then shared it with congressional representatives who were known to have an interest in such objectives and to be "friends of ophthalmology" (members who have supported Academy issues in the past). Two members of Congress agreed to introduce the legislation, and the Academy publicized the effort by issuing public statements backing the bill and the sponsoring members. Academy Governmental Affairs staff and volunteer advocates helped by meeting with other members of Congress to garner their support as co-sponsors for the bill.

Committee Action and Floor Vote

Although the exact route a bill takes toward legislation differs slightly between the House and the Senate, the processes have some essential similarities. Once a bill has a respectable number of co-sponsors from both parties, it can be brought up for consideration by the committee that has jurisdiction over the proposed legislation. The children's vision screening bill discussed above was sent to the House Energy and Commerce Committee. Major legislation is often preceded by a committee hearing to examine the issue carefully and to determine whether further action is necessary (Figure 20-1).

Whether held in subcommittee or full committee, hearings provide the opportunity to put on record the views of the executive branch, various experts, other public officials, and supporters and opponents of the legislation. A committee or subcommittee may

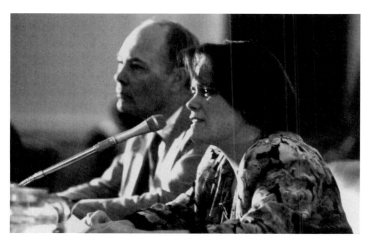

Figure 20-1 Ophthalmologists testifying at a congressional hearing. *(Courtesy of Museum of Vision & Ophthalmic Heritage.)*

decide not to act further on a bill, thereby effectively killing it. Otherwise, it may "mark up" the legislation (make improvements and add amendments) and "vote it out of committee," sending the bill to the House or Senate floor for debate and a vote. The bill needs a simple majority vote to pass. It may be necessary for an identical bill to be introduced (with a different bill number) in the other branch of Congress before the legislation can gain sufficient attention and commitment to move forward.

Conference Committee Report, Final Vote, and Presidential Approval or Veto

If the parallel bills passed by the House and the Senate differ, a conference committee is named by the congressional leadership to work out the differences. The purpose of this conference committee is to negotiate and combine the two bills into one conference report, which is sent back to both the House and the Senate for a final vote. If the conference package passes both chambers, it then goes to the president for signature or veto.

The president may either sign the bill or take no action for 10 days while Congress is in session, allowing the bill to become law. The president can also veto the bill, or take no action after Congress has adjourned its second session (referred to as a *pocket veto*). If the president vetoes a bill, Congress may attempt to override the veto, which requires a two-thirds roll call vote of the members, who must be present in sufficient numbers for a quorum.

Policymaking and Lawmaking at the State Level

The American federalist government system, as it is laid out in the United States Constitution, calls for certain powers and responsibilities to be lodged in the federal government, and for those not specifically named in the Constitution to be reserved for state governments. This means that while some overlap occurs, governmental responsibilities are divided among the various levels. More specifically, in a federalist system, the state and federal governments are complementary.

The federal government has broad responsibilities for such important areas as national defense, regulation of interstate commerce, and control of the national economy, as well as for many other "national" interests. State governments have responsibilities for areas such as education, insurance oversight, professional licensure, and regulations regarding health care. Local governments also share some of these responsibilities by providing for the local infrastructure and making provisions for the education of our children.

Like the federal government, state governments are made up of an executive branch (governor and staff), a legislative branch (two houses [one in Nebraska] of elected representatives that go by various names according to each state's tradition), and a judicial branch. Although the process of writing, introducing, and passing legislation in each state is similar to that described earlier for the U.S. Congress, individual state legislative bodies vary in the makeup of their branches and the way legislation gets enacted.

Each state has dozens of departments, agencies, commissions, and other bodies to oversee and fulfill special state responsibilities, such as public health and education. No two states are organized exactly alike in these areas, even regarding names, hierarchies, and responsibilities of these bodies. So many state policy decisions and regulations made by these bodies directly and indirectly affect the practice of medicine, the profession of ophthalmology, and patient care, that understanding who does what and how in your state government is mandatory for the ophthalmology advocate.

A good way to find out how your own state's government is organized and how its legislative process works is to visit its web site. The URL will likely be www.state.(your state's two-letter abbreviation).us; for instance, New York's would be www.state.ny.us, and Oregon's would be www.state.or.us. As with other state-related issues, your state ophthalmological society is an invaluable resource for all of the information you may need.

The most effective way for ophthalmologists to get involved in the crucial area of state affairs is through membership in the state ophthalmological society. Every state, as well as Puerto Rico and Washington, DC, has an ophthalmological society. They will warmly welcome your participation. You can find contact data for your own state society on the Academy web site, www.aao.org/aao/member/state/directory.cfm.

State Regulatory Agencies and Boards

Like the federal government, state governments have a variety of regulatory boards and agencies made up of appointed or, sometimes, elected officials. These boards can have a wide range of powers depending on state law and are a major source of policies and regulations affecting your profession and your patients.

Most states have professional licensing boards for medical doctors, osteopathic physicians, optometrists, and other health care professionals. Many licensing boards have the power to censure, fine, or revoke the licenses of those under their jurisdiction, and they often dictate methods of patient care. To become an effective voice in their decision making, state ophthalmology advocates must familiarize themselves with these powerful entities.

To find out how your state is organized with regard to regulatory agencies and boards, take advantage of your state government's web site (see above). Although many of these regulatory divisions have organizational charts that show the chain of command within the organization, understanding these charts can be frustrating due to the complexity of many state governments, the lack of consistency in naming the various departments and agencies, and the differences where responsibilities are placed. You will get faster results by simply consulting with your state ophthalmological society.

✓ **KEY POINT**

Keeping track of dozens of state agencies, bureaus, committees, and other policymaking groups is daunting. Fortunately, all states require publication of the various rulings and proceedings of their departments. Contact your state ophthalmological society when you need access to this information.

If you want to make yourself visible and easily available to consult on eye health issues with state departmental and regulatory decision makers, the chances of influencing policy in ways that benefit patient eye care are greatly increased. Gaining advisory positions and membership on panels that have regular dealings with those who define and administer public policy at the state level is one of the best methods of ensuring that your professional concerns are heard and heeded. When it comes to state advocacy, you owe it to yourself, your patients, and society at large to become involved.

State Licensing Boards and Commissions

State licensing boards are part of the executive branch of state government. The state's boards of medicine, osteopathic medicine, and optometry are most important to ophthalmology. These boards have varying degrees of authority and autonomy, depending on state law. The organization, membership, and powers of a licensing board are dictated by publicly available documents, such as the state code, and are subject to change by legislative action.

Increasingly, nonmedical limited-license health care professionals have sought to expand their scope of practice by attempting to get legislation introduced that would grant their licensing board the authority to unilaterally determine what is and what is not the practice of their profession. Although you may not always be able to influence the boards of limited-license health care professionals such as optometrists, knowledge of their workings and membership can add credibility to your discussions with legislators on expanding their authority.

Your state's board of medicine can be a forceful ally in dealing with scope-of-practice issues, particularly if you are able to participate in board proceedings. The presence of ophthalmologists on state medical boards reinforces our position as patient advocates. The laws and regulations defining what constitutes the practice of medicine and surgery for physicians, and whether a practitioner has adhered to those guidelines, is often a matter taken up by the board of medicine. Our continuing participation in organized general medical matters serves to better define us as medical doctors—part of the general medical community—first, and ophthalmologists second. This is an effective counterpoint to those who would define and diminish real patient protection issues as mere "turf battles."

State Department of Health

A state's department of health is a complex entity with wide-ranging oversight and administrative responsibilities. The secretary of health and the various bureaus dealing with everything from school health programs to HIV/AIDS registries are often located within this department.

In some states, the secretary of health has final approval to add drugs to the authorized formulary of certain limited-license professionals. Frequently this is done without public notification, input, or hearings.

Other state departments often also have eye care responsibilities. For example, a state's school health division—often found within the state education department—is responsible for school vision-screening standards and, thus, is another important state entity with which ophthalmologist advocates should become familiar.

State Public Welfare Department

The state department that deals with public welfare and the medical assistance program can have a significant effect on the availability of health care for those with limited financial means. This department generally includes a medical director. Divisions within the medical assistance program incorporate fee-for-service and managed care, children's health insurance programs (CHIPs), nursing home care, and long-term care.

In an era of increasing use of these services and decreasing reimbursement, ophthalmologist involvement in these departments and their processes is vital. Depending on your practice location and your area of specialization, patients using some form of financial assistance may constitute a significant proportion of your practice. There are mechanisms for physician influence in the administration of these programs such as meeting with individuals, writing letters, having patients write letters, and getting appointed to advisory committees within the department.

There is also a mechanism to influence Medicare, the major third-party payor for many ophthalmology practices. Most Medicare coverage decisions are made at the local level, and these "local carrier policies" have significant financial ramifications for patients and providers. The majority of regional CMS-contracted carriers have a mechanism for physician input into their medical decision making. Every state ophthalmological society has physician membership on the carrier liaison committee, and it is through your state society's committee that you can be heard.

As new medical procedures become available, local coverage decisions determine when and whether payment will be made in your state. However, as a consensus emerges, a national coverage policy can evolve. Favorable coverage decisions for photodynamic therapy, nerve fiber layer imaging, and pachymetry are just three examples of national successes that began with ophthalmologists' state advocacy efforts.

Private Insurers and Health Plans

In recent years more and more control over the treatment of patients and the payment for patient care has been assumed by organizations and individuals outside of the medical profession and even outside of government. Insurers often require referrals before patients can be seen, and therapy, whether medical or surgical, must be preauthorized, frequently by nonphysicians who may not fully appreciate the medical issues involved.

These changes in clinical practice require physicians to interact with such private entities as insurers, medical facilities, and vendors of medical supplies. Advocacy with these participants in the medical arena is often considerably more personal than advocacy with large governmental bodies, and it takes place on a more local level. You may find yourself in the position of advocating on behalf of your own practice, an individual patient, or even yourself.

When you work to ensure that policies adopted by third-party payors do not adversely affect patient care and safety, you are advocating on behalf of your patients. When you demand that health plans offer fair and equitable payment for your services, you are advocating for yourself and your practice and your partners. Ultimately through this advocacy the entire profession benefits, as norms become established one practice, one health plan, and one locality at a time. You need to be aware, however, that working together with other physicians on some of these problems is limited by law. See the box "Competition and Antitrust Laws."

In contrast to governmental advocacy, financial contributions and the responsibility of elected officials to constituents play no part here. Your ability to affect policy and to effect change with these organizations may instead depend on such factors as the number of ophthalmologists in the area, the relative market strength of payors and hospitals in relation to practitioners, the presence or absence of physician organizations and large group practices, and the willingness of physicians to invest time and energy. It is possible, however, to be effective and to coax changes in policy that can have a significant impact on reimbursement, patient care, and practice efficiency.

Health Plans

The Academy is a member of the Specialty Society Insurance Coalition (SSIC), which works directly with the national medical directors and policymakers of some of the largest insurers in the country. The SSIC communicates regularly with these influential people and can convey the concerns of physicians across the country regarding contract, billing, coding, payment, and other issues. These interactions can result in both the adoption of national policy and changes to rules and directives by local payors. With the continued consolidation of the major insurers both regionally and nationally, this mechanism for access is assuming increasing importance. It is much easier to have influence by working through a larger group of physicians, and practitioners seeking to affect a health plan's national policy should contact the Academy's Washington, DC, office for additional information.

Most efforts to influence policy within a health plan are undertaken at the local level because that is where many interactions take place and rules are crafted. In the structure of a health plan, the person with the most authority over you and your practice is the medical director, and individual ophthalmologists can and should be in contact with the medical directors of the larger health plans in their area, who generally will welcome credible comments from the practitioners in their plans. When problems inevitably arise, it is useful to have established this relationship beforehand.

The process of gaining the ability to give credible advice is a slow and deliberate one. As an advocate for the interests of your profession you can offer to be on the health

Competition and Antitrust Laws

Antitrust laws forbid concerted action among competitors to set prices or to fix quality or output levels of the products or services available to consumers. Because of antitrust laws, ophthalmologists in separate practices cannot collectively negotiate price or price-related terms. Even if a payor has an unfair advantage due to market power, seeking to "level the playing field" by enlisting the support of other practices to jointly put pressure on the payor places you at risk of substantial civil and criminal penalties under the antitrust laws. Proper use of the "third-party messenger model" (see "Action Steps" at the end of Chapter 22) to negotiate health plan contracts is beyond the scope of this chapter, and you should consult an experienced health care attorney.

plan's specialty review and grievance committees, if that option is available. You should be willing to offer advice on payment and coding issues as well as on new technology. Establish your trustworthiness and credibility by being objective and by citing accurate data when offering opinions. Issues such as contract language or pass-through payments for expensive supplies can often be resolved best at this level through your relationships with local health plans. A decision that goes against you can always be appealed to a higher level.

CHAPTER 21

Advocacy Case Studies

The case studies presented here demonstrate a structure for analyzing an advocacy issue, identifying stakeholders, developing and anticipating arguments pro and con, and identifying levers (advocacy methods) that might be employed by either side. Each case study ends with a summary message and action steps for the advocate.

These case studies are based on real-life situations. They are intended to show how knowledge of the history of advocacy, the workings of governmental and private entities, and the advocacy resources and techniques presented in the prior three chapters can be applied to actual issues you might face sometime in your lifelong commitment to advocacy for ophthalmology and the profession of medicine.

Case Study 1

Reimbursement

The Issue

Most practicing ophthalmologists are affected by third-party insurers, from Medicare and Medicaid to managed care organizations. Third-party payors set reimbursement based on their own criteria, which may not necessarily consider the physician's practice expenses and the cost of delivering appropriate medical care. Physicians are bound by contracts to accept these payments either through a Medicare Participation Agreement or a private or managed care contract, written with little recourse to discussion, negotiation, or change.

This system requires immense administrative effort to track data, complete and submit paperwork, and deal with other bureaucratic requirements. Fees for services rendered by physicians are frequently reduced, and many practices are faced with challenges in providing care because the reimbursement received is less than the expenses incurred.

Physicians wonder how they can exercise their best clinical judgment while, at the same time, working with the administrative, informational, and economic needs of a third-party payor. Moreover, if the regulatory process and constant fee reduction is not slowed, many physicians may be forced to opt out not only from Medicare and Medicaid but from all private and managed care insurers as well. This would negatively affect patients' access to appropriate medical care.

History

Since their enactment in 1965, the Medicare and Medicaid programs have gradually expanded their covered populations and benefits. While these expansions and improvements may be socially laudable, concurrently soaring health care costs have resulted in reductions in the payments these third-party payors allow for services. The Resource-Based Relative Value Scale (RBRVS) System, initiated in 1992 to help control costs, incorporated physician practice, work, and malpractice factors in an effort to devise a fair fee for services rendered, based on the tangible and intangible expenditures that physicians incurred in delivering any given medical service. Factors such as time spent, training required, difficulty of decision-making, and the degree of responsibility associated with delivering specific care, as well as the actual costs involved, were included in attempting to establish reasonable reimbursement policies.

Increasing costs can be attributed to factors such as evolving and improved technology, increased use of services by an aging population, and inequities in the tort system. However, legislative efforts to reduce costs have often resulted in the reduction of physician reimbursement.

Private sector insurers have adopted variations of the Medicare RBRVS fee schedules, so that the fees for services from managed care and private insurers also go down when the federal government lowers its reimbursements.

Some physicians are examining the economics of nonparticipation in many of these plans. Others are actively seeking legislative or regulatory relief through their national and state medical societies.

Stakeholders

The parties essential to regulatory reform and reimbursement adjustment include the following:

- Centers for Medicare and Medicaid Services
- Office of Medicaid Management, state department of health, or other appropriate regulatory agencies
- National, state, and local medical specialty and subspecialty societies
- American Association of Health Plans and related managed care or insurance lobby or trade groups, because most managed care organizations are using a variation of the Medicare RBRVS
- Medicare beneficiaries
- American Association of Retired Persons (AARP)

Arguments and Positions

These are arguments in favor of restructuring reimbursement:

- Payments to physicians should be fairly increased consistent with payments to other providers under Medicare. The congressionally mandated sustainable growth rate (SGR) formula, the basis on which annual fee increases and reductions are determined under the Medicare program, is tied (among other factors) to the gross domestic product (GDP). The GDP bears no relationship to patients' health care or physician costs, and an unrelated economic downturn penalizes the medical profession, the only group to have its livelihood tied to the GDP. In addition, the SGR has spending targets based on incomplete and unreasonable assumptions.

- MedPAC (the independent commission advising Congress on physician and hospital payment) recommends that the SGR and the volume target for physician payment be eliminated, as it cannot be implemented fairly. Physicians today are subject to automatic cuts in payment when the use of physician services exceeds the SGR spending target. For the most part, utilization is not under the medical profession's direct control but driven by other factors such as new treatments and pharmaceutical breakthroughs.
- Payment updates need to more accurately reflect changes due to (1) increases in product costs, such as in-office drugs, under Medicare; (2) coverage of new medical technology with improved diagnostic and treatment methods; and (3) program expansions due to law or regulation and not to physicians actively seeking patients or practicing "defensive medicine."
- Payment updates should recognize site-of-service changes from hospitals to physician offices. Medicare continues to pay hospitals for care and costs that have shifted to the office setting.
- The SGR system is a fundamentally flawed concept and inherently inequitable. Most medical practices are small businesses that cannot continue to absorb the sustained losses or the steep payment cuts that have occurred or that are predicted under the SGR system.

These are arguments against restructuring reimbursement:

- Higher fees will increase utilization, spurred on by physicians attempting to increase revenues.
- Physicians can significantly affect volume and must be given incentives to make cost-effective decisions.
- Higher fees will result in higher insurance premium costs to employers and patients; employers will curtail health insurance offerings to employees and retirees.
- Higher fees will increase the U.S. budget deficit.

Levers

As with other advocacy issues, a key lever in resolving the regulatory and reimbursement quandary is through an association of like-minded interest groups and the development of effective coalitions. Elected federal officials are particularly sensitive to the needs of the Medicare population, and alliances with patient advocacy groups, with "access to care" and "quality of care" as focal issues, could be advantageous.

Political action is also essential for convincing legislators and regulatory agencies at both federal and state levels. It is essential to enlist the support of such entities as state commissioners of health and the regional administrator for the Centers for Medicare and Medicaid Services to demonstrate that continuation of the present reimbursement climate will only negatively affect patient access to care and the delivery of quality medicine.

Take-Home Message

Medical doctors are consistently viewed as among the most respected members of society, and their training, dedication, level of responsibility, and commitment to their patients' welfare must be acknowledged. Many physicians are small business entities and, as such, should be protected as would other small businesses.

Legislators need to be educated about what physicians face daily in their interactions with insurers (see "Action Steps" below). The general public as well as employer and business groups should also be engaged to demonstrate the magnitude of obstacles that physicians face in delivering effective health care. It must be shown that patient welfare and physician welfare are interrelated concepts.

Most important, physicians must be enlisted to bring this message home through a broad-based coalition of county, state, and specialty societies. Individual relationships with legislators, regulators, business leaders, and patients form the cornerstone of effective advocacy.

Action Steps

- Build a coalition of like-minded interest groups to include and emphasize patient and employer advocacy organizations, business councils, and similar groups.
- Initiate media campaigns in conjunction with these organizations using cost-effective and demographically targeted outlets, such as radio spots and print ads that stress continued patient access to effective medical care, physicians as the allies for their patients, and physicians as small business operators in the community.
- Use actual condensed physician case files outlining insurer regulatory and reimbursement abuses culled from medical society third-party payor help programs (if available) for forwarding to media outlets.
- Arrange interviews with society officers or with individual members to highlight the above physician case issues to media outlets. Use examples to emphasize that the results would be devastating if other professions were similarly affected, as the medical profession has been by governmental and third-party payor limitations and restrictions.
- Intensify medical society efforts on national and state levels with regard to physician collective bargaining initiatives as they relate to contractual terms and fee schedule negotiations through a "third-party messenger" model.
- Intensify medical society efforts with federal and state legislators to achieve compromise or trade-offs on other less critical issues.
- Initiate a series of legislator and employer briefing sessions, hosted by medical societies, to outline the regulatory and reimbursement challenges encountered by the medical profession, reinforcing why these groups must care about this issue if the public is to continue to have access to appropriate health care.

Case Study 2

Tort Reform

The Issue

Most physicians (and nearly all ophthalmologists) purchase insurance to cover themselves against the risk of financial loss from an alleged act of medical malpractice. This "medical liability insurance" is a variant of professional liability insurance. Rapidly increasing premiums and decreasing availability of insurance coverage in many states have resulted in initiatives to reform the American system of tort law (which includes medical malpractice claims).

History

A professional may be defined as one who possesses the special knowledge and skill necessary to render a professional service. Typically, the special knowledge and skill result from the person's education and experience in a particular branch of science or learning. Professionals are bound by law (1) to perform the services for which they were hired and (2) to perform these services in accordance with the appropriate professional standards of conduct as defined by law and by their specialty organizations. The first duty is primarily contractual; the second duty arises from the common-law principle of tort law.

Tort actions allege a private or civil wrong or injury resulting from the breach of a legal duty that exists by virtue of society's expectations about interpersonal conduct, rather than by contract or other private relationships. A tort action as it applies to alleged medical malpractice refers therefore not to an illegal act or to ordinary business exposure (such as "slips and falls" or business losses) but to inappropriate conduct in the rendering of professional services or in failing to provide proper services.

The societal emphasis on medical professional liability (malpractice) as a means of seeking redress is a relatively recent concern and phenomenon. Although previously physicians had been sued successfully under tort laws, such suits were relatively infrequent and awards were generally not substantial. Insurance premiums were therefore low; insurance was available to nearly every physician and thus not a major professional or business concern for medical doctors. The mid to late 1970s saw a dramatic increase in the frequency and severity of claims and awards, and many insurance carriers left the market. This resulted in a lack of available insurance and a "malpractice crisis." As a result, many physician-run insurance companies—regional, state, and specialty sponsored—evolved. These "doctor companies" now provide much of the physician professional liability coverage in the United States.

In 1975, California passed the Medical Injury Compensation Reform Act (MICRA). That law constituted a comprehensive package of tort reform with (1) limits on noneconomic damages (pain and suffering), (2) a reasonable statute of limitations, (3) a sliding scale for attorney contingency fees, (4) proportionate liability among all defendant parties, and (5) periodic payment of future damages. Between 1976 and 1999 (since MICRA was enacted), average medical liability premiums increased 505% in the United States but only 168% in California.

The late 1980s and the 1990s were a period of relative stability in insurance premiums. Reform of the tort law system became a less crucial advocacy issue for physicians, compared with such issues as patients' rights, managed care, and the restructuring of the physician payment system.

Beginning in about 1999, insurance companies experienced substantially deteriorating financial performance and responded by raising insurance premiums—sometimes more than 100% a year. What caused this rapid and dramatic increase in premiums? The reasons are many and the relative contribution of each is still debated, but they include (1) an increase in the frequency of claims and suits and (2) an increase in the average size of settlements and awards. A U.S. physician was sued an average of once every 6 years. Over a 6-year period the percentage of judgments greater than $1 million doubled. Were physicians suddenly much more prone to medical error, or were other factors at work, such as an expanding pool of tort attorneys, a litigious society, and a national mood of consumerism and rising patient expectations?

Several medical liability insurance companies failed, were taken over by states, fell into receivership, or left the market entirely, with disruptive results. For example, when St. Paul's Insurance Company decided to leave the market, 42,000 doctors were left without coverage. Insurance premiums for first-year occurrence coverage for some specialties in several states exceeded $100,000. There was therefore a simultaneous crisis of both insurance availability and insurance affordability. This was particularly true in specialties such as obstetrics and neurosurgery—areas with both a high rate of claims and high average awards. As a result, in some areas family physicians and obstetriciangynecologists ceased to provide obstetrical care, others refused to provide hospital emergency room coverage, and some doctors even left the practice of medicine entirely.

Stakeholders

Various parties have engaged in attempts to reform the tort system at both the state and federal levels. These include (1) physician organizations, (2) hospital organizations, and (3) insurance companies offering professional liability insurance for those two groups. The principal parties opposing tort reform are organizations representing trial attorneys, state bar associations, and some patient rights groups.

Arguments and Positions

These are arguments in favor of tort reform:

- The current system of tort laws is unfair to physicians and places an unacceptable burden on the practice of medicine.
- The current system of tort laws results in premiums that are unaffordable to many physicians. These high premiums are passed along to patients, thus increasing the cost of health care.
- Tort reform is necessary to avoid forcing physicians in certain high-risk specialties (eg, obstetrics) to limit or entirely abandon their practice.

- Tort reform is necessary to protect physicians who practice in high-risk environments (eg, emergency departments, neurosurgery).
- Tort reform helps amend the practice of defensive medicine, thus lowering health care costs and eliminating the risk associated with unnecessary tests and procedures.
- Tort reform does not reduce objective economic damages actually incurred but attempts to limit the much more subjective and frequently very expensive emotional damages associated with "pain and suffering."
- Most malpractice cases are either dropped by the plaintiff or won by the physician. Despite the questionable validity of these cases, the expense, both in dollars and emotion, of defending these cases is significant.

These are arguments against tort reform:

- Tort reform is unnecessary since most lawsuits are won by physicians anyway.
- Tort reform will result in fewer patient protections.
- Tort reform will be unfair to those patients genuinely injured by medical malpractice.
- Tort reform will make some attorneys unwilling to represent any but the most obvious and egregious cases.
- High medical liability insurance premiums are the result not of the tort system but of poor management by insurance companies, combined with bad investment results.

Levers

An important lever for advancing tort reform is coalition building. This is not an issue for any one specialty but rather for all of medicine. It is also not just a physician issue but an issue for health care facilities and insurance companies. In a broader context, tort reform is important for all businesses, and an effective coalition may include chambers of commerce and business groups, as well as employers sensitive to anything that might raise health insurance premiums. Other effective coalition members would be those groups affected by poor emergency department staffing or by the departure of obstetricians, neurosurgeons, or trauma specialists from rural areas.

Another important lever is advocacy with political parties and elected officials. Which political parties or key legislators have constituencies that include small rural towns worried about losing obstetrical, trauma, and neurosurgical services? How many of their business-community constituents simply cannot afford any further increase in health insurance premiums?

On the opposite side, those opposing tort reform try to build coalitions of patient rights groups, trial attorneys, and state bar associations. Using a public relations lever, they will counter the "obstetrician forced out of practice" with the "pain and suffering of a malpractice victim."

Take-Home Message

Most state legislatures generally include many more attorneys than health care professionals in their membership. Advocacy success for the medical profession will therefore hinge on demonstrating the tangible negatives associated with high premiums that force physicians from practice and that are passed along to patients through rising health care costs. As is generally the case in politics, good arguments and strong logic alone will not prevail. A well-financed, broad-based coalition must accompany the arguments. While federal legislation may not be forthcoming, keeping the issue alive at the federal level will put pressure on the states to solve the problem.

Action Steps

- Contact the Academy, the AMA, your state ophthalmological society, state medical association, or any other medical organization to which you belong for the most recent developments and talking points on tort reform.
- Build coalitions inside and outside the profession of medicine.
- Identify cases demonstrating the need for tort reform.
- Support key legislators, such as those who have seniority or influence or who sit on important committees that can affect tort reform.
- Develop relationships with legislators and their staffs, since support can come from unexpected sources.
- Use the media effectively.
- Build an effective case statement. Use arguments and illustrations that will resonate both intellectually and emotionally with your intended audience. Specific, brief data and human interest examples will help.
- Anticipate trial attorneys' arguments and prepare counter arguments.

Practice Management Resources

Products and Services from the American Academy of Ophthalmology

The American Academy of Ophthalmology is a valuable resource for ophthalmic education, meetings, advocacy, and global eye care. Membership in the Academy is open to any ophthalmologist worldwide as well as to medical doctors currently enrolled in an ophthalmology training program. The following types of products are available: clinical education for ophthalmologist and residents, clinical education for allied staff, patient education materials, practice management materials and information, practice standards and quality, and member periodicals and directory.

Apart from the prestige of belonging to an internationally renowned medical organization, all Academy members receive access to information not available elsewhere, and valuable benefits at no added cost, such as:

- Free Annual Meeting registration
- Subscription to *Ophthalmology* journal
- Subscription to *EyeNet* magazine
- Subscription to *Academy Express* e-mail newsletter
- Access to "Members only" areas of the Academy web site
- Listing in the Academy's Member Directory
- Continuing medical education (CME) credit reporting service
- Discounts on products, programs, materials, and services

To obtain more information and to request the Academy's latest *Product and Resource Catalog,* visit the web site (www.aao.org).

Products and Services from the American Academy of Ophthalmic Executives

The American Academy of Ophthalmic Executives (AAOE), a partner of the American Academy of Ophthalmology, provides products to help your practice in the areas of business operations, coding and reimbursement, compliance and risk management, financial management, human resources, information technology, and professional growth. AAOE also maintains a list of consultants who have qualified for inclusion by virtue of their experience in the field of ophthalmology business.

AAOE is a membership organization addressing the needs of those responsible for managing the business side of the ophthalmic practice. With more than 2,500 members, AAOE provides administrators and managing physicians with the relevant, accurate, and timely information they need to keep pace with changing professional responsibilities. Programs address current issues including coding, technology, and human resources. AAOE's tools and professional development programs are designed to address the key competencies defining the roles of professional ophthalmic administrators, office managers, and managing physicians.

AAOE membership benefits include:

- Subscriptions to *The Coding Bulletin* and *The Executive Update*
- Subscription to *EyeNet* magazine
- E-Talk e-mail distribution list for communicating with administrative colleagues
- Access to AAOE's online member center with content arranged by key competency
- Free registration to the Academy Annual Meeting plus advance registration, early-bird housing, and invitations to members-only events
- Discount pricing on all Academy and AAOE products
- Discount pricing on legal services through national attorneys with a wide range of expertise
- Free use of the Academy's Customized Coding Answer Service. AAOE members may have two questions answered for free each year.

While membership in the American Academy of Ophthalmology will help you remain current on clinical and advocacy issues, by joining partner-organization American Academy of Ophthalmic Executives, you will have access to all of the key practice management and coding information that is so pivotal to the business performance of your practice. For more information and an application form, visit the web site (ww.aao.org/aaoe).

Membership in AAOE is available only to practice management staff and physicians employed in a practice where one or more physicians are members of the American Academy of Ophthalmology.

AAOE Tools and Services

Here is a sampling of AAOE resources for those managing the business side of an ophthalmology practice. Please visit the AAOE web site (www.aao.org/aaoe) for the latest information. The Academy's *Product and Resource Catalog* (referred to in the preceding section) includes fuller descriptions of all AAOE tools and services.

Coding and Reimbursement

- Developed by AAOE, *Ophthalmic Coding Coach* is the most comprehensive coding reference book available, with detailed content on each CPT code affecting ophthalmology.
- The *Ophthalmic Coding Series* offers new and established coders the most comprehensive and up-to-date ophthalmic coding information available. Ensure that the ophthalmologists, technicians, and coding staff in your practice receive proper education to avoid penalties for coding errors. Each module offers one category 1 CME credit or one JCAHPO category B CE credit.

- AAOE and JCAHPO (Joint Commission on Allied Health Professionals in Ophthalmology) have joined forces to develop a certificate of completion in ophthalmic coding. Those who have passed the rigorous open-book Ophthalmic Coding Specialist exam, covering all aspects of ophthalmic coding, will earn the title of Ophthalmic Coding Specialist (OCS). To learn more or to sign up for an exam, contact JCAHPO at 800-284-3937.

CPT and ICD-9 References and Programs

- *Ophthalmic Coding FlipCards,* developed by AAOE, is a handy text that mounts directly on the side of your computer monitor, giving you instant access to the most commonly used codes for CPT, ICD-9, modifiers, denial, and place of service.
- The American Medical Association's *CPT Standard Edition* soft-bound book highlights new CPT codes and CPT description changes.
- The Academy's *ICD-9 for Ophthalmology Coding* book, with multiple cross-references, is invaluable to ophthalmologists and staff for precise diagnostic coding. Quickly locate those codes that correctly reflect your diagnoses.
- CODEquest Coding Seminars: Ophthalmic Coding College is a series of convenient one-day seminars, sponsored with your state or specialty society, that focus on up-to-date state- and specialty-specific coding information. Let CODEquest provide the tools and training you need for correct reimbursement. For information and schedules, call AAOE at (415) 447-0369, or visit www.aao.org/codequest. Category 1 CME credit is offered.
- The *HCPCS* book provides specifics about the health care common procedure coding system not currently found in CPT and ICD-9 books.
- AAOE's Customized Coding Answer Service offers services of coding experts who quickly research and answer your specific coding questions. The cost is $25 per inquiry, and each inquiry may contain two related questions. For more information and a coding question submission form, visit www.aao.org/resources.

Information Technology

AAOE can help you learn about trends, computer systems, and software specifically designed for today's ophthalmic practice:

- *The Ophthalmic Executive's Resource Guide: Making the Most of Your Practice Web Site* offers strategies that can be applied in-house to capitalize on the presence of an already established practice web site or to help launch a new web presence on solid ground.
- *Selecting and Implementing the Right EMR, Practice Management, or Optical System for Your Practice* is a comprehensive book describing the step-by-step process for making these important decisions.

Financial Management

Keeping abreast of income analysis, productivity, tax laws, and third-party contracts is a key area of responsibility for the ophthalmic practice administrator. The following resources will help you manage this responsibility:

- *Financial Management for Medical Groups,* published by MGMA and available through the Academy, is the essential financial management handbook for practice administrators, financial managers, and entry-level administrators. Covers financial management, including financial analysis, budgeting, cash-flow analysis, and cost accounting, as well as managed care, access to capital, financial information systems, and accountability in health care.
- Through the Managed Care Contract Review service, AAOE members can obtain a telephone evaluation or an in-depth written opinion of their contract by submitting information to Academy attorneys, Dorsey & Whitney, LLP. Dorsey & Whitney will bill any balance due directly to the member. This service is available to AAOE and Academy members only. The review fee ranges from $350 to $500 per hour and is subject to change.

Business Operations Products

AAOE's business operations products help you keep your practice running smoothly and plan for the future:

- The Practice Forms Master product contains a library of more than 300 professionally created forms to use as is or easily tailor for your office. Design and customize new forms or scan in your existing favorites with user-friendly OmniForm 5.0 software. To see a demo, visit the Academy web site (www.aao.org/ PFMdemo).
- *Mastering Patient Flow: More Ideas to Increase Efficiency and Earnings,* published by MGMA and available through the Academy, is a leading primer on medical practice efficiency.
- *Protecting Your Practice: What You Need to Know About Buying Insurance* helps you evaluate your current carrier and select the best long-term program for your practice.
- *39 Ways to Raise Revenue and Cut Costs,* gathered from visits to hundreds of practices all over the United States, provides proven ways practices are increasing revenues and lowering expenses in a competitive health care marketplace.
- *Winning Patients and Keeping Them for Life* helps you understand what patients really want from your practice, how to exceed their expectations, and how to create "missionary" referrers who will find new patients for you through "word-of-mouth" advertising.
- The Physician–Employee Contract Review service enables AAOE and Academy members to obtain a telephone evaluation or an in-depth written opinion by experienced legal advisors. Legal fees are billed directly to you by the firm. Contact AAOE at 415-561-8561 for more information. Fees for this service range from $350 to $500, and are subject to change.
- Through the Online Consulting Network, you can use medical practice management consultants to sort out the complexities of practice administration. All consultants listed have been prequalified by AAOE and have many years of experience with ophthalmic practices. For an introduction to their specialized services, you

may e-mail or visit the web sites of consultants in the network. For more information, contact AAOE at 415-447-0335.

Professional Growth

- Professional Choices is the online ophthalmology career center. It's a quick, easy, and reliable way to find opportunities for ophthalmologists, administrators, registered nurses, and technicians; it is free for job seekers. Practices for sale are also listed. Visit the web site for more information (www.aao.org/professionalchoices).
- *Coaching and Mentoring for Dummies,* by Marty Brounstein (published by Wiley and available through the Academy) shows managers how to boost productivity, develop employees, and build morale—without spending hundreds of dollars on training seminars.
- *Communicating Effectively for Dummies,* by Marty Brounstein (published by Wiley and available through the Academy) teaches assertive speaking and active listening skills so that you communicate forcefully without alienating your boss, colleagues, or patients.

Human Resources

The Ophthalmic Executive's Resource Guide series includes titles to help you choose, retain, and motivate staff, actions that are critical to the success of the practice and the retention of patients:

- *Coaching for Top Performance* helps you learn how to manage as a coach rather than as a "doer," drive top performance using constructive feedback, develop employee capability and self-sufficiency, and increase employee productivity and performance through delegating and motivating.
- *Developing Your Employee Handbook: Creating a Protective Shield or Legal Minefield?* helps you evaluate your need for an employee handbook and determine what information should be included and what should be omitted. Use the included CD-ROM to customize the employee handbook template to your practice.
- *Helping New Employees Succeed* provides managers with practical tips and tools for getting new employees off to a good start and helping them sustain good performance.
- *Interviewing to Hire Smart* provides hiring managers with hands-on practical tools and tips that will increase the likelihood of making the right hiring decisions.
- *Solving Performance Problems* provides the coaching tools for constructively addressing and correcting performance problems.

Additional Recommended Reading

Arbinger Institute, The. *Leadership and Self-Deception: Getting Out of the Box.* San Francisco: Berrett-Koehler Publishers, Inc, 2002.

Blanchard K, Bowles S. *Raving Fans.* New York: William Morrow, 1993.

Deming WE. *Out of the Crisis.* Cambridge: The MIT Press, 2000.

Eppler M. *Management Mess-Ups.* Franklin Lakes, NJ: Career Press, 1997.

Gross, TS. *Positively Outrageous Service*. New York: Warner Business Books, 1994.

Johnson S. *Who Moved My Cheese?* New York: GP Putnam & Sons, 1998.

LeBoeuf M. *How to Win Customers and Keep Them for Life*. New York: Penguin Putnam, 2000.

Martin CA, Tulgan B. *Managing Generation Y*. Amherst: HRD Press, 2001.

Maxwell JC. *The 17 Indisputable Laws of Teamwork*. Nashville: Nelson Books, 2001.

Trout J. *Differentiate or Die*. New York: John Wiley & Sons, Inc., 2000.

Yate M. *Hiring the Best*. Holbrook, Mass: Adams Media Corp, 1993.

Sample Materials

This section features a selection of materials related to practice management:

- *Group practice questionnaire:* The form in Figure I-1 can help you assess your options when you are considering joining a group practice (see Chapter 1).
- *CMS-1500 insurance form:* Figure I-2 shows the front of a standard health insurance claim form. Most medical management software can print the CMS-1500 insurance form used for filing a claim with Medicare, Medicaid, and insurance companies (see Chapter 5).
- *Example of a policy and procedures document:* Figure I-3 features an example of procedures that have been set up for handling insurance and patient collections at a practice (see Chapter 5).
- *Insurance plan assessment form:* Figure I-4 shows a form that can help you in conferring with your insurance agent or consultant (and with legal counsel, as appropriate) regarding your insurance program (see Chapter 8).
- *Example of a table of contents for an employee handbook:* Figure I-5 shows topics that can be helpful in formulating your own handbook. It is always advisable to have an attorney review your employee handbook to make sure you do not state anything that could make commitments beyond what you intend (see Chapter 9).

To help you compare different offers, fill out this questionnaire for each practice you are considering.

Name of group: _____

Main office address: _____

Telephone: _____

Addresses of satellite offices: _____

Administrator/key contact: _____ Home telephone number: _____

Group Structure

What is the group's legal structure? [ ] Partnership [ ] Professional Corporation [ ] Limited Liability Corporation
[ ] Individuals sharing space

Who are the group's partners and/or principal stockholders?

Name: _____ Age: ___ Gender: ___ Specialty: _____

Name: _____ Age: ___ Gender: ___ Specialty: _____

Name: _____ Age: ___ Gender: ___ Specialty: _____

Who are the employed physicians?

Name: _____ Age: ___ Gender: ___ Specialty: _____

Name: _____ Age: ___ Gender: ___ Specialty: _____

Name: _____ Age: ___ Gender: ___ Specialty: _____

Are there physicians planning to retire? If so, what is the expected date(s) of retirement? _____

Are there plans to increase the size of the group?Are there plans to add other subspecialists?_____

What is the ultimate goal regarding size? _____

What makes up the group's geographic market area (eg, counties, miles)? _____

What is the population of the group's market area? _____

How many other ophthalmologists are in the market area, not including the doctors in this practice? _____

Area Hospitals

List hospitals where group members have staff privileges:

Name: _____# of beds: _____

Name: _____# of beds: _____

Are there other hospitals in the area? _____

Does the group place restriction on having privileges at other hospitals? _____

List surgery centers in the market area:

Name: _____ Ownership:_____

Name: _____ Ownership:_____

Name: _____ Ownership:_____

Figure I-1 Group practice questionnaire.

Figure I-1 (cont.)

Initial Compensation

Offered salary or draw: _____ Bonus calculation: _____

Benefits offered and paid for by the practice: _ Malpractice insurance _____

Health insurance _____ Disability insurance _____

Life insurance _____ Paid time off: _____

Sick leave: _____ Professional development leave: _____

CME course expenses paid: _____ Moving expenses: _____

Other:_____

Other:_____

Income Distribution

How is practice income distributed for the partners?

[ ] Equal pay   [ ] Equal percent of overhead [ ] Equal overhead   [ ] Equal Resources

[ ] Other:_____

Buy-In Opportunities

Does the group offer partnership to all physician employees? _____

What are the criteria for partnership? _____

How many years of employment are required? _____

Is buy-in required? _____

Are the buy-in requirements written into the original employment contract? _____

Practice Styles

What is the ethical orientation of the group? _____

Is there a feeling of compatibility and cooperation among group physicians? _____

Are all group members Board Certified? _____

Do any group members have a particular skill or certification that sets them
apart from other specialists in the same field? If so, what are these skills? _____

Are academic appointments encouraged? _____

Are there constraints placed on time spent in teaching activities? _____

Do any of the physicians have personal or practice problems or limitations of
which associates should be aware? _____

How many physicians have left the group in the last three years? _____

Were they employees or partner physicians? _____

What were their reasons for leaving? _____

Will the other physicians in the group be introduced before making a decision? _____

Social Interactions

Do the physicians seem to have a good relationship with each other? _____

Is socializing expected or discouraged among physicians? _____

Do spouses socialize with each other? _____

Have the spouses of the group's physicians been introduced? _____

How does my spouse feel about the other spouses that have been introduced? _____

Do any of the physicians have personal/social problems? _____

(cont.)

Figure I-1 (cont.)

Office Facilities

What was the first impression of the office appearance? _____

Is the office clean? Well organized? Well equipped? _____

How long has the group practiced at this address? _____

How many square feet are there in the facility? _____

Are there plans for future expansion? _____

Is the size of the reception area adequate? _____

What ancillary services/tests are provided in office? _____

How accessible is the practice location to patients? _____

Are parking facilities adequate? If not, what plans exist to improve this? _____

Will a personal office be available? _____

How many exam lanes does each physician have available? _____

Is the facility owned by the group, by the physicians personally, or leased from another entity? _____

What is the distance to hospital(s)? _____

Is the practice in a high growth area or in a declining neighborhood? _____

What days and hours are the offices open? _____

If there are satellite locations, are the physicians rotated through each location? _____

What is the rotation schedule? Which office would I be working in? _____

Group Governance

How are decisions made within the group?

[ ] Majority vote   [ ] Governing board   [ ] Senior physicians   [ ] Informal clique

Who makes day-to-day decisions versus long-term decisions or changes? _____

Is there an office manager/administrator? _____

To whom does this person report? _____

Are there regular business meetings? _____

How often are they held? _____

Are all physicians invited to attend? _____

Office Personnel

How many employees in the practice? Clinical:_____   Administrative: _____

What is the staff-to-physician ratio? _____

Are there any employed optometrists? _____

Does each physician have a technician, or is a pool of techs used? _____

How are patients treated by the staff? _____

Does the staff seem efficient, courteous, and professional? _____

How many staff members have left voluntarily within the last year? _____

What were the reasons they left (ask staff members)? _____

How many staff members have been terminated within the last year? _____

Have they been replaced? _____

Is there good communication between staff and physicians? _____

(cont.)

Figure I-1 (cont.)

Financial Overview

What were the total charges last year? _____

What were the total collections, same period? _____

What were the total expenses? _____

What percent of the total expenses were for staff payroll? _____

How many days outstanding are in the accounts receivable? _____

Does the practice have an operational budget? _____

Does the group review financials together every month? _____

What reports will be routinely provided? _____

What is the fee schedule? _____

Do all physicians use the same fee schedule? _____

Are billing and collections done in-house? _____

If not, how is it handled? _____

What software is used for practice management? _____

Does the practice use Electronic Medical Records? If not, any plans to implement EMR in the future? _____

Managed Care/Medicare Participation

Are all physicians participating in Medicare? _____

What percentage of practice is Medicare? _____

How many managed care contracts does the group have? _____

What percentage of total patients are on managed care plans? _____

How many plans have at least 20% of the group's patient base? _____

Does any MCO have more than 20% of the group's patient base? _____

Which ones? _____

Does the group have any capitated contracts? _____

How is information about each managed care contract tracked? _____

Does becoming a part of this group make one eligible to see patients on these contracts immediately? _____

Patient Distribution

How are new patients distributed if no preference is given? _____

How is the patient load distributed? _____

What is the expectation for referring patients to subspecialty physicians within the group? _____

How are managed care patients distributed? _____

What is the current call schedule rotation? _____

Risk Management Issues

What has been the group's malpractice experience? _____

Are any malpractice suits pending? _____

Are any considered to have merit? _____

Are any liabilities retroactive? _____

Are there any other legal actions pending or threatened against the practice or any of its doctors? _____

Does the practice have an active coding compliance plan? _____

Does the practice regularly survey its patients? _____

PLEASE
DO NOT
STAPLE
IN THIS
AREA

CARRIER

	PICA		**HEALTH INSURANCE CLAIM FORM**	PICA		

1. MEDICARE   MEDICAID   CHAMPUS   CHAMPVA   GROUP HEALTH PLAN   FECA BLK LUNG   OTHER
   (Medicare #) (Medicaid #) (Sponsor's SSN) (VA File #) (SSN or ID) (SSN) (ID)

1a. INSURED'S I.D. NUMBER   (FOR PROGRAM IN ITEM 1)

2. PATIENT'S NAME (Last Name, First Name, Middle Initial)

3. PATIENT'S BIRTH DATE MM DD YY   SEX   M   F

4. INSURED'S NAME (Last Name, First Name, Middle Initial)

5. PATIENT'S ADDRESS (No., Street)

6. PATIENT RELATIONSHIP TO INSURED   Self Spouse Child Other

7. INSURED'S ADDRESS (No., Street)

CITY   STATE

8. PATIENT STATUS   Single   Married   Other

CITY   STATE

ZIP CODE   TELEPHONE (Include Area Code) (   )

Employed   Full-Time Student   Part-Time Student

ZIP CODE   TELEPHONE (INCLUDE AREA CODE) (   )

9. OTHER INSURED'S NAME (Last Name, First Name, Middle Initial)

10. IS PATIENT'S CONDITION RELATED TO:

11. INSURED'S POLICY GROUP OR FECA NUMBER

a. OTHER INSURED'S POLICY OR GROUP NUMBER

a. EMPLOYMENT? (CURRENT OR PREVIOUS)   YES   NO

a. INSURED'S DATE OF BIRTH MM DD YY   SEX M   F

b. OTHER INSURED'S DATE OF BIRTH MM DD YY   SEX M   F

b. AUTO ACCIDENT?   PLACE (State)   YES   NO

b. EMPLOYER'S NAME OR SCHOOL NAME

c. EMPLOYER'S NAME OR SCHOOL NAME

c. OTHER ACCIDENT?   YES   NO

c. INSURANCE PLAN NAME OR PROGRAM NAME

d. INSURANCE PLAN NAME OR PROGRAM NAME

10d. RESERVED FOR LOCAL USE

d. IS THERE ANOTHER HEALTH BENEFIT PLAN?   YES   NO   If yes, return to and complete item 9 a-d.

READ BACK OF FORM BEFORE COMPLETING & SIGNING THIS FORM.
12. PATIENT'S OR AUTHORIZED PERSON'S SIGNATURE I authorize the release of any medical or other information necessary to process this claim. I also request payment of government benefits either to myself or to the party who accepts assignment below.

SIGNED _____   DATE _____

13. INSURED'S OR AUTHORIZED PERSON'S SIGNATURE I authorize payment of medical benefits to the undersigned physician or supplier for services described below.

SIGNED _____

PATIENT AND INSURED INFORMATION

14. DATE OF CURRENT: MM DD YY   ILLNESS (First symptom) OR INJURY (Accident) OR PREGNANCY(LMP)

15. IF PATIENT HAS HAD SAME OR SIMILAR ILLNESS. GIVE FIRST DATE MM DD YY

16. DATES PATIENT UNABLE TO WORK IN CURRENT OCCUPATION MM DD YY   FROM   TO MM DD YY

17. NAME OF REFERRING PHYSICIAN OR OTHER SOURCE

17a. I.D. NUMBER OF REFERRING PHYSICIAN

18. HOSPITALIZATION DATES RELATED TO CURRENT SERVICES MM DD YY   FROM   TO MM DD YY

19. RESERVED FOR LOCAL USE

20. OUTSIDE LAB?   YES   NO $ CHARGES

21. DIAGNOSIS OR NATURE OF ILLNESS OR INJURY. (RELATE ITEMS 1,2,3 OR 4 TO ITEM 24E BY LINE)

1. L___ . ___   3. L___ . ___

2. L___ . ___   4. L___ . ___

22. MEDICAID RESUBMISSION CODE   ORIGINAL REF. NO.

23. PRIOR AUTHORIZATION NUMBER

24. A						B	C	D			E	F	G	H	I	J	K
DATE(S) OF SERVICE From			To			Place of Service	Type of Service	PROCEDURES, SERVICES, OR SUPPLIES (Explain Unusual Circumstances) CPT/HCPCS MODIFIER			DIAGNOSIS CODE	$ CHARGES	DAYS OR UNITS	EPSDT Family Plan	EMG	COB	RESERVED FOR LOCAL USE
MM	DD	YY	MM	DD	YY												
1																	
2																	
3																	
4																	
5																	
6																	

PHYSICIAN OR SUPPLIER INFORMATION

25. FEDERAL TAX I.D. NUMBER   SSN EIN

26. PATIENT'S ACCOUNT NO.

27. ACCEPT ASSIGNMENT? (For govt. claims, see back)   YES   NO

28. TOTAL CHARGE $

29. AMOUNT PAID $

30. BALANCE DUE $

31. SIGNATURE OF PHYSICIAN OR SUPPLIER INCLUDING DEGREES OR CREDENTIALS (I certify that the statements on the reverse apply to this bill and are made a part thereof.)

SIGNED _____   DATE _____

32. NAME AND ADDRESS OF FACILITY WHERE SERVICES WERE RENDERED (If other than home or office)

33. PHYSICIAN'S, SUPPLIER'S BILLING NAME, ADDRESS, ZIP CODE & PHONE #

PIN#   GRP#

(APPROVED BY AMA COUNCIL ON MEDICAL SERVICE 8/88)   **PLEASE PRINT OR TYPE**   APPROVED OMB-0938-0008 FORM CMS-1500 (12/90), FORM RRB-1500,
APPROVED OMB-1215-0055 FORM OWCP-1500,   APPROVED OMB-0720-0001 (CHAMPUS)

Figure I-2 CMS-1500 insurance form.

Handling Insurance and Patient Collections

Policy: Practice staff charged with collection of receivables will operate within established legal guidelines and protocols during the pursuit of payment on outstanding patient account balances.

Purpose: To define guidelines for collection of patient account balances.

Procedure:
- Practice staff members DO NOT engage in any conduct that may be construed as harassment, oppression, or abuse of anyone in connection with collection of debt. Conduct disallowed includes, but is not limited to: verbal abuse, threats to inform debtor's employer of debt, disclosure of debt to any third party, and invasion of individual's privacy.
- Telephone collections may occur Monday through Friday, 8:00 am to 9:00 pm, Saturday, 8:00 am to 5:00 pm, unless instructed otherwise by the patient.
- Patients may be contacted at their place of employment, unless otherwise instructed by the patient. However, be careful not to indicate to anyone but the patient the nature of your collection call.
- All accounts must be approved by the physician or practice administrator before referral to a collection agency.
- Threats of legal action may not be used UNLESS such action is likely.

ACCOUNT RESPONSIBILITIES/STANDARDS

Policy: The office staff must pursue collection of outstanding patient account balances and perform all subsequent write-offs without delay.

Purpose: To expedite reimbursements on patient accounts and to reduce outstanding accounts receivable.

Procedure:
- Maintain the standard or better.
- Review Explanation of Benefits (EOBs) daily and pursue unpaid services.
- Report trends regarding changes or delays in reimbursement from payors to Manager.
- Prepare timely write-offs, taking adjustments at the time of posting.
- Take bad debt write-offs as soon as an account is determined to be noncollectible.

Recommendations: Use the collection feature on the practice management system to facilitate timely follow-up, or use a tickler system to remind you.

Figure I-3 Example of a policy and procedures document.

Figure I-3 (cont.)

ACCOUNT FOLLOW UP

Policy: Manager assigns accounts to the appropriate practice staff for timely follow-up and account maintenance.

Purpose: To ensure all patient accounts receive timely follow-up and subsequent account maintenance.

Procedure:
- All accounts over 30 days old are reviewed and pursued for prompt payment, which is accomplished by following up with the patient.
- The tickler system or the practice management system should be used to systematically follow up on accounts. (NOTE: A manual tickler system can simply consist of writing the patient's account number on a designated calendar date to make the return status call.)
- All follow-up calls should be documented in the practice management system, noting the following information: date and time the patient was contacted, brief summary of discussion, indication of commitment on the part of the patient to clear the account, and date payment is expected.

PROBLEM PAYORS

Policy: Accounts receivable issues should be identified and resolved in a timely manner. Problematic issues are documented and should be followed up by management.

Purpose: To ensure all contracted payors are compliant with specific contract terms and that all noncontract payors remit appropriate reimbursement in a timely manner.

Procedure:
- Notify physician or manager of any problem-related issues involving payors.
- Attempt to quantify the scope of the problem (eg, total claims outstanding, the dollar amount, and aging associated with those claims).
- Once the information is quantified, contact the payor's provider representative to discuss resolution of the issue within 15 days. The conversation should be documented and a letter sent to the provider representative confirming the conversation and the expected outcome.
- If no resolution is reached by the 16th business day, contact the provider representative to inform of the intent to send a certified letter to the medical director requesting resolution within 15 days.
- A copy of this letter should also be sent to the patient's employer group, attention benefits manager. You may want to copy your state's insurance commissioner also.
- If resolution has not been received within the stipulated 15 days, the next option will be to consider engaging legal representation or a health care consultant to resolve the issue.

Recommendations: Thoroughly review the payor contracts for all restrictions and stipulations. Before entering any contract with a payor, have a legal representative or consultant review the agreement.

Insurance Assessment

A. Property—Building—Consensus
1. What perils are you insured against?
   - Fire, extended coverage, and vandalism.
   - Sprinkler leakage, if needed.
   - All risk, including burglary and theft.
     Is coverage on a replacement cost basis—no deduction for depreciation?
     Is coverage actual cash value, subject to depreciation?
     What is the deductible?

2. Is coverage limit adequate to comply with coinsurance clause?	Yes	No
3. Does coverage for contents include coverage for building items installed at your expense and in which you have an insurable interest until lease expires?	Yes	No
4. If building coverage is provided, is there any exposure to loss due to condemnation after a fire loss due to nonconforming construction? If so, is policy properly endorsed?	Yes	No
5. Are outdoor signs and awnings covered?	Yes	No
6. Are the named insured and lien holders properly designated on the policy?	Yes	No

B. Time Element

1. Is business interruption or loss of earnings covered?	Yes	No

2. What perils are you insured against?
   - Fire, extended coverage, and vandalism.
   - Sprinkler leakage, if needed.
   - All risk, including burglary and theft
     Is coverage on a replacement cost basis—no deduction for depreciation?
     Is coverage actual cash value, subject to depreciation?
     What is the deductible?

3. Is coverage limit adequate to comply with coinsurance clause?	Yes	No
Does contents coverage include coverage for building items installed at your expense and in which you have an insurable interest until lease expires?	Yes	No
If building coverage is provided, is there any exposure to loss due to condemnation after a fire loss due to nonconforming construction? If so, is policy properly endorsed?	Yes	No
4. If building is owned, is rental income coverage carried?	Yes	No
5. Is extra expense insurance carried?	Yes	No

C. Separate Floaters

1. Is glass coverage required and carried?	Yes	No
2. Is accounts receivable records coverage carried?	Yes	No
In absence of coverage are records properly protected in a fire-resistant safe or cabinet and/or are records duplicated and kept off premises?	Yes	No
3. Is there any fine arts coverage?	Yes	No
4. Is there any valuable papers and records coverage to cover cost or research and development necessary to reproduce records destroyed?	Yes	No
5. Is data processing coverage needed	Yes	No
6. Do lease requirements of leased personal property require "all risk" floater insurance?	Yes	No
7. Are instruments, cameras, portable lasers or other equipment scheduled for specific off-premises coverage?	Yes	No

D. General Liability (Excluding Professional)

1. Is coverage on a comprehensive form?	Yes	No
2. Is coverage included for personal injury, including suits involving employment?	Yes	No
Is coverage provided without participating in loss?	Yes	No
3. Is coverage provided for liability assumed under contract?	Yes	No
4. Is coverage provided for fire, legal liability for leased premises?	Yes	No
5. Are special extensions or coverages required for owned or nonowned watercraft or aircraft?	Yes	No
6. Host liquor (not sale) liability coverage?	Yes	No
7. Additional insured employees? Products?	Yes	No
8. Independent contractors?	Yes	No

Figure I-4 Insurance plan assessment form. *(Source: The Business Side of Medical Practice, pp. 53–57, American Medical Association, 1989, Chicago, Illinois.)*

Figure I-4 (cont.)

E. Auto Liability and Physical Damage

1. Are all owned autos insured for:

Liability—bodily injury and property damage?

Medical payments?	Yes	No
Uninsured motorists?	Yes	No
Collision?	Yes	No
Comprehensive?	Yes	No
Towing and replacement auto?	Yes	No

2. Is coverage provided for the liability of employee vehicles used on your behalf or hired vehicles through a nonowned and hired auto endorsement? Yes No

3. What are deductibles for comprehensive and collision coverage? Yes No

4. Is an endorsement necessary to make corporate-owned vehicle coverage as broad as a personal policy? Yes No

F. Excess Umbrella Liability (Excluding Professional)

1. Is coverage carried? Yes No

2. Is limit adequate? Yes No

3. Do underlying policy (Items D and E) limits meet umbrella requirements? Yes No

4. Is coverage provided on a first dollar defense basis for those suits not covered by underlying policy? Yes No

5. Any special exclusions that require further explanation? Yes No

G. Crime

1. Is employee dishonesty coverage carried with adequate limit? Yes No

2. Is employee dishonesty coverage carried or required by ERISA-1974? Yes No

3. Is coverage required for other crime areas? Yes No

Money and securities on and off premises?	Yes	No
Depositor's forgery?	Yes	No
Credit card forgery?	Yes	No
Contents burglary and theft if not provided under Item A?	Yes	No

H. Workers' Compensation

1. Is coverage required and carried? Yes No

2. Are certificates of insurance requested for all independent contractors performing work in your behalf to prevent additional premium charges? Yes No

3. Any loss frequency or severity that indicates problems, and are you receiving company engineering assistance? Yes No

4. Does policy cover employee injury in other states? Yes No

5. Voluntary compensation exposure? Yes No

   • Sponsored athletic groups exposure? Yes No

I. Boiler Coverage

1. Is coverage required for explosion of steam or hot water boiler? Yes No

2. Is coverage on a replacement cost basis—no deduction for depreciation? Yes No

3. Is limit adequate? Yes No

4. Is coverage provided for other boiler exposure areas such as:

Business interruption or loss of earnings?	Yes	No
Rental value?	Yes	No
Extra expense?	Yes	No

5. Is coverage required for other machinery exposures, particularly if you are the owner of a building, such as but not limited to: Yes No

Air conditioning equipment?	Yes	No
Electrical switchboards?	Yes	No
Transformers?	Yes	No
Unfired pressure vessels?	Yes	No
Electric motors?	Yes	No
Compressors?	Yes	No

J. Miscellaneous: Have exposures been examined for the following areas of coverage?

1. Fiduciary responsibility insurance? Yes No

2. Directors and officers liability—for own corporations and boards on which you may serve? Yes No

K. Make sure the agent reviews ISO (Fire Rating Bureau) inspection reports for rate surcharges due to correctable property conditions.

Employee Handbook Contents

Welcome Letter and Introduction

Letter of Appreciation to Current Employees

Letter of Welcome to New Employees

Purpose of Handbook

Background of Practice

Organization Chart

Physician(s)' Biographical Information

Equal Employment Opportunity Statement

Suggestion and Complaint Procedures

Employment Policies and Procedures

Nature of Employment

Probationary Period

Employment Relations

Supervisor's Responsibilities

Employee's Role and Responsibilities

Work Schedules

Rest and Meal Periods

Overtime Policy

Attendance and Punctuality

Time Cards

Personnel Records

Payday

Payroll Deductions

Performance and Salary Reviews

Resignation/Termination

Telephone Use

Benefits

Holidays

Vacations

Hospital and Medical Insurance

Life Insurance

Pension and Profit-Sharing

Training

Educational Assistance Program

Service Awards

Workers' Compensation

Sick Leave

Disability Leave

Personal Leave

Bereavement Leave

Jury Duty

Witness Duty

Safety

Safety Rules

Emergency Procedures

Personal Protective Equipment

Reporting Accidents

Employee Conduct and Disciplinary Action

Standards of Conduct

Confidentiality Policy

Smoking Policy

Drug, Alcohol, and Substance Abuse Policy (including testing, if applicable)

Sexual and Other Forms of Impermissible Harassment

Security Inspections

Solicitation

Personal Appearance and Dress Code

Corrective Discipline

Summary and Acknowledgment

Disclaimer Statement

Figure 1.5 Example of a table of contents for an employee handbook.

Ethics Resources

This appendix includes a variety of resources available for information and guidance concerning issues of medical ethics. Print and electronic or online publications are included, both from the Academy and other sources. Also reproduced is the full text of the Belmont Report, commissioned by the Department of Health Education and Welfare in 1979. The Belmont Report is the major ethical statement guiding human research in the United States. Ethics courses can be found through various institutions such as bioethics departments of many universities, community hospitals, and medical centers.

American Academy of Ophthalmology

Academy products are available for purchase online. Many Academy electronic publications are available to download for free. For more information on the following Academy materials, visit the Academy's web site, www.aao.org.

Academy Courses

The Ethical Ophthalmologist Series (online CME courses) offers three online courses that cover the effect of ethical issues on everyday decision-making in ophthalmology. The courses use case studies with questions and discussions, providing opportunities to recognize and analyze ethical dilemmas.

- Course 1. Commercial Relationships, Compensation, and Advertising
- Course 2. Informed Consent, Doctor–Patient Relationship, and Delegated Services
- Course 3. Research, New Technology, and Collegiality

These courses are also available as audio CDs. For more information, visit the Academy's web site (www.aao.org).

Academy Opinions and Statements for the Code of Ethics

Advisory opinions:

- *Communications to the Public*
- *Delegated Services*
- *Clinical Trials and Investigative Procedures*
- *Postoperative Care*
- *Unnecessary Surgery and Related Procedures*
- *Informed Consent*
- *Advertising Claims Containing Certain Potentially Misleading Phrases*
- *Employment and Referral Relationships between Ophthalmologists and Other Health Care Providers*
- *Appropriate Examination and Treatment Procedures*
- *Release and Confidentiality of Patient Records*
- *Disclosures of Professionally Related Commercial Interests*
- *Ethical Obligations in a Managed Care Environment*
- *Learning New Techniques after Residency*

Policy statements:

- *An Ophthalmologist's Duties Concerning Postoperative Care*
- *Ophthalmic Care for Patients in Residential Care Centers*
- *Pretreatment Assessment: Responsibilities of the Ophthalmologist*
- *Gifts to Physicians from Industry*

Information statements:

- *The Moral and Technical Competence of the Ophthalmologist*
- *Unique Competence of the Ophthalmologist*

Recommended Reading

Angell M. The doctor as double agent. *Kennedy Inst Ethics J*. 1993;3:279–286.

Aristotle. *The Nichomachean Ethics (Oxford World's Classics)*. Ross D, trans. New York, NY: Oxford University Press; 1998.

Bayles MD. The Professions. In: Callahan JC, ed. *Ethical Issues in Professional Life*. New York, NY: Oxford University Press; 1988.

Beauchamp TL, Childress JF. *Principles of Biomedical Ethics*. 5th ed. New York, NY: Oxford University Press; 2001.

Berg JW, Applebaum PS, Lidz CW, et al. *Informed Consent, Legal Theory and Clinical Practice*. New York, NY: Oxford University Press; 2001.

Bettman JW Sr. Ethics and the American Academy of Ophthalmology in historical perspective. *Ophthalmology*. 1996;103(suppl):529–539.

Carson RA, Burns CR, eds. *Philosophy of Medicine and Bioethics: A Twenty-Year Retrospective and Critical Appraisal*. Boston, Mass: Kluwer Academic Publishers; 1997.

Christakis DA, Feudtner C. Temporary matters. The ethical consequences of transient social relationships in medical training. *JAMA*. 1997:278:739–743.

Drane JF. *Becoming a Good Doctor, The Place of Virtue and Character in Medical Ethics.* 2nd ed. Kansas City, MO: Sheed & Ward; 1995.

Freidson E. Professionalism and institutional ethics. In: Baker RB, Caplan AC, Emanuel LL, et al., eds. *The American Medical Ethics Revolution.* Baltimore, MD: The Johns Hopkins University Press; 1999:123–143.

Friedman LM, Furberg CD, DeMets DL. *Fundamentals of Clinical Trials.* 3rd ed. New York, NY: Springer-Verlag; 1998.

Garrison FH. *An Introduction to the History of Medicine.* 4th ed. Philadelphia, PA: W. B. Saunders Co.; 1929.

Haakonssen L. *Medicine and Morals in the Enlightenment: John Gregory, Thomas Percival and Benjamin Rush.* The Wellcome Institute Series in the History of Medicine. Atlanta, GA: Clio Medica; 1997.

Himmelfarb G. *One Nation, Two Cultures.* New York, NY: Vintage; 2001.

Hoskins HD Jr. LASIK advertising is testing our profession. *EyeNet.* June 2000:12–13.

Hughes EC. *Professions.* In: Callahan JC, ed. *Ethical Issues in Professional Life.* New York, NY: Oxford University Press; 1988.

Jolly A. *Lucy's Legacy: Sex and Intelligence in Human Evolution.* Cambridge, MA: Harvard University Press; 2001.

Kohlberg L. *The Psychology of Moral Development: The Nature and Validity of Moral Stages.* Vol 2. New York, NY: Harper & Row; 1984.

Kohn A. *The Brighter Side of Human Nature: Altruism and Empathy in Everyday Life.* New York, NY: Basic Books, Inc.; 1990.

Krause EA. *Death of the Guilds.* New Haven, CT: Yale University Press; 1999.

Lynn J, Harrold J, Ayers E, et al. Hearing voices: How should doctors respond to their calling? *N Engl J Med.* 1996;335:1991–1993.

Mill JS. *On Liberty.* Buffalo, NY: Prometheus Books; 1986.

Newton LH. Collective responsibility in health care. *J Med & Philos.* 1982;7:11–21.

Nuland SB. *Doctors: The Biography of Medicine.* New York, NY: Vintage Books; 1995.

Osler W. *The Evolution of Modern Medicine.* New Haven, CT: Yale University Press; 1921.

Packer S, Lynch J. Ethics of comanagement. *Arch Ophthalmol.* 2002;120:71–76.

Pellegrino ED, Thomasma DC. *For the Patient's Good: The Restoration of Beneficence in Health Care.* New York, NY: Oxford University Press; 1988.

Pellegrino ED, What is a profession? The ethical implications of the FTC order and some Supreme Court decisions. *Surv Ophthalmol.* 1984:29:221–225.

Pellegrino ED. The phenomenon of trust and the patient–physician relationship. In: Pellegrino ED, Veatch RM, Langan JP, eds. *Ethics, Trust, and the Professions. Philosophical and Cultural Aspects.* Washington, DC: Georgetown University Press; 1991.

Pellegrino ED. *The Philosophical Basis of Medical Practice: Toward a Philosophy and Ethic of the Healing Profession.* New York, NY: Oxford University Press; 1981.

Rawls J. *A Theory of Justice.* Boston, MA: Harvard University Press; 1999.

Relman AS, Lindberg GD. Business and professionalism in medicine at the American Medical Association. *JAMA.* 1998:270:169–170.

Relman AS. What market values are doing to medicine. *The Atlantic Monthly.* March 1992;03:96–106.

Roter DL, Hall JA. *Doctors Talking With Patients, Patients Talking With Doctors. Improving Communication in Medical Visits.* Westport, CT: Auburn House; 1993.

Rothman DJ. *Strangers at the Bedside.* 2nd ed. New York, NY: Aldine De Gruyter; 2003.

Self DJ, Baldwin DC Jr. Moral reasoning in medicine. In: Rest JR, Narvaez D, eds. *Moral Development in the Professions*. Hillsdale, NJ: L. Erlbaum Associates Publishers; 1994.

Shalit R. When we were philosopher kings: The rise of the medical ethicist. *New Republic*. April 28, 1997.

Starr P. *The Social Transformation of American Medicine*. New York, NY: Basic Books, Inc.; 1982.

The Nuremberg Code. Trials of War Criminals before the Nuremberg Military Tribunals under Control Council Law no 10, vol 2. Nuremberg, October 1946–April 1949. Washington, DC: US Government Printing Office; 1949:181–182.

Thomasma DC. Establishing the moral basis of medicine: Edmund D. Pellegrino's philosophy of medicine. *J Med & Philos*. 1990;15:245–267.

Toulmin S. Medical ethics in its American context. An historical survey. *Ann NY Acad Sci*. 1988;530:7–15.

Veatch RM. *A Theory of Medical Ethics*. New York, NY: Basic Books, Inc.; 1981.

The Belmont Report

Source: National Institutes of Health (http://ohsr.od.nih.gov).

THE BELMONT REPORT: ETHICAL PRINCIPLES AND GUIDELINES FOR THE PROTECTION OF HUMAN SUBJECTS OF RESEARCH

The National Commission for the Protection of Human Subjects of Biomedical and Behavioral Research

April 18, 1979

AGENCY: Department of Health, Education, and Welfare.

ACTION: Notice of Report for Public Comment.

SUMMARY:

On July 12, 1974, the National Research Act (Public Law 93348) was signed into law, thereby creating the National Commission for the Protection of Human Subjects of Biomedical and Behavioral Research. One of the charges to the Commission was to identify the basic ethical principles that should underlie the conduct of biomedical and behavioral research involving human subjects, and to develop guidelines, which should be followed to assure that such research is conducted in accordance with those principles. In carrying out the above, the Commission was directed to consider: (**i**) the boundaries between biomedical and behavioral research and the accepted and routine practice of medicine, (**ii**) the role of assessment of risk-benefit criteria in the determination of the appropriateness of research involving human subjects, (**iii**) appropriate guidelines for the selection of human subjects for participation in such research, and (**iv**) the nature and definition of informed consent in various research settings.

The Belmont Report attempts to summarize the basic ethical principles identified by the Commission in the course of its deliberations. It is the outgrowth of an intensive four-day period of discussions that were held in February 1976 at the Smithsonian Institution's Belmont Conference Center, supplemented by the monthly deliberations of the Commission that were held over a period of nearly four years. It is a statement of basic ethical principles and guidelines that should assist in resolving the ethical problems that surround the conduct of research with human subjects.

By publishing the Report in the Federal Register, and providing reprints upon request, the Secretary intends that it may be made readily available to scientists, members of institutional review boards, and Federal employees. The two-volume Appendix, containing the lengthy reports of experts and specialists, who assisted the Commission in fulfilling this part of its charge, is available as DHEW Publication No. (OS) 78-0013 and No. (OS) 78-0014, for sale by the Superintendent of Documents, U.S. Government Printing Office, Washington, D.C. 20402.

Unlike most other reports of the Commission, the Belmont Report does not make specific recommendations for administrative action by the Secretary of Health, Education, and Welfare. Rather, the Commission recommended that the Belmont Report be adopted in its entirety, as a statement of the Department's policy. The Department requests public comment on this recommendation.

National Commission for the Protection of Human Subjects of Biomedical and Behavioral Research

Members of the Commission

Kenneth John Ryan, MD, Chairman, Chief of Staff, Boston Hospital for Women.
Joseph V. Brady, PhD, Professor of Behavioral Biology, Johns Hopkins University.
Robert E. Cooke, MD, President, Medical College of Pennsylvania.
Dorothy I. Height, President, National Council of Negro Women, Inc.
Albert R. Jonsen, PhD, Associate Professor of Bioethics, University of California at San Francisco.
Patricia King, JD, Associate Professor of Law, Georgetown University Law Center.
Karen Lebacqz, PhD, Associate Professor of Christian Ethics, Pacific School of Religion.
*David W. Louisell, JD, Professor of Law, University of California at Berkeley.
Donald W. Seldin, MD, Professor and Chairman, Department of Internal Medicine, University of Texas at Dallas.
Eliot Stellar, PhD, Provost of the University and Professor of Physiological Psychology, University of Pennsylvania.
*Robert H. Turtle, LLB, Attorney, VomBaur, Coburn, Simmons & Turtle, Washington, D.C.

* Deceased.

Ethical Principles & Guidelines for Research Involving Human Subjects

Scientific research has produced substantial social benefits. It has also posed some troubling ethical questions. Public attention was drawn to these questions by reported abuses of human subjects in biomedical experiments, especially during the Second World War. During the Nuremberg War Crime Trials, the Nuremberg Code was drafted as a set of standards for judging physicians and scientists who had conducted biomedical experiments on concentration camp prisoners. This Code became the prototype of many later codes[1] intended to assure that research involving human subjects would be carried out in an ethical manner.

The codes consist of rules, some general, others specific, that guide the investigators or the reviewers of research in their work. Such rules often are inadequate to cover complex situations; at times they come into conflict, and they are frequently difficult to interpret or apply. Broader ethical principles will provide a basis on which specific rules may be formulated, criticized and interpreted.

Three principles, or general prescriptive judgments, that are relevant to research involving human subjects are identified in this statement. Other principles may also be relevant. These three are comprehensive, however, and are stated at a level of generalization that should assist scientists, subjects, reviewers and interested citizens to understand the ethical issues inherent in research involving human subjects. These principles cannot always be applied, so as to resolve beyond dispute particular ethical problems. The objective is to provide an analytical framework that will guide the resolution of ethical problems arising from research involving human subjects.

This statement consists of a distinction between research and practice, a discussion of the three basic ethical principles, and remarks about the application of these principles.

A. Boundaries Between Practice and Research

It is important to distinguish between biomedical and behavioral research, on the one hand, and the practice of accepted therapy on the other, in order to know what activities ought to undergo review for the protection of human subjects of research. The distinction between research and practice is blurred, partly because both often occur together (as in research designed to evaluate a therapy), and partly because notable departures from standard practice are often called "experimental," when the terms "experimental" and "research" are not carefully defined.

For the most part, the term "practice" refers to interventions that are designed solely to enhance the well-being of an individual patient or client and that have a reasonable expectation of success. The purpose of medical or behavioral practice is to provide diagnosis, preventive treatment or therapy to particular individuals.[2] By contrast, the term "research" designates an activity designed to test an hypothesis, permit conclusions to be drawn, and thereby to develop or contribute to generalizable knowledge (expressed, for example, in theories, principles, and statements of relationships). Research is usually described in a formal protocol that sets forth an objective and a set of procedures designed to reach that objective.

When a clinician departs in a significant way from standard or accepted practice, the innovation does not, in and of itself, constitute research. The fact that a procedure is "experimental" in the sense of new, untested or different, does not automatically place it in the category of research. Radically new procedures of this description should, however, be made the object of formal research at an early stage, in order to determine whether they are safe and effective. Thus, it is the responsibility of medical practice committees, for example, to insist that a major innovation be incorporated into a formal research project.[3]

Research and practice may be carried on together when research is designed to evaluate the safety and efficacy of a therapy. This need not cause any confusion regarding whether or not the activity requires review; the general rule is that if there is any element of research in an activity, that activity should undergo review for the protection of human subjects.

B. Basic Ethical Principles

The expression "basic ethical principles" refers to those general judgments that serve as a basic justification for the many particular ethical prescriptions and evaluations of human actions. Three basic principles, among those generally accepted in our cultural tradition, are particularly relevant to the ethics of research involving human subjects: the principles of respect for persons, beneficence and justice.

1. Respect for Persons

Respect for persons incorporates at least two ethical convictions: first, that individuals should be treated as autonomous agents, and second, that persons with diminished autonomy are entitled to protection. The principle of respect for persons thus divides into two separate moral requirements: the requirement to acknowledge autonomy, and the requirement to protect those with diminished autonomy.

An autonomous person is an individual capable of deliberation about personal goals and of acting under the direction of such deliberation. To respect autonomy is to give weight to autonomous persons' considered opinions and choices, while refraining from obstructing their actions, unless they are clearly detrimental to others. To show lack of respect for an autonomous agent is to repudiate that person's considered judgments, to deny an individual the freedom to act on those considered judgments, or to withhold information necessary to make a considered judgment, when there are no compelling reasons to do so.

However, not every human being is capable of self-determination. The capacity for self-determination matures during an individual's life, and some individuals lose this capacity wholly or in part, because of illness, mental disability, or circumstances that severely restrict liberty. Respect for the immature and the incapacitated may require protecting them as they mature or while they are incapacitated.

Some persons are in need of extensive protection, even to the point of excluding them from activities which may harm them; other persons require little protection beyond making sure they undertake activities freely and with awareness of possible adverse consequences. The extent of protection afforded should depend upon the risk of harm and the likelihood of benefit. The judgment that any individual lacks autonomy should be periodically reevaluated, and will vary in different situations.

In most cases of research involving human subjects, respect for persons demands that subjects enter into the research voluntarily and with adequate information. In some situations, however, application of the principle is not obvious. The involvement of prisoners as subjects of research provides an instructive example. On the one hand, it would seem that the principle of respect for persons requires that prisoners not be deprived of the opportunity to volunteer for research. On the other hand, under prison conditions they may be subtly coerced or unduly influenced to engage in research activities for which they would not otherwise volunteer. Respect for persons would then dictate that prisoners be protected. Whether to allow prisoners to "volunteer" or to "protect" them presents a dilemma. Respecting persons, in most hard cases, is often a matter of balancing competing claims urged by the principle of respect itself.

2. Beneficence

Persons are treated in an ethical manner not only by respecting their decisions and protecting them from harm, but also by making efforts to secure their well-being. Such treatment falls under the principle of beneficence. The term "beneficence" is often understood to cover acts of kindness or charity that go beyond strict obligation. In this document, beneficence is understood in a stronger sense, as an obligation. Two general rules have been formulated as complementary expressions of beneficent actions in this sense: (1) do not harm and (2) maximize possible benefits and minimize possible harms.

The Hippocratic maxim "do no harm" has long been a fundamental principle of medical ethics. Claude Bernard extended it to the realm of research, saying that one should not injure one person, regardless of the benefits that might come to others. However, even avoiding harm requires learning what is harmful; and, in the process of obtaining this information, persons may be exposed to risk of harm. Further, the Hippocratic Oath requires physicians to benefit their patients "according to their best judgment." Learning what will in fact benefit may require exposing persons to risk. The problem posed by these imperatives is to decide when it is justifiable to seek certain benefits despite the risks involved, and when the benefits should be foregone because of the risks.

The obligations of beneficence affect both individual investigators and society at large, because they extend both to particular research projects and to the entire enterprise of research. In the case of particular projects, investigators and members of their institutions are obliged to give forethought to the maximization of benefits and the reduction of risk that might occur from the research investigation. In the case of scientific research in general, members of the larger society are obliged to recognize the longer term benefits and risks that may result from the improvement of knowledge, and from the development of novel medical, psychotherapeutic, and social procedures.

The principle of beneficence often occupies a well-defined, justifying role in many areas of research involving human subjects. An example is found in research involving children. Effective ways of treating childhood diseases and fostering healthy development are benefits that serve to justify research involving children—even when individual research subjects are not direct beneficiaries. Research also makes it possible to avoid the harm that may result from the application of previously accepted routine practices that on closer investigation turn out to be dangerous. But the role of the principle of beneficence is not always so unambiguous. A difficult ethical problem remains, for example, about research that presents more than minimal risk without immediate prospect of direct benefit to the children involved. Some have argued that such research is inadmissible, while others have pointed out that this limit would rule out much research promising great benefit to children in the future. Here again, as with all hard cases, the different claims covered by the principle of beneficence may come into conflict and force difficult choices.

3. Justice

Who ought to receive the benefits of research and bear its burdens? This is a question of justice, in the sense of "fairness in distribution" or "what is deserved." An injustice occurs when some benefit to which a person is entitled is denied without good reason or when some burden is imposed unduly. Another way of conceiving the principle of justice is that, equals ought to be treated equally. However, this statement requires explication. Who is equal and who is unequal? What considerations justify departure from equal distribution? Almost all commentators allow that distinctions based on experience, age, deprivation, competence, merit and position do sometimes constitute criteria justifying differential treatment for certain purposes. It is necessary, then, to explain in what respects people should be treated equally. There are several widely accepted formulations of just ways to distribute burdens and benefits. Each formulation mentions some relevant property on the basis of which burdens and benefits should be distributed. These formulations are (1) to each person an equal share, (2) to each person according to individual need, (3) to each person according to individual effort, (4) to each person according to societal contribution, and (5) to each person according to merit.

Questions of justice have long been associated with social practices such as punishment, taxation and political representation. Until recently, these questions have not generally been associated with scientific research. However, they are foreshadowed even in the earliest reflections on the ethics of research involving human subjects. For example, during the 19th and early 20th centuries the burdens of serving as research subjects fell largely upon poor ward patients, while the benefits of improved medical care flowed primarily to private patients. Subsequently, the exploitation of unwilling prisoners as research subjects in Nazi concentration camps was condemned as a particularly vagrant injustice. In this country, in the 1940s, the Tuskegee syphilis study used disadvantaged, rural black men to study the untreated course of a disease that is by no means confined to that population. These subjects were deprived of demonstrably effective treatment in order not to interrupt the project, long after such treatment became generally available.

Against this historical background, it can be seen how conceptions of justice are relevant to research involving human subjects. For example, the selection of research subjects needs to be scrutinized in order to determine whether some classes (e.g., welfare patients, particular racial and ethnic minorities, or persons confined to institutions) are being systematically selected simply because of their easy availability, their compromised position, or their manipulability, rather than for reasons directly related to the problem being studied. Finally, whenever research supported by public funds leads to the development of therapeutic devices and procedures, justice demands both that these not provide advantages only to those who can afford them and that such research should not unduly involve persons from groups unlikely to be among the beneficiaries of subsequent applications of the research.

C. Applications

Application of the general principles to the conduct of research leads to consideration of the following requirements: informed consent, risk/benefit assessment, and the selection of subjects of research.

1. Informed Consent

Respect for persons requires that subjects, to the degree that they are capable, be given the opportunity to choose what shall or shall not happen to them. This opportunity is provided, when adequate standards for informed consent are satisfied.

While the importance of informed consent is unquestioned, controversy prevails over the nature and possibility of an informed consent. Nonetheless, there is widespread agreement that the consent process can be analyzed as containing three elements: information, comprehension, and voluntariness.

Information. Most codes of research establish specific items for disclosure intended to assure that subjects are given sufficient information. These items generally include: the research procedure, their purposes, risks and anticipated benefits, alternative procedures (where therapy is involved), and a statement offering the subject the opportunity to ask questions and to withdraw at any time from the research. Additional items have been proposed, including how subjects are selected, the person responsible for the research, etc.

However, a simple listing of items does not answer the question of what the standard should be for judging how much and what sort of information should be provided. One standard frequently invoked in medical practice, namely the information commonly provided by practitioners in the field or in the locale, is inadequate since research takes place precisely when a common understanding does not exist. Another standard, currently popular in malpractice law, requires the practitioner to reveal the information that reasonable persons would wish to know in order to make a decision regarding their care. This, too, seems insufficient, since the research subject, being in essence a volunteer, may wish to know considerably more about risks gratuitously undertaken than do patients who deliver themselves into the hand of a clinician for needed care. It may be that a standard of "the reasonable volunteer" should be proposed: the extent and nature of information should be such that persons, knowing that the procedure is neither necessary for their care nor perhaps fully understood, can decide whether they wish to participate in the furthering of knowledge. Even when some direct benefit to them is anticipated, the subjects should understand clearly the range of risk and the voluntary nature of participation.

A special problem of consent arises where informing subjects of some pertinent aspect of the research is likely to impair the validity of the research. In many cases, it is sufficient to indicate to subjects that they are being invited to participate in research of which some features will not be revealed until the research is concluded. In all cases of research involving incomplete disclosure, such research is justified only if it is clear that (1) incomplete disclosure is truly necessary to accomplish the goals of the research, (2) there are no undisclosed risks to subjects that are more than minimal, and (3) there is an adequate plan for debriefing subjects, when appropriate, and for dissemination of research results to them. Information about risks should never be withheld for the purpose of eliciting the cooperation of subjects, and truthful answers should always be given to direct questions about the research. Care should be taken to distinguish cases in which disclosure would destroy or invalidate the research from cases in which disclosure would simply inconvenience the investigator.

Comprehension. The manner and context, in which information is conveyed is as important as the information itself. For example, presenting information in a disorganized and rapid fashion, allowing too little time for consideration, or curtailing opportunities for questioning, all may adversely affect a subject's ability to make an informed choice.

Because the subject's ability to understand is a function of intelligence, rationality, maturity and language, it is necessary to adapt the presentation of the information to the subject's capacities. Investigators are responsible for ascertaining that the subject has comprehended the information. While there is always an obligation to ascertain that the information about risk to subjects is complete and adequately comprehended, when the risks are more serious, that obligation increases. On occasion, it may be suitable to give some oral or written tests of comprehension.

Special provision may need to be made, when comprehension is severely limited—for example, by conditions of immaturity or mental disability. Each class of subjects that one might consider as incompetent (e.g., infants and young children, mentally disabled patients, the terminally ill, and the comatose) should be considered on its own terms. Even for these persons, however, respect requires giving them the opportunity to choose, to the extent they are able, whether or not to participate in research. The objections of these subjects to involvement should be honored, unless the research entails providing them a therapy unavailable elsewhere. Respect for persons also requires seeking the permission of other parties in order to protect the subjects from harm. Such persons are thus respected, both by acknowledging their own wishes and by the use of third parties to protect them from harm.

The third parties chosen should be those who are most likely to understand the incompetent subject's situation and to act in that person's best interest. The person authorized to act on behalf of the subject should be given an opportunity to observe the research as it proceeds in order to be able to withdraw the subject from the research, if such action appears in the subject's best interest.

Voluntariness. An agreement to participate in research constitutes a valid consent only if voluntarily given. This element of informed consent requires conditions free of coercion and undue influence. Coercion occurs when an overt threat of harm is intentionally presented by one person to another in order to obtain compliance. Undue influence, by contrast, occurs through an offer of an excessive, unwarranted, inappropriate or improper reward or other overture in order to obtain compliance. Also, inducements that would ordinarily be acceptable may become undue influences if the subject is especially vulnerable.

Unjustifiable pressures usually occur when persons in positions of authority or commanding influence—especially where possible sanctions are involved—urge a course of action for a subject. A continuum of such influencing factors exists, however, and it is impossible to state precisely, where justifiable persuasion ends and undue influence begins. But undue influence would include actions such as manipulating a person's choice through the controlling influence of a close relative and threatening to withdraw health services to which an individual would otherwise be entitled.

2. Assessment of Risks and Benefits

The assessment of risks and benefits requires a careful arrayal of relevant data, including, in some cases, alternative ways of obtaining the benefits sought in the research. Thus, the assessment presents both an opportunity and a responsibility to gather systematic and comprehensive information about proposed research. For the investigator, it is a means to examine whether the proposed research is properly designed. For a review committee, it is a method for determining whether the risks that will be presented to subjects are justified. For prospective subjects, the assessment will assist the determination whether or not to participate.

The Nature and Scope of Risks and Benefits. The requirement that research be justified on the basis of a favorable risk/benefit assessment bears a close relation to the principle of beneficence, just as the moral requirement that informed consent be obtained is derived primarily from the principle of respect for persons. The term "risk" refers to a possibility that harm may occur. However, when expressions such as "small risk" or "high risk" are used, they usually refer (often ambiguously) both to the chance (probability) of experiencing a harm and the severity (magnitude) of the envisioned harm.

The term "benefit" is used in the research context to refer to something of positive value related to health or welfare. Unlike "risk," "benefit" is not a term that expresses probabilities. Risk is properly contrasted to probability of benefits, and benefits are properly contrasted with harms rather than risks of harm. Accordingly, so-called risk/benefit assessments are concerned with the probabilities and magnitudes of possible harms and anticipated benefits. Many kinds of possible harms and benefits need to be taken into account. There are, for example, risks of psychological harm, physical harm, legal harm, social harm and economic harm, and the corresponding benefits. While the most likely types of harms to research subjects are those of psychological or physical pain or injury, other possible kinds should not be overlooked.

Risks and benefits of research may affect the individual subjects, the families of the individual subjects, and society at large (or special groups of subjects in society). Previous codes and Federal regulations have required that risks to subjects be outweighed by the sum of both the anticipated benefit to the subject, if any, and the anticipated benefit to society in the form of knowledge to be gained from the research. In balancing these different elements, the risks and benefits affecting the immediate research subject will normally carry special weight. On the other hand, interests, other than those of the subject, may on some occasions be sufficient by themselves to justify the risks involved in the research, so long as the subjects' rights have been protected. Beneficence thus requires that we protect against risk of harm to subjects and also that we be concerned about the loss of the substantial benefits that might be gained from research.

The Systematic Assessment of Risks and Benefits. It is commonly said that benefits and risks must be "balanced" and shown to be "in a favorable ratio." The metaphorical character of these terms draws attention to the difficulty of making precise judgments. Only on rare occasions will quantitative techniques be available for the scrutiny of research protocols. However, the idea of systematic, nonarbitrary analysis of risks and benefits should be emulated insofar as possible. This ideal requires those making decisions about the justifiability of research to be thorough in the accumulation and assessment of information about all aspects of the research, and to consider alternatives systematically. This procedure renders the assessment of research more rigorous and precise, while making communication between review board members and investigators less subject to misinterpretation, misinformation and conflicting judgments. Thus, there should first be a determination of the validity of the presuppositions of the research; then the nature, probability and magnitude of risk should be distinguished with as much clarity as possible. The method of ascertaining risks should be explicit, especially where there is no alternative to the use of such vague categories as small or slight risk. It should also be determined whether an investigator's estimates of the probability of harm or benefits are reasonable, as judged by known facts or other available studies.

Finally, assessment of the justifiability of research should reflect at least the following considerations: (i) Brutal or inhumane treatment of human subjects is never morally justified. (ii) Risks should be reduced to those necessary to achieve the research objective. It should be determined whether it is in fact necessary to use human subjects at all. Risk can perhaps never be entirely eliminated, but it can often be reduced by careful attention to alternative procedures. (iii) When research involves significant risk of serious impairment, review committees should be extraordinarily insistent on the justification of the risk (looking usually to the likelihood of benefit to the subject—or, in some rare cases, to the manifest voluntariness of the participation). (iv) When vulnerable populations are involved in research, the appropriateness of involving them should itself be demonstrated. A number of variables go into such judgments, including the nature and degree of risk, the condition of the particular population involved, and the nature and level of the anticipated benefits. (v) Relevant risks and benefits must be thoroughly arrayed in documents and procedures used in the informed consent process.

3. Selection of Subjects

Just as the principle of respect for persons finds expression in the requirements for consent, and the principle of beneficence in risk/benefit assessment, the principle of justice gives rise to moral requirements that there be fair procedures and outcomes in the selection of research subjects.

Justice is relevant to the selection of subjects of research at two levels: the social and the individual. Individual justice in the selection of subjects would require that researchers exhibit fairness: thus, they should not offer potentially beneficial research only to some patients, who are in their favor, or select only "undesirable" persons for risky research. Social justice requires that distinction be drawn between classes of subjects that ought, and ought not, to participate in any particular kind of research, based on the ability of members of that class to bear burdens and on the appropriateness of placing further burdens on already burdened persons. Thus, it can be considered a matter of social justice that there is an order of preference in the selection of classes of subjects (e.g., adults before children) and that some classes of potential subjects (e.g., the institutionalized mentally infirm or prisoners) may be involved as research subjects, if at all, only on certain conditions.

Injustice may appear in the selection of subjects, even if individual subjects are selected fairly by investigators and treated fairly in the course of research. Thus, injustice arises from social, racial, sexual and cultural biases institutionalized in society. Thus, even if individual researchers are treating their research subjects fairly, and even if institutional review boards are taking care to assure that subjects are selected fairly within a particular institution, unjust social patterns may nevertheless appear in the overall distribution of the burdens and benefits of research. Although individual institutions or investigators may not be able to resolve a problem that is pervasive in their social setting, they can consider distributive justice in selecting research subjects.

Some populations, especially institutionalized ones, are already burdened in many ways by their infirmities and environments. When research is proposed that involves risks and does not include a therapeutic component, other less burdened classes of persons should be called upon first to accept these risks of research, except where the research is directly related to the specific conditions of the class involved. Also, even though public funds for research may often flow in the same directions as public funds for health care, it seems unfair that populations dependent on public health care constitute a pool of preferred research subjects if more advantaged populations are likely to be the recipients of the benefits.

One special instance of injustice results from the involvement of vulnerable subjects. Certain groups, such as racial minorities, the economically disadvantaged, the very sick, and the institutionalized, may continually be sought as research subjects, owing to their ready availability in settings where research is conducted. Given their dependent status and their frequently compromised capacity for free consent, they should be protected against the danger of being involved in research solely for administrative convenience, or because they are easy to manipulate as a result of their illness or socioeconomic condition.

Notes

[1]Since 1945, various codes for the proper and responsible conduct of human experimentation in medical research have been adopted by different organizations. The best known of these codes are the Nuremberg Code of 1947, the Helsinki Declaration of 1964 (revised in 1975), and the 1971 Guidelines (codified into Federal Regulations in 1974) issued by the U.S. Department of Health, Education, and Welfare. Codes for the conduct

of social and behavioral research have also been adopted, the best known being that of the American Psychological Association, published in 1973.

[2]Although practice usually involves interventions designed solely to enhance the well-being of a particular individual, interventions are sometimes applied to one individual for the enhancement of the well-being of another (e.g., blood donation, skin grafts, organ transplants) or an intervention may have the dual purpose of enhancing the well-being of a particular individual, and, at the same time, providing some benefit to others (e.g., vaccination, which protects both the person who is vaccinated and society generally). The fact that some forms of practice have elements other than immediate benefit to the individual receiving an intervention, however, should not confuse the general distinction between research and practice. Even when a procedure applied in practice may benefit some other person, it remains an intervention designed to enhance the well-being of a particular individual or groups of individuals; thus, it is practice and need not be reviewed as research.

[3]Because the problems related to social experimentation may differ substantially from those of biomedical and behavioral research, the Commission specifically declines to make any policy determination regarding such research at this time. Rather, the Commission believes that the problem ought to be addressed by one of its successor bodies.

Advocacy Resources

This appendix highlights resources from the American Academy of Ophthalmology.

Academy Advocacy Information Online

The Advocacy section of the Academy web site is a key resource for breaking news, descriptions of state and federal issues, action alerts concerning issues needing your vocal support, and names of and e-mail links to legislators. The URL is www.aao.org/aao/advocacy, or click on the Governmental Affairs section from the Academy web site home page www.aao.org. The online advocacy pages include tips on what to say in a phone call and what addresses and salutations are appropriate in correspondence to legislators. Continually updated, the web site is an important tool for those just starting in advocacy as well as for seasoned ophthalmology advocates.

The Advocacy Action Center on the web also allows you to send a letter to your members of Congress on an important issue for which the Academy is lobbying. Form letters are available either to e-mail to your representatives directly from the Action Center or to download onto your practice letterhead and fax to members of Congress or other public officials. If you don't know who your representatives are, you can simply type in your ZIP code and the names will appear. In addition to the Action Center, the Governmental Affairs section of the Academy web site contains information on the federal and state issues that the Academy has identified as important to patients and the profession.

Legislative and regulatory events and news and their effect on ophthalmology appear in the Academy's biweekly *Washington Report* newsletter and the Washington Report section of the weekly *Academy Express* e-newsletter. Each regularly suggests specific, timely advocacy actions and opportunities.

Governmental Affairs Division

The Academy has a Governmental Affairs Division in Washington, DC, with staff lobbyists exclusively representing and working for the interests of ophthalmology. The office is led by an individual who is a respected lobbyist and a vice president of the Academy. In addition, the office has established and nurtured relationships with regulatory agencies to ensure that regulations are properly implemented and that policy proposals have adequate input from and represent the interests of ophthalmologists and their patients.

OPHTHPAC and the Congressional Advocacy Committee

OPHTHPAC is the Academy's voluntary, nonpartisan political action committee. With one of the largest medical specialty PACs in Washington and full-time lobbyists representing our interests, our voice is heard.

The Academy has also developed the Congressional Advocacy Program, the mission of which is to establish a relationship with every member of Congress by identifying and training 535 "key contact" ophthalmologists as lobbyists. With this mechanism in place, when an issue of importance arises, a contact can be made with each legislator almost immediately by an ophthalmologist who has a relationship with that legislator, to directly communicate the concerns of organized ophthalmology. More than 80% of congressional representatives already have such advocates. If you have an established relationship with a legislator or are willing to build one, call the Academy's Washington office at 202-737-6662.

State Affairs Activities

The Academy's State Affairs Secretariat has committee members from around the United States and expert lobbyists in Washington to represent the interests of ophthalmologists on state issues. The main area of focus at the state level has traditionally been optometric scope-of-practice concerns, and much Academy staff energy has been devoted to assisting state ophthalmological societies in working on these issues. The Academy provides precise and detailed information, references, expert testimony, and political strategy to all states on a continuing basis and when specific needs arise. In addition, the establishment of a national Surgical Scope Fund has made financial resources available to state societies when additional lobbying efforts and major legal challenges become necessary.

The Academy has also started a Leadership Development Program that identifies young potential leaders from throughout the United States. These ophthalmologists participate in a formal program designed to teach them leadership and organizational skills and approaches that enable them to return to their state and subspecialty society sponsors and rapidly become an asset in the political process.

Abbreviations and Acronyms

A/R	accounts receivable
AAOE	American Academy of Ophthalmic Executives
AARP	American Association of Retired Persons
ABO	American Board of Ophthalmology
ACGME	Accreditation Council for Graduate Medical Education
ADA	Americans with Disabilities Act
ADEA	Age Discrimination in Employment Act
AMA	American Medical Association
AOS	American Ophthalmological Society
ASC	ambulatory surgery centers
ASP	application service provider
BBRA	Balanced Budget Refinement Act
BCBS	BlueCross and BlueShield
CDC	Centers for Disease Control and Prevention
CEO	corporate executive office
CF	conversion factor
CGL	commercial general liability
CHIPs	children's health insurance programs
CLIA	Clinical Laboratories Improvement Act
CME	continuing medical education
CMS	Centers for Medicare and Medicaid Services
COA	certified ophthalmic assistant
COMT	certified ophthalmic medical technologist
COT	certified ophthalmic technician
CPA	certified public accountant
CPT	current procedural terminology (as in codes)
CV	curriculum vitae
DEA	Drug Enforcement Agency
DOJ	Department of Justice
DOL	Department of Labor
DPA	diagnostic pharmaceutical agent
EEOC	Equal Employment Opportunity Commission
EIN	employer identification number
EMR	electronic medical records
EMTALA	Emergency Medical Treatment and Active Labor Act

EOB	explanation of benefits
ESRD	end stage renal disease
FDA	Food and Drug Administration
FDCA	Fair Debt Collection Act
FLSA	Fair Labor Standards Act
FTC	Federal Trade Commission
FTE	full-time equivalent
GDP	gross domestic product
GPCI	Geographic Practice Cost Indices
HCFA	Health Care Financing Administration
HEW	Health, Education, and Welfare [Department of, now HHS]
HHS	Health and Human Services [Department of]
HIPAA	Health Insurance Portability and Accountability Act
HMO	health maintenance organization
IOL	intraocular lens
IPA	independent practice associations
IPO	individual practice organization
IRS	Internal Revenue Service
JCAHO	Joint Commission on Accreditation of Healthcare Organizations
JCAHPO	Joint Commission on Allied Health Personnel in Ophthalmology
LASIK	Laser in situ keratomileusis
LCD	local coverage determination
MCO	managed care organization
MEI	Medicare Economic Index
MICRA	Medical Injury Compensation Reform Act
MMA	Informal term for Medicare Prescription Drug, Improvement and Modernization Act (also known as Medicare Modernization Act)
MOC	maintenance of certification
MSO	management service organization
NCD	national coverage determination
NEI	National Eye Institute
OCS	Ophthalmic Coding Specialist
OIG	Office of the Inspector General
OMB	Office of Management and Budget
OMIC	Ophthalmic Mutual Insurance Company
OSHA	Occupational Safety and Health Administration
PAC	political action committee
PhRMA	Pharmaceutical Research and Manufacturers of America
POS	point of service plan
PPO	preferred provider organization
PTO	paid time off
RBRVS	resource-based relative value scale
RCPSC	Royal College of Physicians and Surgeons of Canada
RFP	Request for Proposal

RVU	relative value unit
SCHIP	State Child Health Insurance Program
SGR	sustainable growth rate
SRA	Social and Rehabilitation Service
SSA	Social Security Administration
SSDI	Social Security Disability Insurance
SSIC	Specialty Society Insurance Coalition
TPA	therapeutic pharmaceutical agent
UCR	usual and customary reimbursement
UPIN	universal provider identification number (assigned by CMS)

Index

(*b* = box; *f* = figure; *t* = table)